THE DOCTORS
BLACKWELL

ALSO BY JANICE P. NIMURA

Daughters of the Samurai: A Journey from East to West and Back

THE DOCTORS
BLACKWELL

~

HOW TWO PIONEERING SISTERS
BROUGHT MEDICINE TO WOMEN—
AND WOMEN TO MEDICINE

JANICE P. NIMURA

W. W. NORTON & COMPANY
Independent Publishers Since 1923

For information about permission to reproduce selections from this book, write to
Permissions, W. W. Norton & Company, Inc., 500 Fifth Avenue, New York, NY 10110

For information about special discounts for bulk purchases, please contact
W. W. Norton Special Sales at specialsales@wwnorton.com or 800-233-4830

Manufacturing by Lake Book Manufacturing
Book design by Chris Welch
Production manager: Lauren Abbate

Library of Congress Cataloging-in-Publication Data

Names: Nimura, Janice P., author.
Title: The doctors Blackwell : how two pioneering sisters brought medicine to women—
and women to medicine / Janice P. Nimura.
Description: First edition. | New York : W.W. Norton & Company, 2021. |
Includes bibliographical references and index.
Identifiers: LCCN 2020023919 | ISBN 9780393635546 (hardcover) | ISBN 9780393635553 (epub)
Subjects: LCSH: Blackwell, Elizabeth, 1821–1910—Health. | Blackwell, Emily, 1826–1910—
Health. | Women physicians—United States—Biography. | Women in medicine—United States—
Biography. | Sexism in medicine.
Classification: LCC R692 .N56 2021 | DDC 610.92 [B]—dc23
LC record available at https://lccn.loc.gov/2020023919

W. W. Norton & Company, Inc., 500 Fifth Avenue, New York, N.Y. 10110
www.wwnorton.com

W. W. Norton & Company Ltd., 15 Carlisle Street, London W1D 3BS

3 4 5 6 7 8 9 0

FOR CLARE AND DAVID,

SCIENTISTS AND FEMINISTS

Contents

THE DOCTORS
BLACKWELL

PROLOGUE

On May 14, 2018, a cheerful crowd of activist New Yorkers blocked the sidewalk at the corner of Bleecker and Crosby streets. Before them stood an elderly and unremarkable building: four stories topped by a pair of attic dormers, battered brick facade obscured by a fire escape, pre-hipster neighborhood bar on the ground floor. After a parade of speakers, all but one of them women, the Greenwich Village Society for Historic Preservation unveiled a commemorative plaque, the newest stop on its Civil Rights and Social Justice Map. "In this building," it read, "the first female doctor in America, Elizabeth Blackwell, established the first hospital for, staffed, and run by women."

Applause erupted, VIPs grinned, cameras clicked. There was a triumphant sense of reclaiming a hero; of restoring a story of female agency; of lifting, for just a moment, the grim political mood. Someone was selling eye-popping T-shirts, black and hot pink on white: ELIZABETH BLACKWELL: OG MD. The celebrants dispersed into the balmy evening, imagining the first female doctor: saintly and sepia-toned, bending solicitously over her grateful patients; or maybe a fiercer version, Original Gangster of medical women, crusading feminist. Both images were satisfying. Neither was accurate.

～

On May 12, 1857, in a room overlooking that same corner of Bleecker and Crosby, Dr. Elizabeth Blackwell—petite, unsmiling, soberly dressed—moved into the light slanting through tall sash windows to address a small audience of ladies and a sprinkling of gentlemen. Two rows of iron bedsteads filled the space, made up with mismatched but carefully smoothed white linens. The assembled guests had settled themselves with a waggish chuckle or two about the impropriety of mixed company gathering in a room that was, strictly speaking, a ladies' bedchamber. It would never be so pristine again, but for now, stethoscopes and scalpels, opium and mercury, blood and piss and all the unmentionable mess of illness and childbirth and surgery and death were nowhere to be seen.

Elizabeth cleared her throat to be heard over the hoofbeats and clatter of busy Broadway, a short block away, and read with stiff gravity from the document she held: "This institution, which is publicly opened today, is a hospital and dispensary for poor women and children."

Its unprecedented purpose, she read on, was threefold: to allow women to consult doctors of their own sex, free of charge; to provide the growing number of female medical students with the practical experience denied them by established hospitals; and to train nurses. Her tone was level and businesslike, betraying no sense that for most of New York's burghers—not to mention their wives—the idea of a woman doctor was outrageous. She did not mention the loneliness, drudgery, and pain she had transcended to become the first woman in America to receive a medical degree, in 1849. Nor did she acknowledge the taller, equally grave woman by her side, who shared her direct gaze and determined jawline: her sister Emily, who had struggled just as mightily to earn her own degree in 1854, and without whom this moment might not have arrived.

The trustees of the newborn New York Infirmary for Indigent Women and Children, thirteen men and four women, had rejected the suggestion that one of these female physicians should tell her own story that day, fearing she might sound off-puttingly like an agitator for women's rights. But Elizabeth was not a radical, however radical her choice to study medicine might seem. "The full thorough education of women in medicine is a new idea, and like all other truths requires time to prove its value," she continued. "Women must show to medical men, even more than to the public, their capacity to act as physicians, their earnestness as students of medicine, before the existing institutions with their great advantages of practice and complete organization will be opened to them." Then she ceded the floor to a man: Henry Ward Beecher, the heavy-lidded, silver-tongued, irrepressibly libidinous pastor of Brooklyn's Plymouth Church, arguably the most famous man in New York.

"There are none less able to make provision for themselves in this world than women and children," Beecher intoned, and then—with more brio than coherence—insisted that he believed "most thoroughly in woman's accomplishments." Indeed, women might well be better suited to medicine than men. "Her intuition, perception and good mother wit render her so," he explained, surrendering to stereotype and dispensing with science altogether. "The tread of woman in the sick chamber is itself antidote." Their expressions neutral, the Blackwell sisters applauded with the rest. Allowing this patronizing, magnetic man—whom they had known, in fact, long before his fame took hold—to proclaim that "woman was ordained to be a doctor" was the best publicity imaginable.

A dozen years earlier, at the age of twenty-four, Elizabeth Blackwell had selected medicine as a means of proving a truth she believed to be divinely sanctioned: that women could be anything they wished according to the limits of individual talent and toil, and in reaching their fullest potential would raise humanity closer to its ideal. Medicine had not been an obvious choice for a young woman who equated illness with weakness, cared little for anyone beyond the circle of her eight siblings, and preferred the life of the mind to the functions of the body—which she found, quite frankly, disgusting. But God had chosen her, she believed, to pursue this arduous path, and she had chosen Emily, her most capable sister, five years younger, to follow her.

In the decades to come, Elizabeth would make greater use of her pen than her medical instruments, her opinionated eloquence preserved in reams of her own writing, both private and published. It was plainspoken, understated Emily who quietly embraced the challenge of medicine itself, Emily who would spend her life as a practicing physician, surgeon, and instructor—though like her sister, she too fell short of empathy. "There is certainly nothing attractive in the care of miserable forlorn sick people," she wrote to Elizabeth. "It is only as scientific illustration that I can take the least interest in them, unless it were possible to raise them, and that is a difficult matter."

Raising the expectations and ambitions of women, from the slums of Five Points to the salons of Fifth Avenue: a difficult matter indeed. Together the Blackwell sisters managed it. Their story does not fit on a plaque.

~

CHAPTER 1

BRISTOL—NEW YORK— CINCINNATI

The yellowed notebook is inscribed with perfectly straight lines of Elizabeth Blackwell's careful eleven-year-old penmanship. "There lived as my story says a Lady and Gentleman," it begins. The Gentleman, a manufacturer like Elizabeth's father, watches his friends emigrate from England to America,

> and as he knew that his business was a very good one and that he could bring up his children better there than in England he asked his wife what she thoght about going though she was was sorry to leave her native land, yet as she knew, that it was for her chidren's good she consented. [*sic*]

They would embark in "the best vessell in the port," in a cabin "just like a parlour," furnished with "a carpet a sofa some chairs a piano a bookcase with several interesting books in and a number of beautiful plants on the windowseat." Music, books, nature, and nice furniture: everything anyone could want, in a safe cozy space. It is the vision of a child trying to tame her fears.

In August 1832 the Blackwell family left their native Bristol forever. The party of fifteen—Samuel and Hannah, their eight children, a governess, two maids, and two aunts—boarded the *Cosmo* for seven weeks and four days of malodorous misery. Cholera—a plague that had reached England for the first time the previous year—stowed away with the steerage passengers, several of whom died en route. It was a terrifying passage from the predictable comforts of home toward an unimaginable future. Then again, home had recently become less comfortable or predictable.

~

A decade earlier Samuel Blackwell, son of a Bristol cabinetmaker, had claimed his place in the industrial middle class and established his family in a terraced house at the corner of Wilson Street and Lemon Lane. An ambitious young sugar refiner, he dressed in ministerial black with a snowy white cravat, though his wife Hannah was known to indulge her frivolous side—she loved dancing and cherished her china tea service. The family was growing rapidly: first Anna and Marian, and then Elizabeth, her birth in 1821 bracketed by the deaths of two infant brothers, both named Samuel. After this came a third, healthy Samuel, followed quickly by Henry. Soon there would be Emily and Ellen, then Howard and George. The nine Blackwell children thought of themselves in alternating pairs of girls and boys, with Elizabeth the odd one out. Her nickname was "Little Shy."

Hannah Lane Blackwell found her calling in motherhood. Her own childhood was not a time she liked to dwell upon. "I was fitted with a dress of black in expectation of my father being hanged," she remembered. She was a little girl when her father was arrested—along with a female accomplice not his wife—for forgery, his clock-making business apparently not as profitable as he desired. His protestations of innocence during his trial were undermined by the fact that he had tried to eat his counterfeit banknotes when challenged. Escaping execution, he was transported to Australia, and Hannah never saw her father again. She found a husband whose probity—if perhaps not his business acumen—would never be called into question, and devoted herself to managing a stable and upright household.

Samuel and Hannah were idealists as well as capitalists: protestant Dissenters from the established Church of England; advocates of education, temperance, hard work, and self-improvement; staunch Whig reformers and early antislavery activists. Wait: a sugar refiner opposed to slavery? British trade in humans might have ceased in 1807, but on the sugar plantations of the Caribbean, the English still depended on

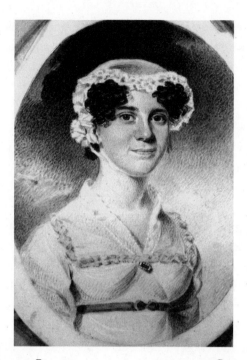

HANNAH BLACKWELL AS A YOUNG WOMAN IN BRISTOL.
COURTESY SCHLESINGER LIBRARY, RADCLIFFE INSTITUTE, HARVARD UNIVERSITY.

enslaved labor. Samuel dealt in a commodity tied to an institution he abhorred, and he dreamed of finding a way to produce sugar without cruelty. Congregationalists in an Anglican society, antislavery activists in the sugar trade: the Blackwells held deeply moral, defiantly unorthodox opinions. In this generation—and more so in the next—they practiced an ideological contrarianism, striving toward a moral high ground that the placid mainstream ignored, dismissed, or failed to imagine. From those isolated and inhospitable heights, they aspired to shine as beacons, guiding the unenlightened toward a truer future.

Firstborn Anna, dictatorial and dramatic, persuaded her mother to let her sleep in the garret and invested her pocket money in a spyglass. When she felt generous, she invited Marian and Elizabeth—Emily was too little—to climb out her dormer window onto the leads of the roof. Snug in their "sky parlour," the three girls majestically surveyed the hills and fields beyond the eastern edge of the city—until someone caught them at it. Unabashed, these daughters of progressive reformers did what they had seen the grown-ups do: they wrote a petition—"promising to sit perfectly still & not lean over the parapet"—and delivered it to their father. Samuel, in turn, responded with another Blackwell pastime: he wrote a poem, which began,

Anna, Bessy, & Polly*!
Your request is mere folly.
The leads are too high
For those who can't fly!

After that, the girls had to content themselves with the wooden rocking horse in the back parlor—Anna in the saddle, Marian perched on the rockers behind, and Elizabeth in front.

All but the youngest of the Blackwells were born in Bristol and grew strong on a diet of nature, literature, and political consciousness. Favorite excursions included the double springs of Mother Pugsley's Well at Kingsdown, or the craggy grandeur of St. Vincent's Rocks, tumbling down to the river Avon, the cliff ledges home to plants found nowhere else: whitebeam, speedwell, rock-cress. Samuel and Hannah granted their daughters the same access to knowledge as their sons. Their books were mostly of the pious and improving sort—Mrs. Sherwood's *Stories Explanatory of the Church Catechism* was a perennial—until Anna and Marian, with the help of a nursemaid, got hold of a few volumes of Sir Walter Scott. "There was a dreadful scene, & our beloved novels were seized & carried off to Papa, & we expected some dreadful punishment," Anna remembered. But Samuel, curious to see what had captivated his daughters, sat down to read Scott and was captivated in turn.

Hannah was the less flexible parent. Her faith abjured vanity—as one admired for her beauty, she struggled with it herself—and she was determined to prevent it from taking root in impressionable minds. "The pretty baby makes the ugliest person!" she insisted. Her vigilance had the contrary effect of making her children morbidly self-conscious, and their awkwardness only grew with time. "We were always so shabbily

---

* Polly was Marian's nickname.

dressed that we were always painfully conscious of not looking like other people," Anna remembered. But with so many siblings, there was never a shortage of companionship at home.

They turned toward one another and held themselves apart. Like many Dissenters—intellectually adventurous, politically engaged—Samuel and Hannah prized the moral over the material, shuddering at the lavish pageantry of the Anglican establishment even as it persisted in excluding them. (Until 1828, Dissenters were barred from public office; their sons, however brilliant, were not permitted to take degrees at Oxford or Cambridge until the 1850s.) The Blackwell children were acutely aware of the contrast between the principled austerity at home and the glittering delights of bustling Bristol.

Though Hannah's marriage was happy, her daughters could not help noticing that the extended family was full of less contented women. Four "poor starveling aunts" lived under their brother Samuel's roof. Mary was the favorite, a "natural lady." Lucy—"very small, kindly, & null"—served as seamstress, though "she had not an atom of taste & knew no more of dress-making than of Greek." Ann, in her namesake niece Anna's unsparing estimation, was "very well-meaning, obstinate, ignorant, & ugly." Barbara was the least popular of all, especially once installed as governess in Wilson Street: Anna called her "one of the most disagreeable, ill-tempered, strict, narrow-minded creatures alive." Yet the girls understood that what their aunts lacked was not intelligence but opportunity. Hateful Aunt Barbara "was very clever, & education might have had its full course of usefulness in her case," Anna mused. "But she straggled up, like the rest of her family, ignorant as a broomstick."

Uneducated and unpartnered, the aunts had no choice but to fill whatever roles were available in their brother's household. Marriage, however, was no guarantee of anything better. Grandmother Blackwell, tiny and gentle, lived in the shadow of her tyrannical husband, a man so unpleasant his family must occasionally have wished it were he, and not Hannah's father, who had been transported to Australia. Anna could not remember Grandmother Blackwell "putting forth an opinion on any subject beyond house-work & meals," but before her death, she startled her eldest granddaughter, warning her,

how careful girls ought to be before they listened to the flatteries of
a man, seeing that all *that* ceased when they'd got a woman to marry
them, & then the poor girl found what a dreadful master marriage
had given her, what a slave she was, & what a world of care & labour
& worry she had got into; adding that those were wise who did not
marry, & that if it were to do over again, most certainly she would
not marry Grandpapa.

None of the five Blackwell girls would marry. All of them, at various
times, would earn a living as teachers.

In the Blackwell household, the terms *master* and *slave* were not used
lightly. In 1823 the abolitionist Thomas Clarkson stopped to speak in
Bristol—a port at the center of Britain's sugar trade—carrying with him
a polished wooden chest from which he produced a display of the arts
and produce of African peoples. Inspired, Samuel Blackwell joined Bristol's Auxiliary Anti-Slavery Society and studied the tantalizing promise of
sugar beets, which could be farmed in temperate climates without slave
labor—an innovation in which the French had recently invested, their
access to Caribbean cane sugar blocked by the embargoes of the Napo-
leonic wars. Samuel did not preoccupy himself with bettering the lives
of plantation slaves—his focus had more to do with the moral hygiene
of British sugar consumers—but his beliefs and his livelihood were still
essentially opposed. His offspring took note. "We children had been so
harrowed by the statements about West Indian slavery," Anna remembered, "that we had given up taking sugar in our tea, by way of protest."
Then again, the unsweetened tea had been paid for by sugar.

Sugar refining might have boosted Samuel Blackwell's status, but it
was a tricky foundation on which to build. In 1828 the whole household
watched the "great feathers of flame, & the volumes of sparks, rushing up
into the sky" from across the narrow river Avon as Samuel's Countership
Refinery burned; even from that safe distance, the railings they leaned
upon at the river's edge grew warm from the conflagration. Refineries
received raw sugar from the Caribbean and then boiled, filtered, gran-
ulated, and finally molded and trimmed it into smooth conical loaves;
the combination of roaring boilers and combustible sugar dust meant

that refineries had an alarming tendency to explode. Samuel was able to rebuild his business, but he had to downsize from airy Wilson Street to grittier lodgings attached to his new refinery.

Other disappointments followed. Samuel's brother James, in charge of the Blackwell interests in Dublin, succumbed to violent paranoia and ran the office into the ground. (He was eventually committed to a private asylum, where he felt less threatened by the assassins he believed were trying to kill him.) A Bristol shipping firm that owed Samuel thousands of pounds went bankrupt. And in addition to these financial tremors, a larger political quake shook Bristol in the fall of 1831.

Decades later the Blackwell siblings could still recall the eerie silence of the deserted streets, followed by the roaring tumult of hundreds of angry men pelting past with torches to attack Bristol's seats of power. The rapid rise of industrial cities had made Britain's electoral landscape obsolete, with minimally populated and easily manipulated rural "rotten boroughs" sending members to the House of Commons while the surging populations of urban areas went unrepresented—not that workers could vote anyway, as the franchise was limited to landowners. In October, after the Second Reform Bill was defeated, the city was convulsed by three days of deadly riots. Though the Blackwells were heartily in favor of legislative reform, the violence unleashed around them was terrifying.

At this vulnerable moment, Samuel was unusually susceptible to the glowing reports he had begun to receive from friends who had emigrated to America. It was a nation founded by Dissenters, after all, where the Blackwells' religion would not obstruct their children's prospects. Samuel could bring his antislavery energy to a nation soaked in the blood of slaves—and in the vastness of American agricultural possibility, perhaps he could find a way to root his sugar beets in the same soil. His decision to emigrate was met with horror by his colleagues in Bristol, who offered him a generous loan in an attempt to persuade him to stay. Hannah shared their dismay. She had just given birth to Howard, her eighth living child, and she was already pregnant again.

～

New York, when the Blackwells disembarked from the *Cosmo* at last, was oddly quiet. They soon discovered that the scourge they hoped to leave

behind had leaped ahead of them: the city was in the grip of its first cholera epidemic, and its wealthier residents had fled. An understanding of
the mechanisms by which epidemics spread was still decades away. The
death toll exceeded 3,500, out of a population of 250,000.

For all Samuel's optimism, America was a perilous land where manners were rougher and rules less defined. Would his children and his fortunes flourish in this place full of "active dollar-getting people," hustling
along filthy streets where plain wooden buildings were only just being
replaced with more substantial brick and stone? His wife and children
would never match his zest for the new world. He settled his family in
rented accommodations on Thompson Street, and within a few weeks
Hannah delivered a healthy boy, her ninth and last child. In honor of their
brave beginning, they christened him George Washington Blackwell.

There was a contingent quality to the Blackwell sojourn in New York.
With the help of backers in Bristol, Samuel bought the Congress Sugar
Refinery on Duane Street, one of the largest in the city. Within two years
the family moved from Manhattan to Long Island, near the village of
Flushing, but their enjoyment of a spacious frame house and adjoining
orchard was cut short when Samuel was stricken with malaria. The blame
was placed correctly on their proximity to marshland, though it would be
more than half a century before the mosquito was identified as the true
culprit; as its name proclaimed, *malaria*—"bad air"—was thought to be
caused by the noxious exhalations of stagnant bogs. Malaria was so common in the young United States that illness and recovery were known as
"seasoning," a normal part of settling in. In December 1835 the Blackwells skipped back across Manhattan to Jersey City, a ferry ride across
the Hudson River from Samuel's refinery. There was a reason for every
relocation, but the family's failure to settle in one place prevented deeper
engagement with any community beyond their own clan.

Elizabeth preferred solitude to socializing anyway. Her voracious reading juxtaposed Shakespeare and *Pilgrim's Progress* with the independent
heroines of novels by Maria Edgeworth and Madame de Staël. Books were
a refuge from her own ineptitude in company. "If people will make me
out such a queer being they are very welcome," she declared, "and I shall
take the liberty of caring very little about it." The cultivation of frivolous

feminine charm was beneath her, and though she often found herself on the edge of things, she doubted the center was any better. "How gay the ladies look," she wrote of the passing crowd, "& how miserably their waists are pinched up."

As a teenager, she hungered for recognition and despaired of achieving it. "I fear the brilliant radiance of genius is far from illuminating *my soul*," she confided to her journal. When her younger brother Sam escorted her to the commencement speeches at Columbia College, she was both inspired and frustrated. "The Greek oration called up a multitude of thoughts," she admitted, "and the melancholy reflection that the enchanting paths of literature were not for me to walk in." Although Oberlin Collegiate Institute in Ohio had admitted the first female students to its bachelor's degree course in 1833, it was a startling exception—and anyway Elizabeth daydreamed of claiming a place alongside the men of Columbia, not of joining other women at a tiny and obscure frontier school.

If literature and philosophy were closed to her, what paths were open? "How I do long for some end to act for," she wrote. "To go on every day in just the same jog trot manner without any object is very wearisome." Joining the ranks of the burgeoning temperance movement, she signed the total abstinence pledge. She also ruled out marriage. Upon reading a novel entitled *The Three Eras of Woman's Life*—girl, wife, mother—she complained, "I wish some skillful pen would produce an interesting old maid's life." She was barely seventeen.

Elizabeth's prickliness extended to her sisters. Stormy Anna—nearly five years older—had assumed the role of tutor to the younger children after their governess, Miss Major, became Aunt Eliza, having married Hannah's visiting brother, Uncle Charles Lane. (He already had a wife in England, but the Blackwells, by tacit agreement, forbore from scrutinizing the decisions of "poor, foolish, kind-hearted, void-of-principle Uncle Charley!") Anna's new position of authority heightened the tension between herself and Elizabeth, and their sororal silent treatments could go on and on. "Just as I was getting into bed Anna sent me a most dignified & severe note of forgiveness for my past conduct," Elizabeth recorded, "so I suppose our estrangement of more than 3 months is at an end." Marian, though more retiring than Anna, could be just as critical of Elizabeth's manners.

Sturdy, curious Emily was the beneficiary of her sisters' standoffs, during which Elizabeth might take her "into partnership to her great joy." But Emily was too young to be stimulating company, and when Anna left for a teaching position at a seminary in Vermont, Elizabeth instantly wished her back. "I wonder how Anna gets on," she wrote. "She has hardly been out of my head once, we quite miss her active tongue." And so it would often be with the Blackwells: they liked each other better than anyone else, and they liked each other best with a little distance. Anna's departure marked the beginning of the family diaspora—rarely would the Blackwell siblings all be together again—but until their deaths they never stopped writing to each other. In the early years, when money was tight and postage dear, they filled the page, then rotated it a quarter turn and filled it again, creating dense grids of cramped copperplate.

Elizabeth's brothers Sam and Henry, between herself and Emily in age, enjoyed a livelier social life—Broadway excursions to concerts at Niblo's Garden and a glimpse of the Siamese twins, Chang and Eng Bunker, at Peale's Museum—but the reserved and opinionated Blackwell women spent their leisure time quietly, perhaps more quietly than they wished. On New Year's Day, when ladies were at home to callers, twelve-year-old Sam reported that "Mamma, Anna, Marian, and Bessy sat in the parlour from about ten oclock in the morning, till night, but not one did they receive, save Uncle Charles, until about five oclock in the evening."

Elizabeth preferred more cerebral entertainments, like a visit to the Fowler brothers, Orson and Lorenzo, who had established a thriving practice in the new and fashionable study of phrenology. Its Viennese originator, Franz Joseph Gall, believed that attitudes and aptitudes had their respective organs in the brain, sized in proportion to their strength. One had only to examine the bulges and dents of the cranium to understand deeper truths about an individual's capacity for thirty-seven traits, including steadfastness, prudence, enterprise, humor, and both "amative," or romantic, love, and the "philoprogenitive," or parental, kind. Gall's theory had its origin in his own student days, when he noted that

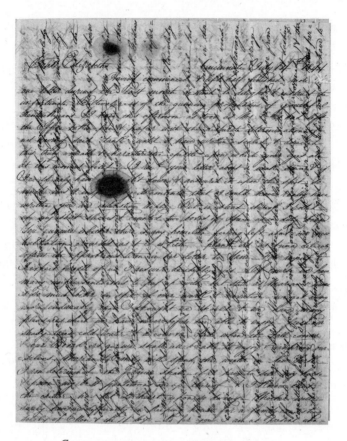

CROSS-WRITING SAVED PAPER AND POSTAGE.
COURTESY SCHLESINGER LIBRARY, RADCLIFFE INSTITUTE, HARVARD UNIVERSITY

the real geniuses among his classmates had high foreheads and protu-berant eyes. Gall, naturally, shared these features.

To enliven a frigid January afternoon, Elizabeth went with a couple of her siblings to be "phrenologized" by the Fowlers and came away intrigued in spite of herself by "the bumpy science." In Elizabeth's case, observed her examiner, "cautiousness" was not large; "veneration" and "imitation" were moderate; "alimentiveness," or hunger, was good; and "ideality," or refinement, was strong. The shape of her skull seemed to justify the misanthropic superiority she sometimes failed to conceal. "Not disposed to trifle, nor will she be trifled with," read the report. "Others do not know how much mind you have." It was all quite gratifying to a girl who longed for confirmation of her own excellence—except for the comment regarding her outsized region of "philoprogenitive love," which had to be a mistake. Elizabeth's ambitions did not include parenthood. She already had six younger siblings to look after.

Antislavery activism was the Blackwells' primary form of social engagement, and in May 1837 every Blackwell sister except nine-year-old Ellen attended the Anti-Slavery Convention of American Women, a groundbreaking meeting that included free black women. Anna was an official delegate, and the proceedings were led by such luminaries as Lucretia Mott and the Grimké sisters, Sarah and Angelina, who would go on to prominence in the women's rights movement. Early murmurs of that cause were audible at the 1837 meeting, when Angelina Grimké proposed a resolution on the imperative for women "to plead the cause of the oppressed in our land"—the implication being that women were among those oppressed. "The time has come for woman to move in that sphere which Providence has assigned her," Grimké announced, "and no longer remain satisfied in the circumscribed limits with which corrupt custom and a perverted application of Scripture have encircled her." The audience was by no means unanimous in its affirmation of this sentiment, and Anna, Marian, Elizabeth, and Emily walked home still discussing whether it was "very ill advised."

Their father, continuing to live a paradox, joined in whenever he could spare time from his sugar refinery. "The spirit of Slavery blackens and curses everything here morally and politically," Samuel Blackwell wrote, "and I fear will work like a Canker until perfect rottenness will be the end and ruin of these States." He befriended William Lloyd Garrison and joined New York's Committee of Vigilance, helping to protect fugitives from recapture. "A colored man came here tonight who said he was a runaway slave," Elizabeth wrote one December night. "We gave him some money to help him on his journey." For a solitary, bookish, uncompromisingly high-minded young woman, antislavery activism added savor to static days: access to famous figures, the thrill of moral righteousness in the face of opposition, and the risky romance of aiding fugitives in the night. There was little actual contact with the pain and peril of black lives, but Elizabeth was happier with the abstract ideal.

She chafed at the limited scope of her life. "What a dearth of incidents," she griped in the summer of 1837. "I wish I could devise some good way of maintaining myself but the restrictions which confine my dear sex render all my aspirations useless." A week later the accession of Princess Victoria to the British throne roused Elizabeth from her torpor. "How ardently I hope our young queen may prove worthy & capable of governing our flourishing kingdom, & may be an honour to our sex," she wrote. A woman ascendant, and just two years older than herself! It lifted Elizabeth's spirits and reignited her English pride. Queen Victoria sounded like a woman worth getting to know.

Meanwhile that spring, the situation in New York had grown precarious. A convergence of economic forces, exacerbated by President Andrew Jackson's ill-advised financial policies, resulted in a panic that shuttered banks, ruined fortunes, and brought soldiers onto the streets to prevent unrest. Samuel's bad luck continued—his refinery had burned again, and he sold out to his foreman, determined to focus his energy at last on the elusive grail of beet sugar. Napoleon's wartime subsidies decades earlier had made France the leader in sugar beets, but American interest in the commodity had recently begun to sharpen. Land was cheap and plentiful, and domestic sugar looked like a promising investment. Samuel was no farmer, but the idea of controlling both ends of the production process, free of the taint of slavery, was powerfully attractive—a chance to do well at last, in addition to doing good.

"I hope Papa is not taking up [his] Michigan beet idea again," Elizabeth wrote, "but his talking so much about beets & bringing home those French books for us to translate is rather suspicious." It was hard not to draw the obvious conclusion when Samuel disappeared into the basement with Hannah's silver saucepan to "make some experiments," only to emerge with a burn on his face from boiling sugar. In the spring of 1838, he left Jersey City for extended explorations into Pennsylvania and Ohio—less distant than Michigan but still dauntingly remote—trying to determine where to plant his beets and his family.

In lengthy, reflective, whimsical letters, Samuel strove to convince his wife and children of the promise of the West, so vast and raw compared to New York, let alone Bristol. "Tell dear Washy,"* his father wrote, "that I have seen a 'possum . . . and squirrels jumping from tree to tree in the woods—and people making holes in trees for sugar to run out—and trees as high as church towers." Cincinnati, more primitive even than Pittsburgh, was a "fine and flourishing place—and though I should not apply the epithet 'glorious' to it, there is certainly much to admire."

～

In May 1838 the Blackwells left New York for Cincinnati, minus Anna and Marian, who remained in their teaching positions. The journey, via ocean steamer to Philadelphia, railway over the Alleghenies, and multiple stages of river travel, took nine days. In the squashed society of the riverboats, Elizabeth looked on as Emily and Ellen, eleven and ten respectively, were indulged by the young men aboard; Emily won consistently at checkers, to the delighted chagrin of her opponents. No one paid Elizabeth much attention, which was both a relief and also a little disappointing. "I suppose I am considered *fixed*," she grumbled, "for a lady asked me while I was ablutionizing Wash, if that was *my son*." She passed the time reading Pascal's *Pensées.*

Perched on the riverbank and ringed with low hills, Cincinnati in 1838 was a rising city of thirty-five thousand, styling itself "Queen of the West" but more accurately known as "Porkopolis." In a best-selling travelogue, the British writer Fanny Trollope, mother of the more celebrated Anthony, had recently shared her appalled impressions of an unlovely frontier town where garbage disposal was entrusted to the free-range pigs. Pork was the engine of Cincinnati's prosperity, and the streams ran red every fall with the effluent of the city's slaughterhouses; butchering, in the era before refrigeration, was a cold-weather industry. But now it was spring. "I saw some very handsome houses & well-dressed people," Elizabeth wrote with determined optimism after her first morning's walk. "There seems an air of respectability & cleanliness about the place." Perhaps her father would prosper here at last. And though Cincin-

---

* The family's nickname for George Washington.

nati stood on free soil, Ohio farmers commonly rented enslaved hands from across the river in Kentucky as seasonal laborers. The need for anti-slavery advocacy was obvious.

The Blackwells found yet another house to rent, and in the absence of Anna and Marian, Elizabeth taught her younger siblings. On Sundays, in the absence of anything resembling cultural diversion, she tried out churches, including the congregation of Lyman Beecher, a theologian renowned for his fiery Presbyterian leadership as well as, eventually, for his famous progeny. It would be another decade before Henry Ward Beecher, Harriet Beecher Stowe, and Catharine Beecher became household names, but the Blackwells were immediately drawn to them. Perhaps Cincinnati wasn't such a muddy backwater—perhaps there was scope for young women whose minds were more impressive than their wardrobes. "If we cannot show off physically, we must mentally, & eclipse them all by the charms of our understanding," wrote Marian to Elizabeth. "I intend to come out a bel esprit, you may be a mentor 'severe in youthful beauty' & Anna shall dazzle them all by her refined wit sharp as a needle's point." Elizabeth, currently making her way through Jane Austen, wholeheartedly approved this vision of intellectual conquest.

But before the family even finished unpacking, Samuel began to show symptoms of an illness that had plagued him for years—possibly the same malaria he had contracted in Flushing. Fevers and fainting fits became more frequent, and soon the doctor was visiting several times a day. "He is just the color of an Indian," Elizabeth wrote. "Aunt M thinks he will never leave his bed."

As Samuel sank, Elizabeth—the oldest child present—recorded her father's symptoms in detail: his distressing restlessness, his irregular breathing, his slowing pulse, the doses of brandy and broth and laudanum, the rubbings with mercury ointment and the spongings with muriatic—better known today as hydrochloric—acid. Unsurprisingly, none of these efforts helped. Though it is tempting to discern in this moment the germ of her medical future, it is perhaps more accurate to see it as the first time she found herself in charge. "I had sat all the evening at the head of his bed with his right hand in mine," she wrote. "As I leant over the sofa weeping, most ardently did I pray that if it was God's will to take him from us that [He] would give him a peaceful & easy passage to another world."

Just after ten o'clock on August 7, 1838, Samuel Blackwell died, his distraught wife and stunned children kneeling at his bedside. "I put my hand to his mouth," wrote Elizabeth, "& never till my dying day shall I forget the dreadful feeling when I found there was no breath." The grief in her words is clear, but so is the sense of a young woman feeling the dramatic power of her own narrative as it flows from her pen. "He is dead," she wrote. "Oh that I should live to write it, the support of our house, the kind generous fond indulgent parent is no more."

The brutal August heat forced a swift burial. The next day Elizabeth and Hannah examined Samuel's papers. He had left his widow and nine children, newly deposited at the edge of the world, with twenty dollars.

～

Fatherlessness produced a sequence of inversions within the Blackwell family. The necessity of earning an income shoved mourning aside, and as the Blackwell sons ranged in age from Sam and Henry, fifteen and thirteen, to Howard and George, seven and five, it fell to their oldest sisters to provide it. Less than three weeks after Samuel's death, the Cincinnati English and French Academy for Young Ladies welcomed its first students. Elizabeth had printed circulars grandly offering a course of study in "Reading, Writing, Sketching and the rudiments of Drawing, Arithmetic, Grammar, Ancient and Modern History, Geography, Natural and Moral Philosophy, Botany, Composition, the French Language and Vocal Music." Classes met in the Blackwells' front parlor.

Having missed their father's funeral, Anna and Marian hurried to Cincinnati just in time for another death. "Aunt Mary exceedingly unwell," Elizabeth wrote on September 24. A week later she too was gone. "It seemed as if whatever arrived I should never feel again," wrote Elizabeth, "not one tear did I shed, the dreadful blow we first received seems to have rendered me callous to everything else." Transatlantic letters arrived from Hannah's brothers, urging the new widow to bring her children home to England. Surely Hannah was tempted—but it had always been her husband who steered the family's course, and now her daughters took the helm. Elizabeth scorned her uncles' implication that their headless family was helpless as well: "They don't know what we are made of." But she hated the long hours, the constant flickering between boredom and anxiety, and the exhausting lack of time to herself. "After school I took my work & sat on the roof in a most delightful wind, how I love that high wind blowing up my hair so boisterously," she wrote. "I always fancy myself on the ocean sailing back to our home."

Sam, earnest and pedantic, found a job as a courthouse clerk. Henry, as ebullient as his brother was sober, managed to escape for a year of school in St. Louis until he too came home to work in a bank. Emily had the happiest position: too young to work but old enough to study. Though younger than Henry, she was taller—which amused everyone in the family except Henry—and she threatened to top him in scholarship as well. "I have cut all my wisdom teeth," she crowed to her closest brother, "and you cannot think how wise I have grown." Life with three opinionated older sisters had taught her to watch and listen; she was already showing scholarly aptitude on a par with Elizabeth's, paired with a steadiness that her family would come to appreciate.

On Sundays, liberated from labor, the Blackwells refreshed themselves with ideas. Hannah, true to her Dissenting roots, aligned herself with Lyman Beecher, president of Lane Theological Seminary, where he trained young men to win the West for God. Fervent revival meetings were less attractive to Hannah's more intellectual daughters, but there was no shortage of pulpits in Cincinnati, where church was the most plentiful form of entertainment. To Hannah's horror—or possibly because of it—Elizabeth announced her intention to be confirmed in the Episcopal Church, the conservative, socially elite American cousin of the Church of England. Its Englishness perhaps fed her nostalgia for Bristol. But within the year she swung to the other extreme, thanks to the arrival of a charismatic young man named William Henry Channing.

Not quite thirty, and with the hooded gaze and dramatic cheekbones of a poet, the Harvard-educated Channing swept into Cincinnati in 1839 as the pastor of the Unitarian Society. Whereas Episcopalians hewed to ornate High Church practices—the Trinity, saints, embroidered vestments, and clouds of incense—Unitarians believed in the oneness of the divine, with an emphasis on reason, a tolerance for doubt, and a capacious attitude toward individual modes of worship. Through Channing, the Blackwells encountered Transcendentalism, which chimed with their own ideas regarding the natural goodness of humans. "I well remember the glowing face with which I found Mr. Channing reading a book just received," Elizabeth wrote. "'Sit down,' he cried, 'and listen to this!' and forthwith he poured forth extracts from Emerson's essays." By 1840— again to their mother's horror—the three eldest sisters were Unitarians.

It was through Channing as well that the Blackwells first became interested in the utopian visions of the Frenchman Charles Fourier. Fourier had imagined planned communities, or phalanxes, in which work, determined by individual passion, would become pleasure, and women would fill any role for which their skills and interests equipped them. His doctrine of Associationism imagined harmonious cooperation unbound by corrupt social constraints—including marriage. Where other girls of twenty might daydream of husband, children, and household, Elizabeth began to plan her own phalanx.

But these radical ideas, in the context of Cincinnati society, were not respectable, and the Blackwells needed to project enough respectability to persuade Cincinnati's leading families to send them their daughters. "I'm sorry to say the school is shrunk very much," reported Sam after only three years of operation. It closed in 1842, but by then Sam and Henry were older, with steady work.

A new chapter was beginning, and with it a second inversion of convention. Samuel Blackwell's death had taught his daughters that a husband—especially a dreamer like their father—was no guarantee of security. Marian, the least robust of the Blackwell women, would become the family's Hestia, tending the family hearth and looking after widowed Hannah as she aged, but Anna, Elizabeth, Emily, and eventually even Ellen would seek fulfillment outside the domestic sphere. During their first fatherless years, the Blackwell daughters had provided for the sons. Now Sam and Henry would remain at home, working at uninspiring jobs while supporting, admiringly and sometimes enviously, their sisters' bolder journeys.

CHAPTER 2

~

BETWEENITY

At the end of February 1844, Elizabeth, now twenty-three, left her family for the first time and boarded a riverboat, watching with growing dismay as it slid west past Louisville and beyond what she recognized as civilization. "Madam, we have reached Henderson," a crew member announced at last, pointing out Elizabeth's new home: "three dirty old frame buildings, a steep bank covered with mud, some negroes & dirty white people at the foot." The town of Henderson, Kentucky—four days down the Ohio River and across the border into slave territory—was in need of a schoolmistress.

Elizabeth was soon installed in the drafty brick house of one of Henderson's first families, who were perhaps too assiduous in their hospitality. "I who so love a hermit's life for a good part of the day," she wrote, "find myself living in public & almost losing my identity." Upon her arrival, they sat her by the fire to warm herself—and then, to Elizabeth's horror, "placed a little negro girl before me as a fire screen."

Her domain was a chilly, dirt-floored schoolhouse and twenty-one girls who regarded their new teacher with some awe. "I give as far as I can learn universal satisfaction," Elizabeth wrote. "Indeed I believe the people are a little afraid of me, particularly when they see me read German." She cultivated this imposing aura, as there was nothing worse than socializing with Henderson's notables or, as she put it, "striving dreadfully to take an interest in their little miserabilities." Elizabeth didn't mind her students, but she was mightily bored by the tobacco-stained provinciality of Henderson, untouched by anything approaching Transcendentalism. "Carlyle's name has never even been distantly echoed here," she complained to Marian, citing her favorite Scottish satirist. "Emerson is a perfect stranger, & Channing I presume would produce a universal fainting-fit."

She found comfort in solitary walks by the river, only to find, as the weather warmed, that her preferred destination was known to courting couples as Lover's Grove. Not that she wasn't courted herself, she was quick to point out. "I had many offers of an escort thither and as many beaux as I might desire," she insisted, but she found carving initials and coy verses on the "unfortunate locust trees" unbearable and had no qualms about saying so. "I laughed at them & their sentimental doings & have had no invitation since," she wrote, defiant. She may have forsworn marriage at seventeen, but as one who hated to be underestimated—or worse, pitied—she continued to assert that the choice had always been hers.

How could she possibly find a soulmate among people who owned human souls? Years of involvement in the antislavery cause had not prepared her for daily life among enslaved people. "To live in the midst of beings, degraded to the utmost in body & mind, drudging on from earliest morning to latest night," she wrote, "blamed unjustly & without spirit enough to reply . . . with *no hope for the future*, smelling horridly & as ugly as Satan—to live in their midst, utterly powerless to help them, is to me dreadful." She was dismayed by her own contradictory feelings—as much as she abhorred the institution of slavery, she found herself more comfortable, or at least less uncomfortable, in the company of Henderson's slave owners, even as they prided themselves on their own benevolence. "I endeavor in reply to slide in a little truth through the small apertures of their minds," Elizabeth wrote, but the effort of controlling her disgust took a toll. "I have an intense longing to scream," she told Marian, "& everybody here speaks in a whisper."

She lasted six months. But the experience of earning a salary, answerable only to herself, was formative. "I feel independent for the first time in my life," she wrote.

~

Just before Elizabeth left for Henderson, Anna set off in the opposite direction, back to New York to teach music at St. Ann's Hall in Flushing, a luxurious new girls' school as grand and elegant as her own self-image. She sent ravishing descriptions of her new situation—a becolumned three-story mansion on grounds that included gardens, a riding ring, and an archery range—back to Cincinnati, mentioning in particular her employer, the Reverend John Frederick Schroeder, a prominent Episcopal figure.

Midway through her first term, Anna summoned Emily, now seventeen and struggling to continue her education in Cincinnati. The eminent Dr. Schroeder, Anna reported triumphantly, had enthusiastically seconded Anna's suggestion that Emily come to St. Ann's, being himself, according to Anna, "very fond of drawing out the talents of girls of Milly's age." Emily consulted Elizabeth in Henderson. Should she continue to teach and help at home or seize this rare chance to study? The Blackwells had moved to a house near the Beechers in suburban Walnut Hills, with more room but also more housework. Lately, Emily confessed to Elizabeth, "I have felt as though caught in a crime, if Marian found me before supper with a book in my hand."

Elizabeth's response was immediate. *"Go by all means,"* she wrote, for the first time expressing her high estimation of her younger sister's potential. "When you've finished your studies, we may perhaps join together in some undertaking, & make the cash come in like a perfect Croton river, what fountains and baths we'll establish in our domestic city, how we'll wash away all trouble & annoyance & make all clean and fresh." The undertaking in question had yet to present itself, but Elizabeth clearly saw Emily as a partner in it, whatever it might be.

And so in the late summer of 1844, just as Elizabeth returned from Henderson, Emily left for New York. Determined not to squander her good fortune, she toiled through compositions and Bible lessons, impressing Dr. Schroeder as a "'crack' Greek pupil" and losing herself in botanizing rambles around the school. ("Alas!" sighed her dutiful brother Sam, "I can but gasp aspirations after such an Elysium.") Cheerful and pragmatic, Emily studied "pretty busily but by no means so as to fatigue myself," she wrote to Elizabeth, "and I adhere constantly and in all things to my favourite proverb, 'most haste worst speed.'" Anna, Emily's patronizing patron, was gratified. "Her progress is really wonderful," she reported to the family. "If she continue as at present, she will be a very different person from the young elephant you lost sight of last Fall."

~

Elizabeth, upon her escape from hated Henderson, resumed the uninspiring Cincinnati routine that Emily had left behind and began to feel what Anna described as "the manifold uncomfortablenesses of such a state of *betweenity*." That Christmas of 1844, short as always on cash but with literary creativity to spare, the Blackwells compiled an anthology of their own writings, to be sent to absent Anna and Emily and read aloud by all on Christmas Day. Henry, the comedian, contributed to this inaugural Annual a caricature of each Blackwell. Volatile, opinionated Anna was "Changeable Earnest"; serious Sam was "Sacred Awe." Wisecracking, ever-hungry Henry dubbed himself "Voracious Noodle." Emily, tall and easygoing, at least for a Blackwell, was "Lymphatic Carrot." And Elizabeth, with her philosophical inclinations and musical abilities, was "Transcendental Nightingale." "She may perhaps be the Lion of the family," Henry added, "being a desperate and energetic sort of female." Everyone recognized Elizabeth's caged force.

It was at this frustrated moment, as Elizabeth remembered it, that "a lady friend," stricken with a terminal illness "the delicate nature of which made the methods of treatment a constant suffering to her," suggested that a woman of Elizabeth's intellectual capacity should study medicine. "If I could have been treated by a lady doctor," the friend confided, "my worst sufferings would have been spared me."

The details of this formative conversation are lost; as an origin story, it is vague and abrupt. Why would a young woman enthralled by literature and philosophy, and painfully aware of her family's financial instability, suddenly apply her considerable ambition to what was, essentially, still just a trade—and not even a particularly lucrative one?

Elizabeth at first scoffed at the idea. There was no such thing as a female physician, at least in any honorable sense. Women who claimed that title were peddlers of patent elixirs—or worse, of abortion, that "gross perversion and destruction of motherhood." Even respectable male doctors, armed with little more than purgatives, laudanum, and lancets, tended to do more harm than good—she had seen this at her father's bedside.

And whereas in Europe the title "doctor" might connote a certain level of education and eminence, egalitarian Americans tended to resist such assumptions of privilege—and the prestige of American medical schools did not yet approach that of European ones. Some patients preferred an experienced lay practitioner to a man with an M.D.

On top of this, the general state of human health had rarely been worse. The explosive growth of cities had accelerated the evils that proliferate whenever too many people occupy too little space: contaminated water, accumulated garbage and manure, and the fleas and rats and lice that were the only beneficiaries of overcrowding. Babies died almost as often as they lived—even with the benefit of education and income, Hannah and Samuel Blackwell had buried at least three. Those lucky enough to survive childhood later succumbed to tuberculosis, cholera, typhoid fever, and influenza. No one had yet figured out why these plagues took hold, or how to help the afflicted. Confidence in the ability of doctors to preserve life had never been lower. In 1845 medicine was a strange choice for anyone who craved professional prestige, let alone a woman.

Besides, Elizabeth's dedication was to the life of the mind. Since childhood, she had always hidden signs of illness from her family: Sickness was for the weak. "My favourite studies were history and metaphysics," she wrote, "and the very thought of dwelling on the physical structure of the body and its various ailments filled me with disgust."

But her metaphysical orientation eventually directed her toward the science of the body. During the winter of Elizabeth's betweenity, Margaret Fuller—editor of the Transcendentalist magazine *The Dial* and confidante of Emerson and Channing—published *Woman in the Nineteenth Century*, a book that spoke directly to Elizabeth's unsatisfied mind. Humanity would achieve a moral awakening, Fuller insisted, only when women enjoyed the same independence as men—a step that women must claim for themselves rather than waiting for men to grant it. "I think women need, especially at this juncture, a much greater range of occupation than they have, to rouse their latent powers," Fuller wrote. "If you ask me what offices they may fill; I reply—any. I do not care what case you put; let them be sea-captains, if you will." *The Dial*, in which Fuller's ideas first appeared, was a fixture among the reading materials in the Blackwell parlor. "I believe that, at present, women are the best helpers of one another," Fuller declared, her words reinforcing the suggestion of Elizabeth's dying friend. Could it be that "doctor" was the office Elizabeth was meant to fill?

The allure of medicine may have been reinforced by her brother Sam, trapped in tedious bookkeeping jobs that left him no leisure for idealism. "If I had some noble, glorious aim, clearly defined before me in life, I think I could be truly happy," he wrote. "I have thought that as a physician I might be happy, & truly well employed in a *daily business* of *beneficence*."

Elizabeth was not drawn to the daily business of beneficence—that would involve uncomfortably intimate contact with individual sufferers—but becoming a doctor as qualified as any man was a noble ideological quest, a way of proving Margaret Fuller's faith in woman's equal aptitude. Elizabeth's attraction to this challenge wrestled with her distaste for human biology and won. There was, moreover, the added incentive of the recognition that such an extraordinary accomplishment might bring. She had no use for most social interaction, but she had no objection to fame. "Eliz. is thinking seriously of studying Medicine," Sam recorded that spring.

Embarking on such a quest would also give Elizabeth a conclusive answer to a tiresome question: what about marriage? Though her solitary circumstances might have been of her own choosing, her pride demanded a narrative that justified the choice. Falling in love, a "common malady" like any physical illness, was likewise a weakness, she decided. "I became impatient of the disturbing influence exercised by the other sex," she wrote—a disturbance, she confessed, to which she felt particularly susceptible. "But whenever I became sufficiently intimate with any individual to be able to realise what a life association might mean," she continued, "I shrank from the prospect, disappointed or repelled." She loved the idea of love, not the reality of emotional connection—and physical connection was even harder to contemplate. Evidence of intimacy with another, at any stage of Elizabeth's life, is scarce in the letters and journals she left behind, but whether her romances were real or imagined, the work of becoming a doctor would both forestall love and explain its absence. "I must have something to engross my thoughts," she wrote, "some object in life which will fill this vacuum and prevent this sad wearing away of the heart." Elizabeth considered medicine as a novice might contemplate the convent: as a noble vocation and a refuge from worldly entanglements.

Having decided what to pursue, the next step was how. Elizabeth visited doctors in Cincinnati and wrote to others in New York, receiving everywhere the same reaction: a female physician was an interesting idea, but given the long years and great expense of study, and the intellectual and physical endurance required to practice, not to mention the basic truth that no female would be welcome among male students in a medical lecture hall or operating theater, it was quite impossible. Frankly, what self-respecting woman would voluntarily expose herself to the naked realities of the body *in the company of men?* And then there was the unmentionable question of such a woman's own body, incapacitated monthly. Bedrest was a common prescription for menstrual complaints, and what would a lady doctor's patients do then? Even Elizabeth's friend Harriet Beecher Stowe was dubious. Certainly a woman doctor would be "highly useful," she conceded, but the forces ranged against Elizabeth, which she must "either crush or be crushed by," were formidable.

Of course, women had always served as healers—whether revered as angels at the bedside, or reviled (though still, quietly, consulted) as uncomfortably powerful initiates into the secrets of witchcraft. American colonists, among whom doctors were scarce, had depended on wives and mothers and sisters to provide first aid and nursing, not to mention assistance at childbirth. But as eighteenth-century Enlightenment ideas introduced empirical science and new techniques into the healing arts—like the use of forceps during delivery—female practitioners were replaced by male professionals. As the establishment of medical schools and societies created new frameworks of legitimacy, women were pushed further toward the margins. However: in the last few decades, as medical schools began to proliferate in the United States, led by physicians who hoped to raise the profession to the same level of dignity it enjoyed in Europe, it was perhaps *easier* to argue for a woman's right to be a doctor.

If she attended the same lectures and passed the same examinations as a man, who could deny her qualifications?

There remained only the daunting fact that no woman had ever gained admittance. It had nothing to do with entrance standards. Newly minted American medical schools, unlike liberal arts colleges and law schools, often had none: any student who could pay the fees was welcome. Any male student, that is. And Elizabeth had no money. As someone who scorned the easy path, however, these apparently insurmountable obstacles only hardened her resolve. "The idea of winning a doctor's degree gradually assumed the aspect of a great moral struggle," she wrote, "and the moral fight possessed immense attraction for me."

꒛

It was Anna, bestowing largesse from the superior vantage of age and secure employment at St. Ann's in Flushing, who propelled Elizabeth forward with word of a teaching position in Asheville, North Carolina. There were better reasons than a teacher's salary to venture so far away. It would be another chance to take abolitionist ideas into slave territory, and more important, the proprietor of the school in question, the Reverend John Dickson, had previously been a doctor. Medical students usually studied with an established physician before enrolling in formal lectures. In Dr. Dickson's employ, with access to his medical books, Elizabeth would be able to save money toward her education even as she began it.

The 350-mile journey, by cramped stagecoach on jolting, ungraded roads over the Alleghenies and the Appalachians, would take more than a week. Elizabeth had heard terrifying reports of "drunken drivers galloping their horses at full speed down perpendicular mountains," and the prospect of unaccompanied nights at lonely roadside inns was unattractive. Sam, however, was only too happy to leave his uninspiring duties, hire a wagon, and drive his sister to her new post. In June 1845, less than three weeks after receiving Anna's suggestion, Elizabeth and Sam were on their way to Asheville, with thirteen-year-old Howard tagging along for the adventure. They packed the wagon with Elizabeth's books and trunks and carpetbags and added a chessboard and two loaded pistols.

It was to Emily, still studying in New York, that Elizabeth wrote the fullest account of her journey, after taking "Miss Student" to task for failing to write. ("What a very unnatural sister you are," she scolded, "to take no more notice of my existence than if I were a toad or President Polk.") The first day on the road, Elizabeth confessed, she had felt "as blue as a forget-me-not," drenched by a torrent of rain and a relentless stream of Sam's painful puns. But her mood lightened with the skies, and she proved a more intrepid traveler than her brothers. Reaching a ford across Kentucky's Cumberland River in the gathering dusk, the little party was dismayed by the expanse of tumbling water, darkened by close-growing trees climbing the valley's steep sides and made eerie by the "goblin groans of myriad frogs." Hallooing across, they heard an answering hail encouraging them to march straight from bank to bank, but Sam couldn't muster the nerve. "Shall I say there's a lady in the carriage?" he asked Elizabeth. In response to this fiction of a frightened female, a boy on horseback splashed over to guide them toward dinner and a warm bed.

Asheville was a tiny dot in the grandeur of the Blue Ridge Mountains. Elizabeth found the landscape inspiring and the people less so: to her critical eye, they were another batch of "country boobies and boobyesses." Though the Dicksons' green-shuttered residence was undeniably attractive, and their Female Academy one of Asheville's proudest institutions, Elizabeth's mood plunged as her brothers' departure approached. "I grew so doleful that I almost meditated suicide, it seemed to me that the world was one vale of gloom," she wrote. "I must lead a cold lonely life, on the confines of barbarism, amid totally uninteresting people." And her mattress was full of fleas, who "all turned out to welcome me, with true Southern hospitality."

Elizabeth would remember this nadir as a catalyst for revelation. "I had many causes of deep suffering that I had never imparted to anyone, & I felt lonely & forsaken by every friend," she wrote.

> I stood one starlight night at my window—I shall never forget it—the mountains stood round black & gloomy, the wind sighed mournfully in the oak trees, & the stars seemed to mock me with their cold quiet twinkling. I cried in deep sorrow, "Jesus have you too forsaken me!" and in the instant a peaceful happiness, that I had

never known before seemed to take possession of me; it was as if some bright spirit had shed its atmosphere around, & entered with every breath I drew.

She echoed the words of Jesus on the cross without apparent irony. Elizabeth had always yearned to see herself as the protagonist of an important story; now, officially embarked on her medical quest, she could. Henceforth "I *knew* that, however insignificant my individual effort might be, it was in a right direction, and in accordance with the great providential ordering of our race's progress."

Whether or not the world yet acknowledged it, she was a medical student. An elderly housemaid thanked her for soothing away a headache—"my first professional cure," Elizabeth wrote gaily—and the household affectionately took to calling her "Dr. Blackwell," a title she penned with an extra flourish in her letter. When someone found a large dead beetle, she decided to perform her first dissection. "I thought it would make a capital beginning," she wrote, but the intention was easier than the act. Spreading out a clean sheet of paper, she staked the insect to her desk with a hairpin, opened her penknife, grasped the mother-of-pearl handle, and—hesitated. The place where the head joined the body, being narrowest, seemed like the easiest place to start, and soon the beetle was in two pieces. Finally, with a shudder of disgust, she sliced the body in half—but the creature having died some time ago, all she found within was yellowish dust. "The anatomy was by no means interesting," she wrote wryly, "but the moral courage exercised was of a high order."

Dr. Dickson borrowed an articulated human skeleton for her to study—"a great treat"—and seemed to support her outrageous plans, though she found it difficult to discuss them. "I only wish he were one with whom I could converse freely," Elizabeth wrote, "but I think it would be too hard a trial to subject him to." It was less daunting to discuss Dickson's politics. Though a slave owner himself, he professed an antipathy to slavery strong enough that Elizabeth deemed him "one of the most *right minded* men I have ever known." It was hard to condemn him for his ideals when he was at that moment helping her to realize her own.

Elizabeth had returned to the south "determined," she wrote, "to teach all the slaves I could to read & write & elevate them in every way in my power, as the only way in which I could reconcile it to my conscience to live amongst them." Dickson applauded her idealism, but it was illegal in North Carolina to teach slaves to read, and he refused to break the law. Instead, with the help of Mrs. Dickson, Elizabeth organized a Sunday school providing "oral instruction" on moral ideas. "I assure you it felt a little odd," she wrote, "sitting down in front of those degraded little beings, to teach them a religion which their *owners* professed to follow while violating its very first principles."

The "strong electric friendship" she craved, the kind of idealized communion "where deep calleth unto deep," would not be found in Asheville, but Elizabeth was not bothered. "I always have had somewhat of the anchorite in my composition," she wrote. As one of her colleagues put it, "Miss Blackwell is never less alone, than when alone." Between her job, her studies, and her Sunday school, Elizabeth's life was, for the moment, satisfyingly full. "I feel very wakeful, just at present," she wrote. "My brain is as busy as it can be, & consequently I'm happy."

~

Emily and Anna were not. On the same late July afternoon when Elizabeth was describing her busy days in Asheville, Anna was writing a grimmer letter home from St. Ann's in New York. "It is so painful to be *convinced* that one whom one has loved and admired is really unworthy of confidence," she began. She had abruptly resigned, she announced, as a result of her employer Dr. Schroeder's inappropriate behavior. "All his kind professions of respect," she wrote, "have been succeeded by a system of petty persecution, general annoyance, and unbearable insolence, which have fairly martyrized me."

Emily scrawled a postscript across Anna's last page. "I assure you that she has not spoken of it half as severely as it deserves," she insisted. "His conduct toward her almost ever since I have been here has been very doubtful, but for the last three weeks it had been equally unworthy of a Christian and a gentleman." Their brother Henry's outraged reaction shed some light on Schroeder's unmentioned transgressions. "A most unscrupulous liar & consummate scoundrel!" he exploded. "In short, a perfect *Onderdonk*." Benjamin Treadwell Onderdonk, Episcopal bishop of

New York, had recently been brought to trial on multiple charges of grop-
ing female parishioners. ("He thrust his hand in my bosom," one plain-
tiff testified.) Whether or not Schroeder's crime matched Onderdonk's,
from this point on Anna would be increasingly debilitated by vague and
chronic ill health, and drawn irresistibly toward whatever new fad promised to relieve her. She never held a classroom teaching job again.

Leaving Emily with friends in New York, Anna retreated to Brook
Farm, the utopian community near Boston founded by Transcendentalists and frequented by William Henry Channing. Brook Farm had
recently embarked on an ambitious plan to remake itself according to
Charles Fourier's principles of Associationism, thanks in part to the
arrival of Albert Brisbane, the man responsible for popularizing Fourier's ideas in America. Unfortunately, this was the beginning of the end
for the Brook Farm experiment, but Anna developed a warm regard for
the persuasive Brisbane. By the fall of 1845, she was back in New York,
and so was Brisbane, taking a personal interest in instructing her on
Fourier's ideas regarding free love.

Emily lingered in New York with Anna, the two women moving
among generous friends and furnished lodgings. Anna was earning a
little as a journalist, writing reviews for magazines, and both women
took private pupils. Having had a taste of concentrated study during her
year at St. Ann's, Emily was desperate to continue her work in languages
and mathematics, and she continued to be intrigued by the utopianism
she was hearing from Anna and her friend Mr. Brisbane. She explored
Fourier's ideas not with Elizabeth's idealism or Anna's impulsive passion
but with her own considerable intellectual focus, "reading," Elizabeth
reported approvingly, "a work in five volumes, of 500 pages each." Emily
was too practical to be swept away by Fourier's vision, but her seriousness resonated with Elizabeth—surely Emily was the most kindred of
her siblings. "Your letters always come to me like a puff of fresh North
wind in a Summer's day," she wrote to Emily. "I generally brush my hair
& straighten my things after reading them."

In the spring of 1846, after nearly two years away, Emily returned to
Walnut Hills, impressing the home folk with her gains in both height
and maturity. "So our young giantess is actually arrived," Elizabeth

wrote. "Why didn't some of you let me know?" She had heard from Cincinnati friends that Emily was now "quite a genius," though "this I won't mention, lest Emily should see it."

‍‍ ~

The Dicksons' school in Asheville closed at the end of 1845, but Elizabeth had accepted an invitation from John Dickson's brother in Charleston. Dr. Samuel Henry Dickson had received his medical degree at the University of Pennsylvania—the oldest and most elite American medical school—and helped found the Medical College of South Carolina. His library held over a thousand volumes, and his sister-in-law ran a fashionable boarding school for girls that was in need of a piano teacher.

Samuel Dickson was the most eminent physician Elizabeth had yet encountered. It took her months to muster the courage to consult him directly about her ambitions. "The more I thought of the conversation, the more nervous I became," she wrote, worrying that she "might perhaps lose a friend without gaining a teacher." But Dickson, when she at last confided in him, surprised her. "He thinks my desire of obtaining a thorough scientific education quite feasible," Elizabeth exulted. "When we finished the conversation my head burned with pleasure, I felt it to be the first step gained, and an all important one." Fueled by optimism, she began to enjoy the pursuit of science. "I trace out the wonderful nervous fibres of the body," she wrote, "with the same interest that I once sought for the links that unite the finite with the infinite." She felt increasingly confident that she could reach the summit of her chosen mountain and become an example to the world; after that, she wrote, "whether I devote my life to the practice is another question that experience must determine." But it was her aptitude for the work that would determine her future, not her gender. "I think I have sufficient hardness to be entirely unaffected by great agony," she mused. "I do not think any case would keep me awake at night."

What did keep her awake was the irritating proximity of giddy schoolgirls. "Do listen," she cried to a fellow teacher, jerked awake again one night by agonized shrieks, "they must be whipping a poor negro; isn't it abominable?" But the noise was coming from across the corridor. Yanking open the dormitory door, Elizabeth was mobbed by "six girls, all screaming at the top of their voices, as pale as their nightgowns, and some of them almost in fits." The original source of their terror, it emerged, was the sound of a hairbrush falling to the floor.

Elizabeth's dim view of females was not limited to teenagers. In Charleston she was introduced to Emma Willard, founder of New York's Troy Female Seminary, the first school to offer girls a secondary curriculum comparable to what their brothers could expect. Now approaching sixty, "the famous Trojan" traveled the country as an advocate for women's education and wrote extensively on history and geography. "I did not know till nearly the close of her short stay," Elizabeth reported with breathtaking scorn, "that she was a pretender to medical knowledge." Willard had spent years investigating the intricacies of the human circulatory system and was about to publish her findings. "I fear however that the book will not add to Mrs Willard's reputation," Elizabeth scoffed. "I should judge her, not very profound, though possessed of much varied information." Willard enjoyed national recognition and was venerable enough to be her grandmother, but Elizabeth dismissed her as a dilettante in danger of undermining her own more serious-minded quest. "A grand discovery by her is not very probable," she wrote, "on a subject to which intelligent men have devoted their whole lives."

Willard, fortunately, felt no such wariness. She referred Elizabeth to her friend Dr. Joseph Warrington, a sympathetic Philadelphia Quaker. Though he was inclined to believe that Elizabeth would find the pursuit of nursing smoother, he added, "I beg thee to believe with me that if the project be of divine origin it will sooner or later surely be accomplished."

In May 1847, after a year and a half among the schoolgirls of Charleston, Elizabeth left for Philadelphia, the first city of American medicine, ready to put all her energy toward the pursuit of medical school admission. Her mentor Samuel Dickson was well connected at the University of Pennsylvania; Dr. Warrington, cautiously encouraging, had declared himself an ally. And Anna was already there.

~

Anna—who, unlike Elizabeth, had no qualms about discussing her aches and pains—had grown enamored of unorthodox routes to well-

ness. Scientific observation and experimentation had fostered a growing skepticism regarding the authority of doctors. Several schools of
alternative practice had emerged in response to the excesses of medical
orthodoxy, dependent as it was on bloodletting and drugs whose effects
were often more debilitating than the original complaint. The body was
as mysterious in its workings as ever, but what if the highest authority
on its well-being was the individual who inhabited it? "Know thyself,"
said the Transcendentalists. While alternative practices might have been
less painful, however, it was unclear that they were any more effective.

The Thomsonians, taking their name from New Hampshire farmer
Samuel Thomson, held that all disease arose in cold and was dispelled
by heat; the Thomsonian pharmacopeia consisted almost entirely of red
pepper, steam, and lobelia, an emetic commonly known as "pukeweed."
Thomson's ideas had been subsumed into the Eclectic school, a botanical approach that aimed to reform the excesses of medical orthodoxy
while preserving its grounding in empirical scientific knowledge and
training, combining the soundest ideas from a variety of perspectives.
Poised to overtake the Eclectics in popularity was homeopathy, which
viewed disease in a more spiritual light and prescribed minute doses
of mostly botanical preparations according to the "law of similars": the
correct medication for a given illness would be the one that caused the
symptoms of that illness in a healthy person.

Other techniques strayed further from convention. Mesmerism—
named for the German physician Franz Anton Mesmer—had emerged
a decade earlier. Mesmer believed that a form of energy he called "animal magnetism" emanated from every creature; illness resulted from
blockage of this flow and could be removed by a practitioner skilled in
directing his or her own vital energy toward the sufferer. Mesmerists
staged popular demonstrations, hypnotizing headaches away and reori-
enting the body's energy with the application of magnets or simply by
touch. While recovering at Brook Farm, Anna had experimented with
magnetic treatments, lamenting in the wake of her trauma at St. Ann's
that she was "thin as an aspen leaf, and just about as nervous." And then
there was hydropathy, or the "water cure," which prescribed restorative

bathing, sweating, and drinking, under the assumption that flooding the body with pure water would flush away whatever might be poisoning it.

Anna had come to Philadelphia to seek treatment at Dr. Schifferdecker's Hydropathic Institute, renting a room in the home of William and Sarah Elder, a Quaker doctor and his wife. Elizabeth liked the encouraging Elders, "a thinking talking couple," but thought Dr. Schifferdecker was a charlatan. "Poor A," wrote her brother Sam. "I am very glad E. is near her with her cool, unimpassioned judgment." Elizabeth's criticism, however, was more for the man than for his method. She remained steadfast in her pursuit of a medical credential from a regular, allopathic school—she could hardly expect to win societal approval otherwise—but her oldest sister's alternative fascinations would have a significant impact on her own approach to medicine. She was, paradoxically, seeking legitimacy in a field whose legitimacy was currently in flux. She would not rule out techniques that seemed effective, whatever their provenance.

While Anna took the water cure, Elizabeth sought interviews with Philadelphia's leading physicians and sent letters of inquiry to medical colleges in both Philadelphia and New York. At the University of Pennsylvania, the oldest and most august American medical school, Dr. Samuel Jackson burst out laughing at her request. Dr. William Darrach stared at her for a disconcertingly long pause, then refused either to admit her to his lectures or to explain why. "The subject is a novel one, madam," he ventured at last. "I have nothing to say either for or against it." Dr. William Ashmead sent word that his feelings on a woman studying medicine were so outraged he would rather not meet the woman in question face to face. All of Elizabeth's applications were rejected.

The objections of the medical establishment followed divergent tracks. On the one hand, no true lady would leave the purity of the domestic sphere to study the corruptions of the human body. On the other, what if female doctors were a resounding success, and female patients preferred them? The dean of one school summed up these fears: "You cannot expect us to furnish you with a stick to break our heads with." Even those rare men who approved of Elizabeth's goal balked at the notion of a woman studying anatomy alongside men. Her only way forward, they told her, was to pose as a man—somewhere far away, perhaps in Paris,

where the excellent medical instruction was free, and attitudes less puri-
tanical. The scandal of a cross-dressing woman, apparently, was nothing
compared to the horror of a female in the lecture room.

But to Elizabeth, achieving a diploma in disguise missed the point.
"It was to my mind a moral crusade on which I had entered," she wrote,
"and it must be pursued in the light of day, and with public sanction, in
order to accomplish its end." If she was to be a beacon, she could not hide
herself. She had never wanted to *be* a man—she wanted, as a woman, to
enjoy the same level of respect and freedom men took for granted.

"I cannot tell you how much I would like you to be studying with
me," she wrote to Emily in Cincinnati. "I have calculated again & again,
but find no way to obtain such an end." She reported excitedly on the
chance to observe Dr. Jonathan Moses Allen's private anatomy class, on
hernia. "That is to be my introduction," she wrote. "Rather formidable is
it not?" (More formidable than she knew: Allen would go on to write *The
Practical Anatomist*, a classroom bible for medical students.) He led her
through a dissection of the human wrist: the eight tiny bones with their
lacing of ligaments that were the mechanism of so much graceful expression, whether the flourish of a paintbrush or the striking of a chord at
the piano. "The beauty of the tendons and exquisite arrangements of this
part of the body struck my artistic sense," Elizabeth wrote, "and appealed
to the sentiment of reverence with which this anatomical branch of study
was ever afterwards invested in my mind."

She also made the acquaintance of Paulina Kellogg Wright, a young
widow known for her lectures on physiology to female audiences, using
a papier-mâché model imported from France. Though Wright's purpose
was different—she promoted basic knowledge of the body as a foundation for public health—she and Elizabeth joined forces briefly in search
of anatomical specimens. The trade in cadavers was largely unregulated,
and the visceral horror most felt at the idea of dissection—linked to a
Christian belief that only intact bodies had a chance at resurrection—
meant that bodies were in chronically short supply. Grave robbers, known
sardonically as "resurrectionists," quietly supplied the most august institutions. A large proportion of the specimens on American dissecting
tables were black: the bodies of both enslaved and free black people,

buried, often uncoffined, in segregated ground outside the security of churchyards, were easier to steal. The bodies of babies, easier to transport and plentiful in an era of high infant mortality, were cheapest. In a letter to Sam in late summer, Elizabeth mentioned casually that she and Mrs. Wright were hoping "to purchase a black baby & dissect." The grisly collision of her two pursuits, abolition and anatomy, went unacknowledged.

Rejected by every institution to which she had applied, Elizabeth acted on a whim and traveled to New York, where Marian was visiting, for a rare holiday with her clear-sighted older sister. "I determined not to study or think or do anything that I had been accustomed to," she wrote, "but walk & bathe eat sleep laugh & flirt." The vacation was refreshing, but self-indulgence—not to mention flirting—was not in Elizabeth's nature. "I must accomplish my end," she had written to Emma Willard. "I would sooner die than give it up."

Upon her return to Philadelphia, she sent off a new flurry of applications to a dozen provincial medical colleges across New England. It was already August, and the next term would start in October; there was hardly enough time for good news she could act upon. But it was too late now to turn back.

CHAPTER 3

❦

ADMISSION

The young men of Geneva Medical College were some weeks into the new term of 1847 when the dean of faculty, Charles A. Lee, visited their lecture hall, a letter in his hand.

The worry lines in his perennially concerned expression deeper than usual, Dr. Lee cleared his throat. He held, he announced with a quaver, the "most extraordinary request which had ever been made to the faculty." A young lady, studying privately with an eminent physician in Philadelphia, had applied, with her mentor's endorsement, for admission to their school. Several prominent medical colleges had already refused her. The faculty at Geneva had decided to put the issue to a student vote, Lee continued, with the stipulation that a single nay could turn the decision against the unusual lady in question. Their prompt attention to this matter would be appreciated. Lee refolded the letter and departed.

Two things were clear to the assembled young men. First, their professors were cowards: too timid to reject this unprecedented request out of hand, not bold enough to embrace it. And second, the students had been handed the power to make serious mischief.

Tucked away among the Finger Lakes of western New York State, Geneva College was a modest institution, founded to offer the young men of the region a classical education in two graceful stone halls, Geneva and Trinity, perched above a prosperous village at the northern tip of Seneca Lake. A third building soon rose between the original two to house the medical department, but no one liked the idea of cadavers at the heart of the college. Middle Building became the library, and a spacious new medical building, topped with a domed skylight, was completed in 1843 at a discreet distance up the street.*

Of the 113 students in the medical class of 1847–48, nearly all were local. They were boisterous boys with more energy than polish; young men with intellectual and social ambition generally migrated to cities and studied law. Medicine, as a profession, was considered more manual than cerebral, vulnerable to the taint of patent-remedy hucksters; surgery, when it was practiced at all, had not long since been the bloody craft of barbers. Though the elite medical colleges of New York and Philadelphia might include gentlemen on their rolls, tiny Geneva did not. It wasn't uncommon for the dean to receive written complaints from townsfolk threatening legal action over the raucous behavior of his students. That fall the silence of the night had exploded when several overeager anatomy pupils, unsatisfied with the college's supply of unclaimed bodies from nearby Auburn State Prison, tried to rob the grave of a recently interred Irishman. The dead man's compatriots had driven them off with gunfire.

There were no absentees at a student meeting on the evening of Dr. Lee's bizarre announcement. In speech after speech, the class clowns topped each other in extravagant support for the admission of a corseted classmate. What could be more ridiculous—or more entertaining—than a lady doctor? When the jokes were spent, the vote was called. All in favor? The roar of "AYE" rattled the windows. The air filled with tossed hats and waving handkerchiefs. Any opposed? There was a bemused silence, broken by a single, tentative "nay."

Decades later a distinguished Geneva alumnus named Stephen Smith was still chuckling at the fate of the hapless dissenter. "At the instant, the class arose as one man and rushed to the corner from which the voice proceeded," he recalled. "Amid screams of 'cuff him,' 'crack his skull,' 'throw him down the stairs,' a young man was dragged to the platform screaming 'Aye, aye! I vote aye.'" The students bore their decision in tri-

---

* Geneva and Trinity Halls are today the oldest buildings on the campus of Hobart and William Smith Colleges. Neither medical building survives. Geneva's medical department merged with Syracuse University in 1871.

umph to the horrified faculty and promptly forgot about it. The whole farce was probably a prank cooked up by a rival school anyway, they told each other.

Three weeks later, on a dreary Monday morning, the yawning, slouching students of Geneva Medical College looked up to see their professor coming through the door of the lecture room followed by a slight feminine figure, dressed without ornament. She had a high smooth forehead, a firm set to her jaw, and fair hair parted in the center. She seated herself, placed her bonnet beneath her chair, and turned her penetrating stare toward the front of the room. A stunned silence fell like a curtain. Spines straightened; feet returned squarely to the floor.

"For the first time a lecture was given without the slightest interruption," Stephen Smith remembered much later, "and every word could be heard as distinctly as it would if there had been but a single person in the room." As if by magic, a classroom full of "lawless desperadoes" had been transformed into models of deportment by Elizabeth's mere presence. Or had they? In the moment, the presence of a woman in the lecture hall was no one's idea of a happy ending. At best, for Elizabeth, it was a vindication and a beginning. At worst, it was a freakish experiment her professors would live to regret.

~

The letter from Geneva College had arrived in Philadelphia at the end of October. Elizabeth opened it with a flickering mixture of resignation and stubborn hope.

"At a meeting of the entire Medical Class of Geneva Medical College, held this day, October 20, 1847," it began, "the following Resolutions were unanimously adopted:

> Resolved—That one of the radical principles of a Republican Government is the universal education of both sexes; that to every branch of scientific education the door should be open equally to all; that the application of Elizabeth Blackwell to become a member of our class, meets our entire approbation; and in extending our unanimous invitation, we pledge ourselves that no conduct of ours shall cause her to regret her attendance at this institution.

Resolved—That a copy of these proceedings be signed by the
Chairman and transmitted to Elizabeth Blackwell.

The faculty, Dr. Lee explained disingenuously, had decided to lay Elizabeth's application before the young men among whom she would study.
"I send you the results of their deliberations," Lee wrote, "and need only
add that there are no fears but that you can, by judicious management,
not only 'disarm criticism,' but elevate yourself without detracting, in
the least, from the dignity of the profession." Elizabeth did not dwell
on the lukewarm endorsement, or the fact that the term had already
started. An acceptance was an acceptance. And if Lee chose to close by
wishing her "success in your undertaking, which some may deem bold
in the present state of society," she would have to assume he wasn't one
of those "some."

She had to tell Emily. "Dear Milly," she began, and quoted all the
best bits at length: principles of Republican government! entire approbation! unanimous invitation! "Isn't that fine and liberal?" she crowed.
"It is accompanied by a few words of encouragement from one of the
Professors—oh really it was refreshing. I fairly jumped for joy—it seemed
to me that I was the luckiest mortal on the face of the earth, & that henceforth no difficulty remained." But giddiness was not Elizabeth's natural
state, and her "fit of rapture" soon subsided. Studying the circular Dr.
Lee had enclosed, she reported to Emily on the college's virtues: "well
supplied museums & cabinet of Natural History, a library, plenty of material for dissection, clinical lectures, & surgical operations—the charges
moderate & boarding reasonable." She heaved a sigh of triumphant relief
("though not surprise," she was quick to insist, "for failure never seemed
possible"), packed her trunk, bought a train ticket, and left for Geneva,
entirely unaware of the farcical circumstances of her acceptance.

Train travel, less than two decades old, was a grueling ordeal: the
wooden cars jolted only slightly less than the stagecoaches they were
replacing, the hard seats were like church pews, the floorboards were
sticky with tobacco juice. A stove perched in a corner belched too much
heat into the cramped box of passengers, but opening a window invited a
choking blast of dust and smoke and sparks. The cars could make about

twenty miles per hour, as long as the tracks remained clear of snow, mud, or wandering cows. Derailments were common.

In the chill and deserted darkness of a rainy Saturday night in November, the exhausted and soot-streaked twenty-six-year-old woman who stepped off the train in Geneva felt somewhat less confident than the one who had left Philadelphia two days earlier. The next day was the Sabbath, but she would have no leisure to observe it. She needed a place to live, she needed to learn her way around a new town, and she needed to present herself to a group of professors who had spent the last week dreading her arrival.

࣫

It was still raining on Tuesday, Seneca Lake a dull gray sheet beyond South Main Street. Now Elizabeth had an upper room at Hamilton's boardinghouse, two doors down from the medical building. Though there were plenty of other lodgers, she had not yet spoken to any of them. A small stove kept off the chill. She shoved another stick of firewood into its belly and sat down to report her progress, this time to supportive Marian. She had no one to talk to and much to tell. "The weather is still gloomy," she wrote, "but I feel sunshiny and happy, strongly encouraged, with a grand future before me, and all owing to a fat little fairy in the shape of the Professor of Anatomy!" The letter is a mixture of proud excitement and protective irony; here and henceforth, Elizabeth used the word *little* as a way of diminishing those who might obstruct her path.

The rotund anatomy professor, James Webster—unlike the ambivalent dean of faculty, Charles Lee—was delighted with his exotic new pupil. Of course she would study surgery, Dr. Webster told his more cautious colleague. "Think of the cases of femoral hernia," he enthused, "only think what a well-educated woman would do in a city like New York." Women with complaints in unmentionable places would flock to her, her success would be ensured, her fame widespread—and her alma mater celebrated. Indeed, members of the public were already showing up at lectures to gawk at the lady student. Would she blush, or gasp—or faint? "Yes," Dr. Lee grudgingly concurred, "we were saying to-day that this step might prove quite a good advertisement for the college; if there were no other advantage to be gained, it will attract so much notice."

The demonstrator of anatomy, Corydon La Ford—Dr. Webster's deputy, in charge of dissections—had at first balked at the idea of a woman
among the specimens; now, following Webster's lead, he showed "the
utmost friendliness" and even met with Elizabeth individually to help
her make up the material she had missed. Working with colleagues on
actual specimens—"Oh, this is the way to learn!" she rejoiced.

Things were looking up. "Today when I came home so happy and
encouraged," she told Marian, "I blessed God most heartily." Whatever
else Elizabeth lacked, self-esteem was never in short supply; where others
might seek God's blessing, she blessed God, who seemed at this moment
less a deity than another kindly old gentleman who might assist her. "I
wanted to throw my arms round him & mend his stockings," she continued, "or do something in return if I only knew what." She felt the same
kind of gratitude for Dr. Webster. "The little fat Professor of Anatomy is
a capital fellow; certainly I shall love fat men more than lean ones henceforth," she wrote. "He gave just the go-ahead directing impulse needful;
he will afford me every advantage, and says I shall graduate with _éclat_."

Éclat did not wait for Elizabeth's graduation. The _Boston Medical
and Surgical Journal_ was already gossiping about the appearance of "a
pretty little specimen of the feminine gender" at medical lectures. The
writer was surprisingly respectful, going so far as to ask, "Why should
not well-educated females be admitted?"—though this may have been a
rhetorical flourish. A month later there was a second notice in the same
journal, confirming that the jury was still out: "Nothing has transpired
as yet to disprove the propriety of the action taken by the Faculty and
class." Geneva College may have been the first medical school to admit a
woman, but who could tell whether such a distinction would prove "meritorious or otherwise"? Other schools were not rushing to follow Geneva's
example. Harriot K. Hunt, a Boston woman in her forties who had been
treating women and children with alternative therapies for more than a
decade, was sufficiently emboldened by Elizabeth's success to apply to
Harvard's medical school. The response was immediate and unequivocal: the president and fellows of Harvard College found the admission of
a woman "inexpedient." Hunt would continue to practice and go on to

prominence in the women's rights movement, but she would never earn a medical degree.

Even Austin Flint—editor of the *Buffalo Medical Journal*, lecturer at Geneva College, and one of Elizabeth's earliest supporters in print—was careful to qualify his enthusiasm. Flint applauded the advent of women in certain "special branches" of medicine—obstetrics and gynecology— and hoped that they might "conduce to the diminution of quackery" by debunking the latest medical fads for their sillier sisters. A woman's "appropriate sphere" was of course "the domestic hearth, and the social circle," though he saw no reason why medicine should be "the exclusive prerogative of the lords of creation." But here his courage failed: "The discussion of the subject would, however, lead us too deeply into the metaphysics of woman's rights, and we therefore waive it for the present."

In England, commentators hailed the achievement of this daughter of Bristol with less discretion. The satirical newspaper *Punch* pounced on the news with acidic glee. "We admire MISS BLACKWELL, though we have never seen her," it announced. "She is qualifying herself for that very important duty of a good wife—tending a husband in sickness." The writer hoped a thorough medical education would provide Elizabeth with "very useful information—a knowledge of the distinction between real and fanciful ailments: also, of the consequences of want of exercise, damp feet, and tight lacing." Such information to be used only within the home, of course.

Elizabeth ignored such publicity as resolutely as she did the smirks of her classmates, and tried to shut out the "flat, heavy feeling" that encroached like a quiet fog. The task she had set herself required a degree of self-control beyond anything she had attempted and more isolation than she had ever felt among the townsfolk of Asheville and Charleston. "I sit quietly in this assemblage of young men," she mused, "and they might be women or mummies for aught I care." In order to reach her goal, she needed to hold herself above the whispers and fidgety curiosity that surrounded her in the tiered rows of the lecture hall. "In the amphitheatre yesterday a little folded paper dropped on my arms as I was making notes; it looked very much as if there were writing in it, but I shook it off," she wrote at the end of her second week. "I felt also a very light touch on my head, but I guess my quiet manner will soon stop any nonsense."

Her determined dignity certainly stopped the nonsense; it also drew a hard line between herself and everyone else. The windows of the medical building looked out onto those of a teaching college across the way, whose young female students were well aware of the lecture schedule at the medical school. The Geneva men passed the time before class clustered at the windows, gawking and catcalling: "See the one in pink!" "No, look at the one with a blue tie." Elizabeth sat to the side in her usual seat, studiously reviewing her notes and pretending not to listen. "I believe the professors don't exactly know in what species of the human family to place me," she mused.

Within the college no one could deny her competence and seriousness of purpose; outside, the residents of Geneva were less accepting. Women stopped and stared "as at a curious animal." A doctor's wife encountered at dinner refused to speak to her at all. She realized, gradually, that people had reached one of two conclusions: she was wicked, and her unscrupulous intent would eventually emerge, or she was insane. Either way she was dangerous. Though her lodgings were just a few steps from the medical building, she walked quickly and rarely ventured farther.

In the third week of Elizabeth's enrollment, the class turned to the reproductive organs. Dr. Webster was a popular professor with an irreverent sense of humor, renowned for his lecture on the male genitalia: a raunchy comedy routine that his audience received each term with hoots of hilarity and the thunderous drumming of a hundred pairs of feet. As the day approached, he suggested that Elizabeth should stay home, for her sake and for his own.

He underestimated her. With calm determination, she picked up her pen to school her professor. "I told him that I was there as a student with an earnest purpose, and as a student simply I should be regarded; that the study of anatomy was a most serious one, exciting profound reverence, and the suggestion to absent myself from any lectures seemed to me a grave mistake." A true medical man, she wrote, one elevated by his exalted calling, would never be derailed by prudishness. And if Dr. Webster couldn't face her in the front row, she would be quite comfortable

in the back. Put it to the class, she suggested, remembering the circumstances of her original acceptance. If they balked, she would respect their
feelings. "I did not wish to do so," she wrote, "but would yield to any wish
of the class without hesitation, if it *was* their desire."

To her delight, Webster applauded her pluck, admitted his error, and
allowed her to attend. At last, a teacher who recognized superior moral
fiber when he saw it. "He could hardly guess how much I needed a little
praise," Elizabeth wrote with relief. Still, her presence during his graphic
explanation of an area no lady should dwell upon brought everyone to
the brink. "Some of the students blushed, some were hysterical, not one
could keep in a smile, and some who I am sure would not hurt my feelings for the world if it depended on them, held down their faces and
shook," she wrote. "My delicacy was certainly shocked, and yet the exhi-
bition was in some sense ludicrous. I had to pinch my hand till the blood
nearly came, and call on Christ to help me from smiling, for that would
have ruined everything."

She felt her professor's predicament as least as keenly as her own: "Dr.
Webster, who had perhaps the most trying position, behaved admirably."
Describing the physiology of the penis in mixed company seemed, even
to Elizabeth, a more daunting challenge than listening to such a lecture
as the only woman in a sea of men. God might be on her side, but her
own sympathies lay, to a surprising extent, with the men who were non-
plussed by her presence. She was determined to prove herself, but not at
their expense.

When the ordeal was over, Dr. Webster asked if he could share her
original letter of protest with the students, "saying if they were all actu-
ated by such sentiments the medical class at Geneva would be a very
noble one." She retired to the hallway while Webster read her words aloud
to the men and declared that Elizabeth was a student in the tradition of
Galen, the Greek physician of antiquity, who said, "The study of anatomy
is a perpetual hymn to the gods." When he opened the door to invite
her back in, the room erupted in applause. "The lectures on anatomy
proceeded in regular order to their conclusion," Stephen Smith remembered, "and it was the universal testimony of the oldest students that they
had never listened to such a complete and thorough course."

~

What passed for "complete and thorough" medical education in 1847 was, even then, being called into question; the American Medical Association was founded that very year in an attempt to raise standards. For now, however, medical schools were only as good as their faculties, and these were often loose groups of independent physician-entrepreneurs, collecting fees directly from each student and issuing admission tickets—ornately engraved pasteboard squares bearing the professor's name and specialty—to lectures in their particular subject for the term. Jolly Dr. Webster adorned his tickets with a mournful-looking skull. The subjects included anatomy and physiology, surgery, pharmacology (or "materia medica"), clinical practice, pathology, chemistry, medical jurisprudence, and obstetrics.

All this was squeezed into a term of sixteen weeks, and the achievement of a diploma required only that students attend the identical course

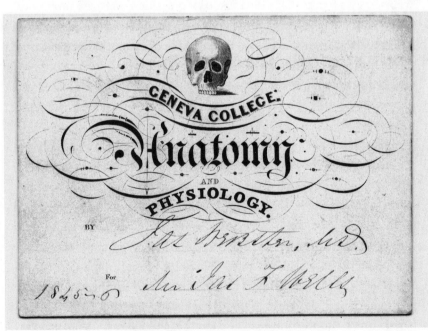

JAMES WEBSTER'S ANATOMY LECTURE TICKET.
COURTESY HOBART AND WILLIAM SMITH COLLEGES ARCHIVES AND SPECIAL COLLECTIONS

of lectures in two successive years, preceded by a few years of study with "some respectable practitioner or practitioners" and supplemented with whatever practical observation they could scrape together in the lengthy interval between the two terms. Often the only method of instruction was the lecture itself: students learned by watching and listening, and rarely touched any instrument other than the pen they used to take notes. If they were lucky, they had access to specimens for dissection; most never got within reach of a living patient. Once past their final examinations— evaluated by their own instructors and not by any objective governing organization—they entered the profession with a terrifying level of ignorance. This was partly due to their sketchy training, and partly to the primitive state of the healing arts.

The first half of the nineteenth century was the high-water mark of what came to be known as "heroic medicine." Doctoring had become an established profession, but the state of medical knowledge had not evolved much beyond the Hippocratic doctrine of the four humors (black bile, yellow bile, phlegm, and blood), the four elements (earth, air, fire, and water), and the four qualities (hot and cold, wet and dry) whose imbalance was thought to be the root of all illness. In the premodern world, governed by agricultural rhythms, human health had drawn its metaphors from the garden, and healers, like gardeners, had seen their role as helping time and nature to correct and restore the body's blooming life force. But as empirical science and then industrialization took hold in the public imagination, the body-as-garden was giving way to the body-as-machine: a mechanism that, when broken, needed to be fixed.

Healers who focused on long-term care—the village midwife, the monk-infirmarian—had been overtaken by doctors fixated on short-term cure. Watching passively while letting nature take its course did not inspire patients to pay their fees; a good doctor, it was thought, produced results you could *see*. Most of those results were painful if not actually dangerous, and few contributed to healing—the importance of hygiene was as yet poorly understood, and the discovery of truly effective pharmaceuticals lay mostly in the future. There were no governmental sanitary commissions to recommend best practices or hold individual practitioners accountable. Physicians built reputations largely on the placebo effect of charisma, with self-assurance substituting for science. They used the same handful of drugs and procedures, trying each in turn, often regardless of the complaint, until the patient either recovered or died.

Thermometers were not yet in use to diagnose fever, and aside from poking, listening, peering, and taking a patient's pulse, there was no accurate way to divine what might be happening inside the body, and even less certainty about why. Treatment was a matter of better-out-than-in: trying to expel the problem with a toxic arsenal of emetics, laxatives, diuretics, and expectorants, not to mention lancets, leeches, and blisters. The more violent the reaction, the more effective the therapy, most doctors—and most patients—agreed. "Medicine is always an evil," Elizabeth noted, "though sometimes a necessary evil." Necessary evils described in Dr. Lee's pharmacology lectures included castor oil, calomel (a powerfully laxative compound of mercury that also caused extreme salivation, not to mention the eventual neurological damage of mercury poisoning), lobelia (the "pukeweed" prized by the Thomsonians), mustard plaster (which could produce first-degree burns), and turpentine (used both externally and internally). Dosages varied not just by age and weight but also by temperament, sex, and even class. "A delicate woman should not be dosed like an Irishman," Elizabeth dutifully recorded. The legacy of the Hippocratic humors persisted, and one's medical complaints were thought to correspond to one's type: sanguine people were prone to inflammation, while spiteful temperaments were more vulnerable to stomach problems.

Bloodletting was relied upon in cases of all kinds, the idea being that "blood is the fuel which feeds the fire of inflammation"—subtract blood, and infection would abate. "The more important the organ, the more necessary to be prompt in bleeding," wrote Elizabeth. For a serious illness involving the brain, forty ounces was not considered excessive. (As reference, modern blood donors in certified good health give no more than a pint—sixteen ounces—at a time.) The production of "laudable pus" was believed to be a sign that the body was expelling infection, so physicians blistered the skin of patients with mustard plaster and then punctured the blisters to release the accumulated fluid. For pain relief, thankfully, there was laudanum, a mixture of alcohol and opium. Opium, Elizabeth's notes record, was "the most valuable article of the Materia Medica—differs from most other narcotics, in being a safe remedy."

Though privately unsure of the efficacy of any of these therapies—they certainly hadn't helped her father back in Cincinnati—Elizabeth threw herself into the task of absorbing all that her professors could teach her about preserving the mechanisms of health. Now was not the time to wonder about phrenology, mesmerism, or the water cure, or about letting time and nature take their course: If she wanted to earn an official diploma from a mainstream medical school, she needed to set her own doubts and interests aside. And much of what she was learning made sense to her. "The human body is a laboratory," she wrote. "The excretions are its refuse; they are both the result and the measure, of the exchanges which go on between the outside world, and our own organization." For a young woman who felt uncomfortable with strong emotion and social interaction, reducing blood, sweat, and tears to scientific secretions was a relief.

Actual sick people were a different undertaking entirely. In early December, barely a month after her arrival, Dr. Webster summoned Elizabeth to his office, where a woman waited to be examined. A poor woman by definition—well-heeled patients summoned doctors to their homes. There is no record of the woman's complaint, but the fact that Webster made a point of including Elizabeth suggests a gynecological problem, a chance for his new prize pupil to gain some practical experience. Geneva, too small to boast a public hospital, afforded little opportunity for its medical students to observe patients.

Elizabeth was shaken to the core by the sight of the woman before her: not a cadaver to be anatomized but a living individual in pain, vulnerable to the gazes of strangers. "'Twas a horrible exposure; indecent for any poor woman to be subjected to such a torture; she seemed to feel it, poor and ignorant as she was," Elizabeth wrote. "I felt more than ever the necessity of my mission." If she achieved her goal, women would at least be able to confide their most intimate ailments to other women. But the encounter unnerved her. "I went home out of spirits, I hardly know why," she wrote. She was abundantly aware of all the noble challenges involved in breaching the male bastion of the medical profession; what she hadn't yet reckoned with was the intimacy of contact with patients. The presence of a partially disrobed stranger in extremis was disturbing. How could she fulfill her destiny as a physician if she recoiled from contact with her patients? "I felt alone," she concluded. "I must work by myself all life long." Even if other medically minded women someday joined her, how could they empathize with a visceral discomfort she could barely articulate to herself?

In letters home, however, she colored her account of this first patient with bravado. "[Elizabeth] says that some of the students begin to develop apprehension at the idea of the precedent they have set," Sam reported with amazement and pride, "& fear lest women should usurp the profession!"

꜀

Elizabeth and Geneva Medical College grew on each other. The facilities were laughably modest compared to the elite institutions of Philadelphia and New York—and had been considerably exaggerated in the circular Elizabeth had received with her acceptance letter—but the humble scale and remote setting allowed Elizabeth to work closely with her professors. Dr. La Ford, the demonstrator of anatomy, selected a quartet of especially level-headed students to form a separate dissecting class with her in the private room of the surgical professor. Far from bridling at this segregation, Elizabeth remembered her evenings with them fondly— "they treated me like an elder sister"—and to her own surprise began to approach her studies with more pleasure than duty. Geneva's lectures on anatomy and physiology were good; in her notes, Elizabeth drew intricate diagrams of branching coronary arteries and the graceful curves of the uterus. Sunk deep in concentration, "tracing out the ramification of parts," she lost track of time, remaining alone in the silent medical building, head bent over a marble-topped laboratory table, until long after the rest of the town had retired for the evening. She would rarely enjoy such unadulterated focus again—outside the sheltering community of the college, few could stomach the idea of a woman with her hands in a corpse.

Elizabeth was now comfortable enough at Geneva to regret the close

ELIZABETH'S DIAGRAMS OF ARTERIES AND THE UTERUS.
COURTESY LIBRARY OF CONGRESS, MANUSCRIPT DIVISION, BLACKWELL FAMILY PAPERS

of her first term in January. After the last lecture, some of her fellow students offered expressions of friendship, which she parried with awkward pride. One asked permission to write to her—a normal request from a young man, but one that solitary Elizabeth found absurd if also gratifying. "It cheered me, funny as it was," she wrote. Another invited her to sit for a daguerreotype portrait—still a novel technology in 1848—"but I told him it had annoyed me so much to see my name in the papers that I certainly could not give my face too." There are no extant photographs of Elizabeth as a young woman.

Anticipating the graduation requirements of the following year, Elizabeth attended the oral examinations of the second-year students. She was unimpressed. "I suppose they were as thorough as most," she wrote dismissively, "but they were certainly not much of a test." Holding her own at this level of difficulty would not be a problem. At the boardinghouse, having warmed to their unusual boarder, they gave her an oyster supper to celebrate the midpoint of her journey through medical school, and Elizabeth packed for her return to Philadelphia, where she would spend the eight months until the next term at Geneva.

After the graduation exercises, she bade her professors farewell. If she expected some gesture of recognition for her impressive success thus far, it was not forthcoming. "They talked over my affairs, but gave me no important advice," she wrote. "To my great disappointment no letters of introduction were prepared for me, but only a promise that they should be sent on at once." It was a pattern—enthusiasm without follow-through—with which Elizabeth would become familiar.

The three months of Elizabeth's first term had been grueling, lonely, and uncomfortable. She was no longer just an ambitious young woman but a public figure. Wherever she went, whatever she did, eyes followed: some shocked, some derisive, some admiring, none indifferent. And that, she began to realize, was how she liked it. She had never made friends easily; she had always been one who would rather impress than endear. She had a mission to fulfill, and a whole town watching. It was exhausting, but it was also exhilarating.

The lawyer and poet William H. C. Hosmer, bard of Avon (a town just a few miles west of Geneva), published a hymn of praise in the *Western*

Literary Messenger just as Elizabeth prepared to depart. "Maiden of earnest thought, heroic heart!" he exhorted her.

> God speed thee on thy way to win the prize,
> And well reward thy struggle *to be wise*:
> Heed not detraction! for thou hast a part
> On the wide, shifting stage of life to play
> That will confer renown on thee for aye.

In later writings, Hosmer would clarify his stance: women should study medicine only in order to rescue their suffering sisters from the terrible shame of exposure to men, not to work alongside men as colleagues. But at this fragile moment, Elizabeth was glad for whatever public support she could find. She saved a handwritten copy of the poem—from the poet himself?—among her most important papers.

~(

CHAPTER 4

BLOCKLEY ALMSHOUSE

The ferry across the Schuylkill River to Philadelphia's Blockley Almshouse had much in common with Charon's across the Styx: for most patients, there was no return trip. Sepsis stalked the wards, which were largely unheated; one winter inspection recorded temperatures between thirteen and eighteen degrees *inside,* with wet linens and standing water frozen solid. From Blockley's walls, meadows stretched down to the riverbank. In winter, the sluice gates were opened, and the river flooded and froze. This ice, bearing all the effluent of a bustling city, was cut for the use of the hospital. Cholera and puerperal, or childbed, fever paid recurring visits from which few recovered. Physicians went from patient to patient—from surgery to postmortem to labor and delivery—without washing their hands or changing their aprons.

Municipal hospitals, evolving from their origins as poorhouses, remained refuges for the destitute, who entered—or were deposited—as a last resort. Four massive yellowish-gray buildings, four stories each, had risen in 1834 as a new home for America's first public hospital, but new construction could not change old attitudes. Fifteen years on, roughly two thousand people lived and suffered within, a grim rebuke to Philadelphia's prosperity.

Outside Blockley's lunatic wards, patients allowed fresh air were chained to iron rings bolted to the courtyard walls; inside, the doors bore the teeth marks and bloodstains of those who remained confined. Wealthy visitors crossed the river to gawk at the insane as a form of entertainment, and persisted in the complacent belief that ill health was the wages of sin rather than the consequence of poverty. "Blockley is the microcosm of the city," wrote one observer. "Here is drunkenness; here is pauperism; here is illegitimacy; here is madness; here are the eternal priestesses of prostitution, who sacrifice for the sins of man; here is crime in all its protean aspects; and here is vice in all its monstrous forms."

Elizabeth's notebooks were full of theory; now she needed practice. Between the two terms of medical school, students were expected to study independently, observing at hospitals or assisting private physicians—but most hospitals would not allow a woman to walk the wards, and Elizabeth wanted to see more than her friends Dr. Warriner and Dr. Elder could show her. In Philadelphia, there was no better place than Blockley to observe illness, if not, perhaps, healing. Young physicians regularly sought experience there, regarding the steady stream of patients more as teaching aids than as people. Its crowded wards were always short-staffed, and its impoverished patients were in no position to take issue with the gender of their doctor. During the empty months before her return to Geneva College, Blockley would be both Elizabeth's home and an intensive course in the social context of disease.

Learning that the hospital's board was riven by political infighting, she plotted a careful strategy. She introduced herself to each party leader in turn—Whig, Democrat, Native American (later known as Know-Nothing)—and impressed them with her modesty and determination. When her petition to enter Blockley reached the trustees, "all were prepared to fight in my behalf, but there was no one to fight!" Her admission was unanimous. "Resolved that permission be granted to Miss Elizabeth Blackwell to enter this Institution, enjoy such accommodations as can be conveniently afforded her and occupy such a position as may be assigned her by the Chief Resident Physician," read the official document, leaving plenty of room for interpretation with each ambiguous "such." By the beginning of March, Elizabeth had moved in as a student, the first woman ever to do so. Official histories of Blockley fail to mention her at all.

Elizabeth reported home with determined cheer, delighting in her airy room with its snow-white walls and large windows, open to the spring breeze and a view of the meadows and the city beyond. "I feel disposed to shut out all business remembrances, listen to the little birds warbling outside, & pay you a spiritual visit," she wrote. "No infection I fancy will travel with the paper."

Her room was located off the female syphilis ward. Today penicillin is effective at the first sign of genital sores, but in 1848, eight decades before its discovery, most women ill enough to end up at Blockley were deep into the debilitating and disfiguring tertiary stage of the disease: seizures, incontinence, blindness, dementia, and necrotic lesions that ate away the bones of jaw and face and skull. The collapsed profile characteristic of advanced cases was known as "saddle nose." Blockley's patients were likely also suffering the effects of earlier attempts to cure them. "One night with Venus, a lifetime with Mercury," went the adage. Mercury—in the form of calomel ointment or pills—was used to burn away syphilitic sores and purge infection, but the intense excretion and salivation it caused led to kidney damage and eroded gums, and then there were the cognitive effects of mercury poisoning. The righteous uninfected saw these afflictions as appropriate punishment for promiscuity. Blockley's syphilis ward was a gallery of misery.

Its inmates had no idea what to make of the studious newcomer in their midst, and Elizabeth, at least initially, was at first equally innocent of the circumstances that might have led to their hospitalization. "Most of the women are unmarried, a large proportion having lived at service and been seduced by their masters," she noted. "I found no instance of a married woman living with her husband entering." She could hear them lurking outside her door; in response, she moved her desk to a position in line with the keyhole, in full view of the curious. "It was thought that my residence there might act as a check on these very disorderly inmates," she wrote, but their impact on her was more profound. Her awareness of their plight, once she came to understand its origins in prostitution and "the hideousness of modern fornication," would resonate later in her career.

Nothing in her peripatetic past had prepared her for the agony she beheld at Blockley. "Within one week," she wrote to her teenaged brother George, "a lunatic scalded himself to death, one woman cut her throat, another fell down a cellar opening and broke both legs, they died the following day, another jumped over the banisters, breaking both ancles [*sic*]." Just the night before, she had been roused from sleep by screams and running footsteps; throwing open her window, she looked down. "There in the moat that surrounds the building, a depth that made me dizzy, lay a white heap, covered with blood, uttering a terrible sound, half groan, half snort." Elizabeth recognized the crumpled form: a young patient who had been locked in the room next door as punishment for fighting. She had tried to escape down a rope made of bedsheets. Elizabeth's account of the scene—the moonlight, the jangling of keys and creaking of hinges as the great gates of the hospital opened and the shrieking woman was borne inside, the voices raised in wonder or pity or scorn—is both clinical and fascinated, the doctor writing with the relish of a gothic novelist.

Blockley was vast, and at first Elizabeth was lost. Like a language student who has only conversed in a classroom, she found her studies of little use, and no one at Blockley volunteered to guide her. "I see a great deal without understanding it, pass over what is important, & dwell upon circumstances of trifling moment," she wrote to Emily with uncharacteristic candor. "Sometimes I feel certain that I see just so & so, & find out afterwards, I was entirely wrong." There was so much she had never witnessed: "Today, for the first time, I saw a person bled—only think of it—& that is a fair specimen of my practical knowledge in general."

The resident physicians watched her with a volatile mixture of scorn and insecurity. Elizabeth was clearly "stepping out of woman's sphere"; at the same time, they feared she might catch them in a moment of ignorance or even malpractice. None of them had any interest in teaching her: "When I walked into the wards they walked out." They evaded her efforts to watch them, listen to them, or even read their decisions regarding their patients; though it was routine to write notes on diagnosis and treatment at the head of each bed, after her arrival this practice was quietly suspended. The physician-in-chief, Nathan Dow Benedict, was an exception—Elizabeth gratefully thought him "the very loveliest man the Almighty ever created"—but she saw him so rarely there was never time to ask all her questions. "I glean a little from him," she told Emily, "but oh how different it would be, with intelligent, interested instructors, & companions to share study"—in other words, with the benefit of what any male medical student of her caliber could expect to find. "You would laugh to see me wandering eagerly about those great wards, timidly enquiring into symptoms, & peering about for useful knowledge," Elizabeth wrote.

She found it easier to avoid the doctors entirely, reading in her room until midmorning, when their rounds were over, and only then venturing onto the wards, feeling like an intruder. "I find that some of the patients like to detail their symptoms," she remarked with surprise. She watched the nurses apply poultices and perform injections, and she sometimes dared to auscultate, listening for a heartbeat with the monaural stethoscope of the time, a straight wooden tube with trumpet-shaped ends, one pressed to the patient's chest, the other to the doctor's ear. She was unable to deduce much from what she heard. Talking to patients, even if she didn't understand their symptoms, did have one benefit. "I believe the practice will be of great service to me morally as well as intellectually," she wrote, "& teach me to go about with that authority & *manner* essential to the physician."

Elizabeth often sought the company of the matron, the woman with the most intimate understanding of the institution. "Ensconced in her armchair, with feet propped on a velvet footstool, she dispenses orders from morning to night, gives out clothing, raves at the paupers, and dooms the refractory ones to a shower-bath," she wrote. "I like to talk with her occasionally, for she is shrewd and has seen much of life through dark spectacles." Separated from Elizabeth by a gulf of class and education—and thus posing no threat—the Blockley matron was a bulwark against discouragement. Here was a woman of authority, surrounded by men, unafraid to raise her voice, and accustomed to being obeyed. Most important, she liked Elizabeth. "I drank tea with her lately & had a very pleasant evening," Elizabeth wrote. "She is a remarkably strong independent woman, full of energy & quick decision—she braces me up, excites me, I never talk so well as in her company." It was a relief, away from the hostile stares of the physicians, to discuss patients with this capable woman—so different, in Elizabeth's opinion, from the lowly nurses, whom she dismissed as "mere *hands*" who "never think."

Blockley was Elizabeth's first deep dive into doctoring. Unlike the empathetic Dr. Benedict, with his "voice as gentle, his touch as kind to each patient as if she were his sister," she walked the wards as if they were the pages of a textbook, and the patients illustrations for intensive study. Waves of refugees from Ireland's Great Famine were arriving in American ports, many of them ill with typhus, known as "ship fever." They filled the beds at Blockley and overflowed onto pallets on the floor, often still infested with the body lice no one yet recognized as the carrier of the disease. Choosing epidemic typhus as her graduation thesis topic—avoiding obstetrics and gynecology in favor of a gender-neutral focus—Elizabeth took meticulous notes on patients' dying agonies. Her letters home contain no reference to them, only an urgent request to send books—"one, 'Letters from Ireland at the Time of the Famine in '47,' the other, on the health of large cities."

At Geneva College, Dr. Lee's materia medica lectures had offered little on why epidemics killed some and left others unscathed. His best guess suggested that "fear predisposes to disease"—a theory Elizabeth used to explain the infection rates of the Irish arrivals, as she imagined their flight, packed into stinking steerage quarters. "Without employment or exercise, their minds had time to brood over the fearful scenes they had left," she wrote. "Fear, sorrow, anxiety joined with the physical evils of their condition to depress the vital energy, & the seeds of disease sown in their constitutions were thus nourished into life."

The precise mechanism of infection was equally mysterious—it would be more than a decade before Louis Pasteur proposed the germ theory of disease. The prevailing wisdom held that "miasma" was responsible for contagion: poisonous air, arising from swamps or other rot-filled places, like the malarial neighborhood of the short-lived Blackwell residence in Flushing. Elizabeth, never one to accept convention without scrutiny, was not afraid to question this, eloquently, in the first draft of her thesis:

In truth we know so little of disease that we are not prepared to state
the manner of its production; we see a certain set of symptoms,
grouped together, and we give a particular name to the state of the
patient, but these symptoms do not constitute the disease, they are
simply indications of a hidden power, whose connexion with the
symptoms, we are unable to trace—of the disease itself we are in
complete ignorance.

Given the general tendency of medical men not to admit what they did
not know, this was bold; coming from a woman attempting to win herself
a place among them, it was ill advised. In the manuscript, the passage is
crossed out with heavy strokes.

Elizabeth laid out a methodical explication of the symptoms of ship
fever, its progression, possible treatments, and onward, whether to convalescence or autopsy. "The following sketch which I made by the bedside
of a woman dying," she wrote, "will serve as an illustration of the general
termination of the fever."

The eyes were bloodshot filmy & nearly closed; the mouth half open,
drawn on one side, the saliva trickling down; the teeth & gums were
covered with hard sordes*; the tongue dry, with black crusts, & incapable of protrusion; the breath of a peculiar and offensive smell; res-
piration labored, the chest heaving violently; the movement of the
heart extremely feeble, the pulse almost extinct; the patient lay in a
comatose state, with entire loss of voluntary power, medicine could
no longer be swallowed, the head slipped down on the chest; there
were now involuntary passages of a dark green colour; the neck &
other parts of the body were swollen & of a livid hue; sometimes a
furious delirium occurred in the last stage; and occasionally the
vomiting of black sooty fluid, continued until death.

It was all dispassionately recorded by a woman who, not three years earlier, could hardly bring herself to touch a dead beetle.

* Encrustations on the mouths of fever patients.

Elizabeth's dissertation made it clear that no one really knew how to treat typhus. She describes the use of virtually every preparation in the apothecary's cabinet, up to and including a heavy reliance on brandy and, as a last resort, the rubbing of cayenne pepper on the inner thighs. Indeed, it seemed more useful to resort to her sister Anna's recent preoccupation: the water cure. In her manuscript, she addressed at some length the findings of the Scottish doctor James Currie, who at the turn of the century had doused fever patients with cold water and won fame for his remarkable success rate: "well worthy of careful consideration," Elizabeth insisted. But no self-respecting medical school—founded, after all, to defend the profession against quacks—would accept a thesis that endorsed an alternative therapy. Between the first and final drafts, this passage also disappeared. Elizabeth did, however, slip in the suggestion that a patient fortunate enough to survive typhus might benefit from "the practise of washing the body in cold water," though she attributed the idea to a male physician, carefully protecting herself from any critic ready to dismiss a woman's laughable attraction to fads.

It was becoming obvious to Elizabeth that a hospital was not a healthy place, and doctors were as likely to do harm as to help. Just a year earlier, in 1847, a physician in Vienna named Ignaz Semmelweis had noticed a connection between contact with corpses and puerperal fever, and he insisted that his students wash their hands when moving between the morgue and the labor ward. The mortality rate among new mothers immediately plummeted. But the universal acceptance of germ theory was decades in the future, and his colleagues jeered, offended by the suggestion that their own habits were to blame. Semmelweis was eventually committed to an insane asylum, still insisting upon his insight, and died there in obscurity—from an infection, no less. Elizabeth remained ignorant of his discovery, though given her growing conviction that simple hygiene was at least as effective as anything she saw prescribed at Blockley, she would not have laughed.

"I am not afraid myself of sickness," she wrote to Marian, "but it is very certain, if I should be ill, none of their nostrums would go down my uncontaminated throat. I should trust to fresh air, cold water, & nature, & live or die as the Almighty pleases." Classing herself neither with patients nor with physicians, she saw no contradiction in her attitude. The work was larger than that.

〜

Six months at Blockley taught Elizabeth formative lessons about the limitations both of her chosen profession and of women, in whose name she had pledged her determination to practice. About doctors, she was skeptical; about women, she was scathing. She was bluntest in her letters to Emily. "Oh Milly, what is to be done with the women," she wrote.

> Alas for woman she seems to me inexpressibly mean—it is not her intellectual inferiority I lament—I believe as a rule, an intellectual difference will always be—but if she were only grand in those qualities attributed to her, all might be well, but the petty, trifling, priest-ridden, gossiping, stupid, inane, women of our day—what can we do with them!

Surrounded by wretched female patients crushed by the weight of ignorance, poverty, and disease; ill-trained nurses who performed their duties mechanically, when not helping themselves to the medicinal brandy; and doctors who dismissed them all as a lesser order of beings, Elizabeth grew ever more convinced of her own strength and the responsibility it placed upon her. "There are a few strong ones—a sort of exceptional eighth[*] perhaps," she allowed. "If they could be united, it would be a good beginning—you are one Milly, and sometime or other, we must work together, though the way does not seem clear yet."

If Elizabeth did not admire most women, neither did she blame them. Living with the syphilitic inmates of Blockley—and discussing Fourier's communal phalanxes at Associationist meetings across the river in Philadelphia on her days off—had opened her eyes. "As I learnt to realize slavery & hate it, deeply eternally, while living amongst slaves—so I am learning to curse from the bottom of my soul this heathenish society

---

[*] Her words carry a prophetic resonance. Half a century later, in his essay "The Talented Tenth," W. E. B. Du Bois would call for college education for Black students, writing, "The Negro race, like all races, is going to be saved by its exceptional men."

of the nineteenth century, surrounded here by its miserable victims," she wrote. The conundrum of woman's lot had never seemed clearer: women could not rise until the attitudes of their society shifted, but social mores would never change without women's leadership, "so there seems to me, no opening in the circle." Even among the educated women of her acquaintance, few seemed formed for noble causes—"there is a great deal of the sweet flower, & bright butterfly about them." How to undergird these "bright loving qualities" with "a foundation of truth & earnestness"?

Her answer, as confided to Emily, was breathtaking in its conviction. "[W]omen will have to save women after all, they have the truer love & understanding for their own sex," she began, reasonably enough. Then her tone intensified:

> I do strongly admire & deeply love, the beautiful weak women, who now occupy so unworthy a place in society, I see into them & feel their lovely qualities but I know they need my eye to guide them & my arm to keep them in a true position, a friendly insight to correct their faults & make them as good as beautiful—what a blessed thing it would [be] to act Providence for the helpless, all unseen but omnipotent to shape their destinies, & create their highest happiness . . . truly to be co-worker with God, to catch a glimpse of his design . . . is reward enough for a life of toil & gloomy effort.

Elizabeth regarded women with the calm superiority of a benevolent deity. Unattributed, her words could pass as the musings of a profoundly paternalistic man. Women were not her peers or her equals, and she had little desire to work alongside them. Empowered by her own divine gifts, she meant to guide them toward better versions of themselves.

This attitude went for all women, including those crusading openly for the newborn cause of women's rights. That summer of 1848, the first formal meeting of these reformers had convened at the squat brick Wesleyan chapel in Seneca Falls, not far from Geneva, where in July the attendees adopted a "Declaration of Sentiments," written mostly by Elizabeth Cady Stanton and modeled on the familiar Declaration of 1776, with certain key edits: "We hold these truths to be self-evident: that all men *and women* are created equal . . ." Laying out "a history of repeated injuries and usurpations on the part of man toward women," the declaration asserted women's moral and intellectual equality, demanded greater opportunity in education and employment, and—though some delegates thought it shockingly radical—called for woman suffrage. A second Woman's Rights Convention followed on August 2 in Rochester, where the Declaration of Sentiments was approved and further resolutions proposed, including one that praised Elizabeth's "persevering and independent course" through medical school as "a harbinger of the day when woman shall stand forth 'redeemed and disenthralled,' and perform those important duties which are so truly within her sphere."

A different sort of woman might have responded to such unsolicited applause with grateful pride, but Elizabeth did not consider herself in thrall to anyone, nor in any particular need of redemption. It was flattering that they had heard of her, but she had no interest in becoming their emblem or their mascot, let alone in joining their ranks. "I don't sympathize with these reforming ladies," she wrote. "I'm very sorry my name was mixed up with the Rochester absurdity. I understand all the good that's in them & esteem it for as much as it's worth, but they mistake the matter & make themselves very foolish." Though Elizabeth was undoubtedly a reformer and a lady, she placed herself in a separate category. She sympathized with the general goals of the women's movement, but she chuckled dismissively at its tactics.

One of the reforming ladies, she reported incredulously, had written her an admiring letter "full of enthusiastic sympathy, at my 'bold resistance of man's outrageous tyranny.'" Responding to the woman with appropriate courtesy, Elizabeth nevertheless proceeded to set her straight. The problem was not the tyranny of men, she wrote, but the disappointing weakness of women. "Women are feeble, narrow, frivolous at present, ignorant of their own capacities, and undeveloped in thought and feeling," she lectured her well-wisher. "The exclusion and constraint woman suffers, is not the result of purposed injury or premeditated insult. It has arisen naturally, without violence, simply because woman has desired nothing more." Once women awoke to their untapped powers, Elizabeth believed—encouraged by the growing respect of her medical school classmates—men would welcome them as equals. The full development of women would then enable "the consequent redemption of the whole human race."

Quoting Margaret Fuller, Elizabeth invoked an idea at the heart of Associationism: "Earth waits for her queen." The limited goal of woman suffrage—winning the vote for women who were still enslaved by their own ignorance—was, she believed, woefully premature. What good was a vote if one didn't know how to think independently? It was more important to prove the capacities of women and show them the way forward into the light, out of the shadow of their menfolk. For women, just as for the enslaved, the first step must be freedom. "The study and practice of medicine is in my thought but one means to a great end," Elizabeth wrote. Caring for suffering individuals had never been the engine that drove her. In becoming a doctor, she meant to heal humanity.

Elizabeth had no interest in joining her strength to the emerging women's movement. "I have curious glimpses into the American female world just now," she wrote:

> There are several little eddies of women, in various places, that whirl & froth so furiously that . . . one would think the whole of womankind, was about to rise in general rebellion, & trample down all the common rules of society. Standing on the bank however, these little eddies assume their relative value, & that I fancy is a very small one.

The metaphor places Elizabeth, godlike, on high, gazing down at the women's rights movement as something directionless and frivolous, bubbly and easily popped, laughably "little." She watched the chaotic eddies whirl away, and kept her feet dry. The only true sisterhood she felt, at this stage of her journey, was with her actual sisters: Anna, Marian, Ellen, and especially Emily.

～

As the heat of summer waned and her months at Blockley drew to a close, Elizabeth took a break from her studies to welcome her cousin Kenyon

Blackwell, visiting from England. With him was her second-youngest brother, Howard, now seventeen and planning to return with Kenyon to Birmingham and join him in the iron trade. After more than four years without seeing her brother—four years of unremitting intellectual intensity for Elizabeth—she thought Howy disconcertingly "dreamy & indifferent." She was unsure whether to admire his gentle, poetic apathy or give him a good shake.

Kenyon she found well read and sympathetic. He had brought her two expensive medical textbooks, gratifying proof of his confidence in her success. "They form a substantial foundation for my future library, & will cut quite a dash in the little office (that is to be)," she reported to Henry. "I consider them a good omen." A decade older than Elizabeth, Kenyon stepped naturally into the role of the solicitous older brother she lacked, and he made it clear that he would be proud to lend her money in support of her admirable goal. With her usual horror of debt, she neither accepted nor declined, but felt "all the safer for the offer"—"it is a very different matter to receive willing aid from friends, for the promotion of a noble object."

The moment was full of promise. On the first night cool enough for a fire in Philadelphia, she drew her chair close to the hearth to write in her journal. "As I watched the beautiful sunset from my great window," she wrote, "I *almost* regretted that I was going to leave."

~(

CHAPTER 5

DIPLOMA

The dissecting room at Geneva College was in an attic, exposed beams crisscrossing the space. The subject was stretched on a narrow wooden table, head and feet exposed, the rest draped with a sheet. Dr. Corydon La Ford, the demonstrator of anatomy, stood at the head, wrapped in a black apron, scalpel in one hand and forceps in the other. He had drawn a chair next to him for Elizabeth's use, "while all around," Elizabeth wrote to Emily, "sitting, standing, leaning on each other's shoulders, on tops of benches, holding onto the rafters, were piled the students."

After the nightmares at Blockley, Elizabeth's return to Geneva for her second term in the fall of 1848—even when confronted, as she was now, with a human brain lying exposed in the bowl of a sawed-open skull—was a relief. The professors were comfortable enough to allow her greater access, and for the first time she joined the rest of the class at a dissection.

Some of Elizabeth's classmates wore aprons, and others protected their clothes with dressing gowns; many were smoking or chewing tobacco in an attempt to hold the stench of a decomposing body at bay. None of them had washed their hands, nor would they when the demonstration was over. Jostling and jockeying for vantage, they somehow preserved a circle of calm around Elizabeth's chair: "if a hand or a shoulder came in the slightest contact, it was instantly withdrawn, & perfect attention & good order prevailed."

The scene was typical of Elizabeth's student days: hours of intense study surrounded by raucous human interaction that never quite touched her. Within the college, among men who had come to recognize her competence, the distance was a respectful one; outside, Genevans continued to regard her with horror. "People still gossip freely," Elizabeth wrote to Sam, "report my intended marriage, if an unlucky student happen to walk home with me, & still consider me a sort of eccentric monster."

She did have one friend, George White Field, one of the steady fellows from her tutorial group. Five years her junior, Field would go on to become a demonstrator of anatomy at the college. "I've never met with a young friend who lets my life flow out so freely," she wrote. "Most people have a *styptic* effect on me." The fact that Field had an older sister named Elizabeth, and Elizabeth a younger brother named George, can only have reinforced the familial comfort. But even this sustaining friendship fell victim to scandalized scrutiny. "Of course," she continued, "all manner of stories have gone abroad about us, which oblige me now, to see scarcely anything of him."

She proclaimed herself grateful for the isolation, as it relieved her of the burden of feigning affection. To Marian, she described a classmate given to gazing at her during lectures, ambushing her on the walk home from church, and blushing when she caught his eye. "He is to me utterly repulsive," she wrote. "Though a handsome fellow, I should be very sorry to let him touch my hand." Chemistry as an academic subject was straightforward, but chemistry between individuals was mystifying: "it is strange that love cannot always excite love." She preferred the noble goal of harmony between Man and Woman to the messy reality of men and women.

As her friendship with Field suggested, what Elizabeth craved most was the unconditional support of a younger sibling: a fellow Blackwell, superior to others but subordinate to her. Her hopes veered again toward Emily, who remained at home in Cincinnati, teaching where she could. "Your life interests me particularly, as it seems more nearly related to my own, than that of any other member of our family," Elizabeth wrote to her. "Emily I claim you, to work in my reform—will you answer to the call, & let us sketch our future together?" She had forced open the door to a new field of study for women; now she invited—or instructed?—Emily to walk through it. The mixture of commendation and command, superiority and supplication, would mark Elizabeth's demeanor toward Emily throughout their entwined careers. "I've taken it into my head that you will lecture on anatomy someday in our college," she told Emily. And Emily, who shared Elizabeth's voracious intellect but not her polestar certainty, began to orient herself toward the future Elizabeth described.

A visit to Geneva from her brother Howard provided a small dose of Blackwellian comfort. Elizabeth skipped lectures to enjoy his company. "I did more laughing than I've done for months," she wrote. "His visit did me real good, for I have been so lonely." But the reunion marked a more permanent parting—Howard had come to say farewell before seeking his fortune with the Blackwell cousins in Birmingham. And Anna, who had a special maternal fondness for Howard, and had been pining for her mother country since the day the Blackwells left Bristol, would return with him. Anna had found an outlet for her fascination with radical ideas in translating the work of the cross-dressing novelist George Sand and the Blackwells' beloved Charles Fourier, progenitor of Associationism. Once abroad, she would also serve as a correspondent for American magazines, reporting on manners and mores in England and France. Neither Anna nor Howard would live in the United States again.

Elizabeth felt intensely the pressure of her task: just a couple of months until her final examinations, and beyond that, a future consecrated to "the accomplishment of a great idea." Alone in her room, she practiced lecturing to an audience of her bed, desk, and washstand, frustrated by her inability to translate the fire in her mind into words. "I would I were not so exclusively a doer," she wrote. "Speech seems essential to the reformer, but mine is at present a very stammering, childish utterance." In December a heavy snowfall made even the few steps between her room and the college treacherous; upon reaching the lecture hall chilled and breathless, she was warmed to the core by the attentions of her classmates. One brought her a chair, several made small talk about the extreme weather, Dr. Webster arrived with his usual jovial energy— everyday pleasures, but to Elizabeth, nothing to be taken for granted. "How little they know my sensitiveness to these trifling tokens!"

Her brother Henry thrilled Elizabeth with the promise of a Christmas visit. Christmas was the high holiday of Blackwell family solidarity, and the compilation of the literary Christmas Annual continued even as their diaspora widened. It had been years since Elizabeth shared Christmas with another Blackwell, and she was especially eager to see Henry, who had been making alarming noises about decamping to California, where the scramble for gold was just beginning—a commodity even riskier than sugar. "Believe me, brother mine," she had written sternly, "nothing lasting, nothing that will mark the Age enduringly, can be accomplished without a persevering effort, that is proof against temptation, & undazzled & unblended by the brilliant bursting meteors, which are accidents not elements of strong life." Just a month from the diploma that she had trudged through so many years to attain, the thought of her own brother galloping after a get-rich-quick scheme was mortifying. The family, equally concerned, had dispatched cousin Kenyon to New York to talk some sense into Henry.

On Christmas Day, Elizabeth garlanded her walls with hemlock boughs and stuck candles into four turnips, heaping more evergreens around her improvised centerpiece. She laid in a supply of almonds and raisins, "told everybody my brother was coming, & then sat down, dressed in best bib & tucker, to await his arrival." But when the knock sounded, at her door stood not Henry but generous Kenyon. Not relishing a Christmas scolding, Henry had decided to stay in New York.

Elizabeth spent New Year's alone, listening to the sleigh bells and shouts of greeting as Geneva's wealthier residents paid their New Year's calls among its trim brick row houses and grand Greek Revival homes. Lacking social or financial capital, she took comfort in her own abilities. In her journal she recorded a postoperative visit to a "pretty blind girl" recovering alone, whose "simple heart and idle fancy" Elizabeth found appealing. "Such are the women I long to surround with my stronger arm," she wrote. She paid a house call to a flu-stricken family outside town and stayed two days amid "a constant concert of coughing." Upon her return, she too fell sick. She prescribed herself sleep, baths, and walks in the cold. "I was *amused* & *gratified*," she wrote, "to see how my body threw off the influenza to which it was exposed." Having questioned the fruitless remedies in the materia medica—"the very thought of the drugs disgusts me"—she was heartened to see her hunch play out successfully.

A month shy of becoming a qualified physician, it appeared she had doctored herself with nothing stronger than water and fresh air.

"I have the strengthening conviction that my aim is right, & that I too am working after my little fashion, for the redemption of mankind," she wrote. "I have a most perfect conviction, that holy influence surrounds me. I know that I am one of the Elect." Her mother, passionate devotee of Presbyterian revivalism, would have embraced this echo of Calvin in the words of her skeptical daughter. But although Elizabeth's soul might be in peril, her self-esteem was fine. Though she was careful to modulate her tone in public, in letters home her faith in her own righteousness could be breathtaking.

Elizabeth finished her final examinations at the top of the class. Though the outcome was no surprise to her—"the examinations were slight as they always are & in no case would the Faculty have rejected me"—her own sense of relief was. She left the examination room with her face aflame and her nerves singing, and was greeted with warm applause by the students still waiting their turn. "They all seem to like me," she wrote, "and I believe I shall receive my degree with their united approval; a generous and chivalric feeling having conquered the little feelings of jealousy." The respect of this group of male peers was a laurel wreath. "I often feel when I am with them how beautiful the relations of man and woman might be under a truer development of character, in nobler circumstances."

～

On January 23, 1849, Elizabeth Blackwell received her diploma from Geneva Medical College. The day was full of sunshine, lake and sky competing for bluest blue, and all of Geneva was trying to get a glimpse of the unprecedented event. An hour before the commencement exercises, the best seats in the First Presbyterian Church on Pultney Square were already taken—by the very townswomen who had been horrified at Elizabeth's arrival. "Nothing but a vast expanse of woman's bonnets and curious eyes," wrote twenty-five-year-old Margaret DeLancey, daughter of the local bishop, eager to glimpse "the Lioness of the day."

At half past ten, Elizabeth left for the church, dressed in black silk brocade trimmed with white lace, swathed in a fringed cape, and conspicuously hatless, the spectators noted, though this had more to do with Elizabeth's limited budget for new millinery than anything else. The dress itself was an unavoidable extravagance, but "I can neither disgrace womankind, the College, nor the Blackwells, by presenting myself in a shabby gown," she insisted. By her side walked Henry, successfully dissuaded from his California dreams and currently honoring his late father's paradoxical ambitions by pursuing an education in the New York sugar trade. Come to visit her at last, he had bought a new handkerchief and cravat and borrowed a cloth cloak from a friend "for the purpose of striking terror & admiration into all beholders."

Henry had arrived in time to cheer Elizabeth through her examinations and had entertained himself by sitting near the stove at the medical building, listening with amused pride to the chatter of students unaware of who he was.

"Well boys," one remarked, "our Elib feels first-rate this morning. Do you notice how pleased she looks?"

"Yes indeed," answered another, "and I think she well may after the examination she passed yesterday."

"So Lizzie will get her diploma after all," said a third. "If any member of the class gets one, *she* is sure of it."

The pageantry of the day gave Elizabeth the opportunity both to demonstrate her unimpeachable modesty and to satisfy the ego that lay just beneath it. Accompanied by the faculty and Bishop William DeLancey, the students walked the short distance around the square from the medical building to the columned portico of the church in grand procession. Dr. Webster—gleeful both at Elizabeth's success and at the commotion it was causing—had sent more than one message inviting her to join the parade, but she had demurred. He intercepted her on the church steps and begged her to change her mind.

Pausing in her ascent, Elizabeth turned to him with eyebrows raised. "It wouldn't be ladylike," she told him, in a tone that left no room for argument.

"Wouldn't it indeed?" exclaimed the doctor, his smile slipping. "Why, no, I forgot—I suppose it wouldn't."

Elizabeth and Henry took their seats in a side pew. The rest of the class filed into the rows front and center, their coats a dark island in a sea of color, as the rustle of whispers and crinolines rose from an audience composed largely of women. After an interlude of choral music and prayer, Geneva's president, Benjamin Hale, conferred the diplomas. Calling up the graduates four at a time and addressing them briefly in Latin—the solemn effect marred by repeated glances downward to remember his lines—he doffed his velvet cap but remained seated as he handed over the sheepskins to the bowing young men. Elizabeth, last to be called, approached the altar alone, a bit of choreography that was meant to underline her propriety but had the happy side effect of highlighting her individual achievement. In comporting herself with such elaborate decorum, she managed to attract the undivided attention of every member of her audience.

This time President Hale rose to his feet. For each quartet of graduates, he had intoned the same formula of address: "*Domine Doctor . . .*" Now, for the first time, he began with "*Domina.*" Placing the precious diploma in Elizabeth's hands, Hale bowed, and she bowed in return. "A silence deep as death pervaded the assembly," wrote an overexcited reporter from the *Geneva Gazette*. "Her bosom heaved, almost too full for utterance." But this was not a romance, and she was not heaving, simply drawing breath for a characteristically measured response. "Sir, I thank you," she began. "By the help of the Most High, it shall be the effort of my life to shed honor upon this* diploma." She bowed once more and descended, her self-possession betrayed only by the rising color in her cheeks as the assembly applauded and Dr. Webster rubbed his hands together and beamed. As Elizabeth reached the last step, her friend George Field stood and beckoned her into the first pew. The row of graduates shifted over to make room, and she took her place with them for the rest of the program, "feeling more thoroughly at home in the midst of these true-hearted young men," she wrote, "than anywhere else in the town."

She had ample time to slow her drumming pulse during Dr. Lee's

---

* Different witnesses recorded Elizabeth's words differently; tellingly, Henry reported her saying "your" diploma, while she remembered it as "my" diploma. Others heard "this" diploma.

lengthy valedictory address. Lee congratulated his students on the first step of their journey. "You have learned how to learn, and what to learn—how to observe, and what to observe," he declared; now the work of actually learning and observing could begin. He roamed in his remarks from the heights of the Hippocratic Oath to the mundanities of daily doctoring: don't pad your bill with unnecessary house calls; don't offer a pessimistic prognosis in order to burnish your reputation with a miracle cure; don't degrade your good name with crackbrained therapies and patent medicines; don't drink. "It has been said that the surgeon should have an eagle's eye, a lion's heart and a lady's hand; but none of these can he have, who habitually indulges in the intoxicating cup," Lee instructed. None of the newly minted physicians before him, even if possessed of eagle eyes and lion hearts, could check off as many of these ideal qualities as the teetotaling woman in the front row.

Lee's respect for female fine-motor skills, however, exceeded his regard for the gender in general. To his mind, credulous women "who would be better employed in their domestic duties" were largely to blame for the success of quacks, against whose schemes the scientific young men of Geneva Medical College were now mobilized. The era of "witches and impostors," Lee announced, was drawing to a close.

Elizabeth, on the other hand, was a disciplined and persevering hero, a "ministering angel" armed with science, clearly not a witch. She was, however, an exception. "Such cases must ever be too few to disturb the existing relations of society," he concluded, "or excite any other feeling on our part than admiration." To men like Lee, Elizabeth was a comet, a single brief streak of light across the sky: impressive, but leaving the eternal order of the stars unchanged.

Up in the gallery, young Margaret DeLancey, the bishop's daughter, joined the applause, thoroughly satisfied with her day's entertainment. And just think! Dr. Lee himself had said Dr. Blackwell "would have more practice than she could attend to—that he would insure her *six thousand* dollars the first year!! Nearly as good as going to California, is it not?" Which, in the year that gave the prospecting forty-niners of the gold rush their nickname, was saying something.

As the audience dispersed, Bishop DeLancey, himself a trustee of the college, was among those who came to congratulate Elizabeth, "to the great astonishment of the conservatives," wrote Henry with amusement. The vestibule of the church was crowded with women hoping for a closer look at the "lioness." As Elizabeth approached on Henry's arm, they parted to make way, still staring, but most with tentative smiles instead of the scowls she had faced upon her first arrival. "I was glad of the sudden conversion thus shown," Elizabeth wrote, "but my past experience had given me a useful and permanent lesson . . . as to the very shallow nature of popularity."

~

Within the Blackwell tribe, Elizabeth's graduation was hailed with fierce approbation. "Beloved Relations," wrote hyperbolic Henry. "The important crisis is past, the great occasion over, the object of so much and so justifiable anticipation has been attained, and proud as I always feel of the Blackwells, my familism never seemed to me so reasonable and so perfectly a matter of course as it did this morning." In Cincinnati, brother Sam awaited the news with characteristic earnestness: "God be with our dear & noble sister! He has made her what she is & enabled her to accomplish so far, the will He has wrought in her; & precious in His sight will she be, in all her ways." The most incisive endorsement came from Marian, whose mild manner belied a clear eye and a keen sense of irony. Elizabeth "has thousands of warm friends," she wrote, "especially now that her exertions have been crowned with success," and in spite of the grumbling physicians who continued to insist that medicine was the privilege of men. "The good sense of the community is beginning to wake up to the *barbarousness* of the custom of permitting men to attend on women during sickness," she continued, her own fragile health making her all too familiar with an invalid's indignities. "And in this way as in everything else if women begin to desire it they will end by carrying their point & having it their own way."

Hannah Blackwell's pride in her third daughter's achievement was tinged with baffled concern. In the decade since her husband's death, she had ceded the family's affairs to her grown children, narrowing her focus to home and God. Elizabeth had ventured far beyond anything her mother could fathom. "I trust her life will be a very useful one. She has very exalted ideas of the profession," Hannah allowed. "But oh what a life of labor it will be." She wrote Elizabeth long querulous letters full of concern for the state of her soul—between medicine and Association-ism, what would become of it? Elizabeth thanked her for her "affection & sympathy in my eccentric course" and tried to reassure her. "You urge upon me the importance of religion—why bless the dear Mother what am I doing else but living religion all the time?" she insisted. "Do you think I care about Medicine—nay verily—it's just to kill the Devil, whom I hate so heartily."

Outside the family, Elizabeth Blackwell, M.D., received a more ambiv-alent reaction. Her thesis on ship fever was published in the *Buffalo Med-ical Journal*—"partly to give a little notoriety to the College, partly to be an introduction to me abroad," Elizabeth wrote. "I disliked the notoriety of the thing, as the thesis is quite an ordinary student's composition," she continued, "but they said it would do me credit, & pressed the matter, so I complied." "They" were presumably her professors Charles Lee and Austin Flint, who gave Elizabeth's work pride of place as the first item in the issue.

Her thesis, as printed, announced not just Elizabeth's competence as a scientific observer of epidemic typhus but also her broader vision for humanity. "When the laws of health are generally understood and practiced," she concluded in ringing tones, "when a social providence is extended over all ranks of the community, and the different nations of the earth interlinked in true brotherhood—then we may hope to see these physical evils disappear, with all the moral evils which cor-respond to, and are constantly associated with them." In an era before germ theory, upright behavior seemed at least as viable a pathway toward physical health as anything else. Elizabeth would never let go of this early conviction.

The *Boston Medical and Surgical Journal* reprinted a "glowing account" of the graduation ceremony and added its own gratifying comment on "Ship Fever": "Its literary merits are above the average of such produc-tions, and it manifests persevering and praiseworthy research." This rec-ognition, and the decidedly unfeminine confidence of Elizabeth's voice in an established medical journal, proved too much for some. A writer signing himself D.K. (a pun on Dike, classical goddess of moral order) sent a blistering letter to the editor condemning the recent commencement—"or what might more properly be called the farce, enacted at the Geneva Medical College"—that seemed to herald "the nefarious process of amalgamation."

Amalgamation was a loaded word, lifted from metallurgy to denote the mixing of races rather than alloys. The issue at hand was coeducation, not miscegenation, but D.K. saw Elizabeth's trespass as equally taboo. A woman who dared to penetrate the medical lecture hall surely "perverts the laws of her Maker." How could the grace and virtue of womanhood possibly be compatible with the rougher realities of the world of men? "The distaff, the needle and the pencil look better in her hand than the hoe or the scythe, the trephine or the gorget,"* wrote D.K. "If a clique of pseudo-reformers, or some mushroom Thomsonian or hydropathic association, had conferred this degree, it would have been a matter of no surprise, because it would be in perfect keeping with their transactions." And with that parting shot, he neatly and inadvertently vindicated Elizabeth's insistence on a degree from a regular medical school.

A letter in response to D.K. seemed to side with Elizabeth's cause—up to a point. Surely, wrote "Justus," D.K. was "decidedly behind the age." There had always been female midwives, and who could argue against the benefits of a well-educated one? Think of Marie-Louise Lachapelle or Marie Boivin, both renowned authorities on midwifery at the largest public hospitals in Paris fifty years earlier. However: "As to females engaging in the general practice of medicine," Justus continued, "the idea is absurd." The letter echoed Charles Lee's perception of Elizabeth: "From all we have been able to learn respecting Miss B.," it concluded, "she is emphatically an exception."

Lee himself added a startling footnote to the published version of his commencement address. He acknowledged the criticism that had

---

* A trephine is a circular bone saw used to cut holes in the skull. A gorget is a gutter-shaped instrument used to guide forceps during surgery to remove gallstones or repair fistulas.

appeared in print and even agreed with it in the case of women in general, though having witnessed Elizabeth's undeniable success, he reasserted his belief that it was appropriate to admit to the medical brotherhood an exceptional woman who possessed the proper "moral, physical, and intellectual qualifications." But his final sentence revealed just how fragile Elizabeth's accomplishment was. "While he holds this opinion," Lee wrote, using the third person to distance himself from hypocrisy, "he at the same time feels bound to say, that the inconveniences attending the admission of females to all the lectures in a medical school, are so great, that he will feel compelled on all future occasions, to oppose such a practice, although by so doing, he may be subjected to the charge of inconsistency." Charles Lee, whom Elizabeth counted among her strongest allies, was still the equivocating administrator who had left her admission up to the students. He would be happy to celebrate her success, but if the world was not ready for a woman doctor, he did not want the blame.

～

Elizabeth didn't linger in Geneva. The day after graduation, she and Henry boarded a train accompanied by Charles Lee, who like many provincial medical professors was in residence only during the sixteen weeks of the term. Soon Elizabeth was back in Philadelphia with her solicitous Quaker friends, the Elders, determined not to slacken the pace of her study while she waited for her plans to become clear.

The men who had blocked her entrance to Philadelphia's medical schools proved more welcoming now that she had achieved her M.D. somewhere else. "About a week ago I had quite a morning of triumph," Elizabeth wrote to Henry. Eager to audit the lectures of the most illustrious physicians of the day, she had presented herself at prestigious Jefferson Medical College. She was invited to sit alone in an anteroom off the lecture hall, where she could listen without intruding her presence. "The lectures were good, & I was glad to hear them, but I felt a little mean at hearing a lecture secretly," she wrote. The next day she returned with an escort of sympathetic professors, including Charles Lee; entering the hall together, they were greeted with warm applause from the five hundred students in attendance.

After that it was easy. One by one, the professors invited her to listen, and the students cheered every time she appeared among them. "Dr Lee was quite in spirits, for he had been blamed in N.Y. for giving me an M.D. & this pleasant recognition from the first college in the country was a support as unexpected as agreeable," she exulted. "I was delighted that all went so smooth, & felt a little pride too in my triumph," she continued more soberly, "perhaps this was why I received rather a rude message of refusal from another professor in the afternoon—a providential punishment." As usual, Elizabeth did not blame her male detractor—pride goeth, after all. Still, it stung: "I am so careful always to avoid intruding, that an ungentlemanly repulse, makes me feel a little bitter," she confessed. "I have not yet recovered from it sufficiently to visit the Museums to which I was invited." It was a rare admission of emotional vulnerability.

Days not spent at medical lectures were still busy; Charles Lee was not the only Genevan now in Philadelphia. "My mornings I spend dissecting with George Field—he is a real good hearted little fellow, & I like to be with him," Elizabeth wrote. Afternoons were for "rubbing up my French" in anticipation of her next goal: practical training in Paris.

For half a century, Paris had been the best place in the world to study medicine. The Enlightenment and the French Revolution had together created perfect conditions for the rapid advancement of medical knowledge: an embrace of skepticism and empiricism; a clearing away of old ideas and authorities; the reorganization of major hospitals as state-supported educational institutions rather than simply charitable refuges for the incurable; a meritocracy of innovative doctor-professors; and an abundant supply of indigent patients, victims of war and industrial displacement. French medical students learned at the bedside—it was not uncommon for a professor to lead a hundred pupils through the wards—and French hospital patients were routinely seen as offerings on the altar of science, their symptoms considered teaching tools as much as illnesses to be cured. This utility extended after death: the French did not share the Anglo-American horror of dissection. With deceased patients providing a steady stream of specimens, French physicians became leaders in investigating the pathology of disease. American medical students were frequent visitors to the "Paris School" in order to burnish their professional prestige at home.

If training in Paris gave a young doctor an extra gleam of legitimacy, then to Paris Elizabeth would go. Her new allies in Philadelphia would, she hoped, be willing to introduce her to their colleagues in France; indeed, they would be only too glad, she suspected, to make her someone else's uncomfortable responsibility. And providential help was at hand in the form of cousin Kenyon, who offered to escort her on his homeward trip across the Atlantic.

But first a quick family reunion, something she had not managed since her departure for Asheville in 1845. Elizabeth's loyalty to the Blackwell tribe burned as true as ever, but Cincinnati lay in the wrong direction, geographically and intellectually. It would be good to renew old ties with the influential Beechers and Stowes in Walnut Hills, though, and fulfilling her filial duty would give her a chance to see—and counsel— the sister she had chosen to follow her. "Is Emily teaching busily, & did she receive my message in relation to certain books I want her to look at, before my return?" she asked. She worried that Emily was spending too much time on German and not enough on anatomy.

Elizabeth stayed in Cincinnati for less than a fortnight. Her impatience was clear. "Obstacles overcome thus far only make her more resolute in her course," Sam wrote in his journal. "She told me I 'could not conceive how intensely she desired to be at work.' Even the 2 weeks at home seemed like lost time." On April 2, 1849, Elizabeth boarded a river steamer for the journey east. The remaining Cincinnati Blackwells— Hannah on Sam's arm, with Marian, Emily, and Ellen on one side, and Henry and young George on the other—waved as she receded. "I could not keep down the tears as I caught the last glimpse of those dear, true ones," she recorded in her journal. As the narrator of her own story, she lingered on the bittersweetness of the moment. But she itched to be gone.

Elizabeth stopped in Philadelphia to bid her friends farewell but also to complete a symbolic errand. On April 13, with Sarah Elder as her witness, Elizabeth Blackwell, M.D., became a naturalized citizen of the United States. For seventeen years, she had thought of herself less as an immigrant than as a semipermanent expatriate. Her attachment to her own Englishness remained strong, but it was in the New World that she had managed to achieve the first step toward her goal. Perhaps this parting gesture was a grateful one—or perhaps it was more strategic. France had long felt more warmly toward America than it did toward England; defining herself as an American might help smooth her path in Paris. For now, having pledged her allegiance to her adopted country, she promptly left it. Within a week she joined Kenyon in Boston and sailed for Europe.

~

CHAPTER 6

PARIS

As the majestic copper dome of the Massachusetts State House receded in the sunset, and the first whiff of bilgewater reached Elizabeth's nose through the stiffening breeze, all thoughts of her noble mission were replaced by more immediate preoccupations. "I gave myself a little convulsive twist," she recorded later, "& told Kenyon in a very loud voice, that I had no expectation of being sea-sick."

When the ship's bell rang for dinner, she marched resolutely into the saloon, but the flash of mirrors and the clash of dishes; the waiters rushing to pour wine; the chattering diners, like "a herd of pigs come to be fed"—it was all overwhelming. She managed one bite, rose from her seat, and rushed to her tiny stateroom, reaching the washstand just in time.

As she collapsed into her berth, the door burst open to admit her assigned cabin mate: an elderly woman, staggering with each lurch of the ship, too overwhelmed by nausea to locate the necessary basin. "After a few minutes violent exertion," Elizabeth recounted, "she tumbled upon a box, declared she had never been so ill in her life, & believed she was going to die." The newly credentialed doctor clung mutely to her lower bunk, leaving the unfortunate old lady to call for the overworked stewardess's help in boosting her up into bed. It was nearly a week before Elizabeth felt well enough to venture out on deck. Throughout the ordeal she maintained a stoic silence, though the poor soul in the upper bunk moaned loudly enough for two.

Too queasy to study, but well enough to feel the weight of idle hours, Elizabeth contemplated the uninspiring society on board. The gentlemen smoked and discussed horse racing and money, their voices rising with each glass of brandy. The ladies "gathered themselves into groups, & turned their backs on all solitary individuals," talking of titles and dresses and the opera. "I listened in vain for one thought, one noble sentiment, or one mark of true refinement," Elizabeth complained. "Oh I grew very very weary of those uncongenial people, who never spoke to me, but were all the time with me." Kenyon, himself bedridden with an attack of rheumatism, was little help.

At last Elizabeth woke to see the banks of the Mersey on either side with Liverpool ahead, the ships at anchor in the harbor seemingly right up among the houses. At the customs house, Elizabeth held her breath anxiously for a moment—partly because she didn't have the money to spare for duties, and partly because she had stashed her two largest and most expensive medical textbooks under her clothes to avoid paying tax on them. But the officials took little notice of the plainly dressed young woman and her ailing cousin. She exhaled, and on they went.

There wasn't much time before the train that would take them to Birmingham, where Howard and Anna were now settled near Kenyon's branch of the Blackwell family. Elizabeth could hardly bear to blink, there was so much to take in. The last time she stood on English soil, she had been a girl of eleven. She might have come of age among Americans, but despite her new citizenship, she still wasn't sure she wanted to *be* one. She was ready to fall in love with England again. Liverpool was built on a noble scale; the buildings seemed so substantial, defying the march of centuries. But as her gaze descended from Liverpool's elegant architecture to its consumptive-looking residents, ambivalence crept in. "Many of the people looked watery to me," she wrote. "I wanted to expose them to a bright American sun & dry them."

Still, as they rattled toward Birmingham, the countryside—neat hawthorn hedges and ancient stone churches, gardens full of cowslips and primroses—seemed verdant and perfect compared to the raw American towns Elizabeth had known. A chaise carried them the last few miles west from Birmingham to Portway Hall, home of Kenyon's brother Sam Blackwell, an iron refiner, and his father, Uncle John Blackwell. Even here in the "Black Country," Britain's coal-fueled industrial heart—where the very leaves on the trees were darkened with soot, and the sun through the smoke "gave a pale light that resembled an eclipse"—Elizabeth found plenty to admire. Portway Hall, built in 1674, was like a castle from a fairy tale: entered through an arched door in a central tower ornamented with a sundial, festooned with ivy, and crowned with battlements. Three stories of mullioned windows commanded a view of lawns sloping down to gravel paths and a fishpond. There were greenhouses, galleries hung with paintings, and a sweeping stone staircase. For Elizabeth, veteran of drafty boardinghouses, daughter of a family eternally on the edge of penury, Portway Hall felt like the beginning of a better story.

It was joyful to see her little brother and eldest sister again. Howard seemed to be flourishing, though Anna was her usual valetudinarian self. "This morning she stood for 10 minutes, rubbing a magnetized dollar over the back of her neck, to cure nervousness, & drank a tablespoon of magnetized water, which has a special tendency to the heart," Elizabeth wrote, bemused but open-minded.

Kenyon, still ailing, had meanwhile become a lesson in the limitations of heroic medicine. The doctor from the neighboring town of Dudley arrived daily with "all manner of drugs & absurd directions" that only weakened the patient. In the doctor's absence, Elizabeth and Anna took matters into their own hands: "For a few days the medicines were regularly thrown away, & bread pills & flavored water substituted, & with judicious diet, cleanliness, & kind cheerful nursing he improved rapidly." But then, disaster: "Uncle Blackwell discovered the plot & all was over, with the unfortunate effect of making Kenyon suspicious of his kind nurses—he gives himself up with the strangest blindness to the Doctor." It didn't occur to anyone that the Dudley physician was unnecessary. There was already a doctor in the house—still green but possessed of good instincts.

A visit to Dudley Castle was an opportunity for Elizabeth to express the pent-up energy that drove her. The ruined keep stood at the top of a hill, its thick curving walls pierced by arrow slits. "I began to imagine how grandly an army would approach, & how noble a defence the Castle would make," she wrote, "till I longed to revive one of the antient conflicts, & almost frightened my companion by my martial demonstrations." The excursion inspired her to resume her own crusade. Touring Birmingham's hospitals, she found a familiar mixture of shock and gratifying courtesy. "Mr. Parker, Surgeon to the Queen's Hospital, had some difficulty in believing that it was not an ideal being that was spoken of," Elizabeth wrote dryly, "but when he found I was really & truly a living woman, he sent me an invitation to witness an amputation." She borrowed Anna's velvet and sables for the occasion—modern crusaders' armor—and was pleased to see young male faces "peeping through doors & windows" to catch a glimpse of the fabled lady doctor.

Impatience for the work ahead soon overwhelmed Elizabeth's limited appetite for family reunions. By the middle of May she had moved on to London, accompanied by her cousin Sam's friend, the amiable Charles Plevins. "I parted from Portway friends with great regret," she wrote home. "We are getting used to one another, a home feeling was growing up there to me, & so—it was time to be off." Domestic contentment was the enemy of progress.

~

London was wonderful. Charles Plevins took Elizabeth to Sunday luncheon at the home of his formidable aunt near Regent's Park, where they were announced by a footman in velvet breeches, white stockings, and a burgundy vest with gold buttons—Elizabeth wasn't sure whether to curtsy or laugh. Museums and hospitals, paintings and pathology; one day she was admiring a Rembrandt at the National Gallery, the next attending a dinner party thrown by a doctor with an exquisite collection of microscopes, through which Elizabeth beheld "the lung of a frog most minutely injected" and the innumerable tiny teeth of a piece of sharkskin. The attention was intoxicating, though Elizabeth, dressed in serviceable black, felt uncomfortably outshined by the begowned beauties she met at soirées. "The English ladies have very beautiful busts," she wrote, with mingled irony and awe, "as round & white & full as gelatinous marble." If this was more human interaction than she had ever sustained in her life, the former teetotaler had luckily discovered a helpful social solvent. "Iced champagne," she told her family, "is really good."

She felt more at home at the Royal College of Surgeons, among the jars of preserved limbs and organs at the Hunterian Museum, where she was unintimidated by the towering forehead and protuberant stare of its notoriously difficult curator, Richard Owen: "Mr. Owen is a man of genius, & the hour passed away like a minute." Racing through the galleries of the British Museum at top speed, she had time only to regret that "a certain Emily B" couldn't be there to enjoy the cultural riches on display. Elizabeth walked the wards with a senior physician at St. Thomas's, one of London's most illustrious hospitals, and proudly heeded his insistence that she sign her name followed by the hard-won "M.D." in the hospital ledger. She received more medical invitations than she could possibly accept during her week's visit. "I thought such excitement would have bothered me intensely—it did at first bewilder, but now I've roused to meet it," Elizabeth exulted. "The more I have to do, the more I can—I believe I've never yet even begun to call out my power of working."

To work, then—though the best place for that was not London. Elizabeth might have enjoyed a warm reception among the city's most open-minded physicians and surgeons, but they considered her an American oddity, not a medical pioneer. Her sober dignity and unique achievement made her a piquant presence at dinner or in a lecture hall, but even the most genial of her hosts would have blanched if she had asked for a place to hang her shingle.

In France, however, the February Revolution of 1848 and the birth of the Second Republic had renewed a commitment to *liberté, fraternité,* and above all, *égalité.* It was time to push onward to Paris, where the already arduous pursuit of medical training would have to be conducted in Elizabeth's rudimentary French.

~

Elizabeth parted from the generous and genial Charles Plevins with heartfelt gratitude. "He must be no longer a stranger to you all," she wrote home. "I could not thank him, words seemed too absurd." Absurd or not, her words suggested an unprecedented depth of feeling. Plevins escorted her all the way to Dover and onto the boat that would carry her across the Channel. "He would neither let me thank him for the great pleasure his companionship had been to me," Elizabeth wrote, "nor would he admit that he had rendered me the slightest service."

Her letter, circulated to siblings and friends, raised eyebrows. William

Elder in Philadelphia, among the staunchest of her supporters, reacted immediately. "I have not time to make any remarks upon Elizabeth's letter," he wrote with bemused alarm, "except to intimate my jealousy of that Mr. Charles Plevins, whom she has grown so very poetical about." What was the man doing, escorting Elizabeth all over England? How dare he distract her from her destiny? "Women are not reliable," Elder continued, exposing the limits of his own liberal-mindedness. "If Elizabeth bolts from the course, the starch is taken out of the enterprise and the cause will be at a discount for good." There was no room for a romantic partner on Elizabeth's narrow and perilous path. "Plevins!" Elder spluttered. "Why the word sounds like swearing—it's a very bad word, we must see to it."

He needn't have worried. If Elizabeth's departure caused either Charles Plevins or herself pain, it was not enough to deflect her from her course. She sailed from Dover in the rain on May 21, 1849. "I cannot give any patriotic description of the white cliffs of England," she wrote, having had "just sufficient sensation of a queer nature to make me wish to lie down on my berth." It was her nose rather than her eyes that told her she had arrived at Calais: "a strong smell of fish." The downpour continued as she stumbled over the stone pier in the dark, the lighthouse above raking the night. For the first time—as gruff bewhiskered officials checked her passport, demanding *"où allez-vous, Madame?"*—Elizabeth felt herself truly among strangers. Sticking closely to an Englishwoman from the ferry who had warned her of the French predilection for cheating foreigners, she spent a night in Calais ("miserable little town") followed by a day on the train, and then finally, alone, "launched boldly into the sea of Paris."

She was not impressed. London had exceeded expectations, but Paris, which she had expected to embrace, repelled her. "I am utterly disappointed in Paris as far as I have yet seen it," she reported, having found "small & gloomy" rooms on the narrow rue de Seine, not far from the medical institutions she intended to explore. Her rosy-cheeked landlady cheerfully volunteered to help with everything from breakfast to French pronunciation but could not dispel Elizabeth's sense of anticlimax. Where was the sophistication, the beauty, the intellectual sparkle she had expected to find? "Paris is a place altogether overrated," she announced after one day of residence. "The city looks as if it had *suffered*." Her out-look was perhaps colored by the sudden absence of her companion. "I miss my friend Charles very much," she wrote to Anna.

For the next few days, Elizabeth set aside medical pursuits in favor of her garrulous landlady's company. They walked together through the neighborhoods of the Left Bank, the noble dome of the Panthéon appear-ing and disappearing as they turned corners. Elizabeth tried to tune her ear to Parisian chatter—"I have great trouble in expressing myself with any elegance"—and took advantage of her companion's help in buying a decent bonnet. This proved unexpectedly challenging. "I found that my unfortunate organs were totally unable to squeeze themselves into a Parisian headdress," Elizabeth wrote with a touch of phrenological humble-brag. In the end, she had a milliner make one in gray silk, ignor-ing horrified protestations that *no one* in Paris wore that color. She had not come for the fashion.

Once in possession of her new headgear, she was ready to resume her campaign. The consul at St. Germain invited her to Sunday dinner and took her for a stroll on the Grande Terrasse with his daughters; it seemed likely he would provide useful letters of introduction. A visit from another official bearing a form for Elizabeth to complete was a more awkward encounter: when she listed herself as *étudiante,* the man's eyes widened "until the whites showed all round them." Noticing her discomfort, he explained his own.

"*Mon enfant,* you must not put yourself down as student," he instructed her. "*Rentière* is the word you must use!" A female student was a contra-diction in terms, but a *rentière* was a woman of independent means—far more respectable. Elizabeth declared herself a *rentière* without delay. No one in Paris knew her well enough to question it. Then again, no one in Paris knew her well enough to be of much help, either.

It was discouraging. "I have nothing as yet to tell you of Paris medi-cine," Elizabeth wrote to Emily, "though I have been here three weeks." Maddeningly, medical instruction was everywhere—free lectures at the imposing École de Médecine and the Jardin des Plantes with its endless twisting beds of exotic specimens; dozens of eminent physicians offer-ing private instruction; vast and venerable hospitals full of patients to observe—as long as you were a man. There were more students at the École de Médecine than there were in all the medical schools in America combined, yet there was no room in the Grand Amphithéatre, with its gorgeous coffered ceiling, for a woman. And for Elizabeth, concealing her sex remained out of the question. It wasn't enough for a woman to study medicine in secret—the world needed to witness her doing it. "Well," she sighed to Emily, "we must have patience with the age while we work hard to bring about a juster arrangement."

The medical community of Paris reacted to her determination along a spectrum with which Elizabeth was growing familiar: "Some of them are certain that Miss Blackwell is a Socialist of the most furious class, and that her undertaking is the entering wedge to a systematic attack on Society by the fair sex," reported the correspondent for the *New York Journal of Commerce*. "Others who have seen her, say that there is nothing very alarming in her manner." It was the women who were most appalled. "Oh, it is too horrid!" one lady was quoted. "I'm sure I could never touch her hand! Only to think that those long fingers of hers had been cutting up people." The correspondent's favorable verdict had little to do with Elizabeth's medical skill. "She is young, and rather good-looking; her manner indicates great energy of character; and she seems to have entered on her singular career from motives of duty."

Welcome encouragement arrived in the form of Anna, seizing the opportunity of her sister's residence in Paris to escape the gritty damp of Birmingham and pursue another adventure in medical tourism. This time she sought the attention of Jules Denis, Baron du Potet, an owlish and renowned mesmerist. Frustrated for the moment in her pursuit of conventional medicine, Elizabeth joined Anna at Baron du Potet's magnetic séances, held in a darkened room "hung round with curious pictures & lined with very curious people." The motley assemblage of "believing heretics" vied for a chance to regard themselves in du Potet's magic mirror and whispered about the last meeting, during which a young man had actually floated up toward the ceiling!

Fully aware of the absurdity of the scene, Elizabeth refused to dismiss it completely—du Potet might claim to be able to communicate with the dead, but he had also successfully demonstrated his magnetic therapies at the Hôtel-Dieu, the largest hospital in Paris. "I am obliged to laugh at it," she wrote, "& yet I have a true respect for M. Du Potet." She might not share his faith in "antient magic," but she honored his single-minded passion—as did many of the most prominent thinkers of the day. Who could say that magnetism wasn't a promising addition to the pharmacopeia? Or at the very least, she recognized wisely, a comfort for her chronically unhappy sister. "He will pursue a mild soothing treatment for her," Elizabeth reported, "& I think her residence here will be beneficial."

Anna was not the easiest roommate—Elizabeth wished it could be Emily at her side instead—but it was good to have a sister near as she contemplated her next step. At Geneva College, she had grown accustomed to pursuing her strange quest with an audience; the anonymity of Paris had caused her momentum to waver. Having another Blackwell at hand helped dispel her self-consciousness, and her rising spirits enabled her to embrace a new plan: to surrender her freedom and enter La Maternité, France's largest public maternity hospital, not as a qualified doctor but as a student.

Every year each territorial department in France—in 1849 there were eighty-six of them—sent two female students to La Maternité to train as midwives at government expense. It was a more progressive approach to obstetric training than anything to be found in England or America, and an unusual benefit of France's high degree of state control in the field of education. A stay of several months would expose Elizabeth to a thousand cases—vastly more than she might see anywhere else—as well as the tutelage of Paul Antoine Dubois, a distinguished professor of obstetrics. In this one branch of medicine, there was no better practical education.

But neither would there be any allowance for Elizabeth's accomplishments or her maturity. She would enter as an *élève* like any other, subject to the same constraints: sleeping in a dormitory when she wasn't on call through the night, eating in a refectory, working long hours at menial tasks, and forbidden to leave. The other students were country girls, "ignorant and degraded" in Elizabeth's estimation. The patients, like the ones she had known at Blockley Almshouse in Philadelphia, were society's outcasts. After all her insistence on studying medicine on the same terms as men, she now seemed to have no choice but to study obstetrics and gynecology among women. Then again, this particular opportunity would not have been available had she been male. La Maternité was housed in the old walled convent of Port-Royal, and the setting hadn't changed much. "I shall take the veil on the first of July," Elizabeth wrote sardonically, "& be seen no more in the world."

She devoted the rest of June to enjoyment of the freedom she was about to surrender. Paris was not as overrated as she had first thought. She visited Notre Dame, imagining the "fearful descent" of Victor Hugo's hunchback, and spent two hours completing one circuit of the main gallery at the Louvre—"you stand at one end, and the other is lost in the distance." Versailles seemed to her a "living church," wherein all French citizens could refresh themselves at the altar of history, art, music, and nature. And no one touched any of the treasures, she marveled, or even picked a flower in the gardens! Surely this was a manifestation of a better society. Indeed, Elizabeth told her cousin Kenyon, "there is a constant effervescence of life in this great city," although she found Parisians at once "the most brilliant and the most conceited people in the world."

The early summer of 1849 was a tense moment to be a tourist in Paris. With the unseasonable heat—thirty-two degrees, though the centigrade measurement meant nothing to Elizabeth—came cholera, the "summer complaint," killing thousands. (Five years later the English physician John Snow would at last connect the disease to contaminated drinking water.) The political temperature was rising as well, as the city's workers began to agitate against a government that had failed to deliver on its revolutionary promises. The Louvre and the Tuileries were full of soldiers, with more lining the streets, bayonets fixed. Agitators shouted on street corners. "We passed through hurrying crowds full of excitement," Elizabeth wrote, "hearing fearful reports of what had happened and what was to come." It was not a bad moment to retreat behind the walls of La Maternité.

Elizabeth could remove herself from society with the satisfaction of knowing that her reputation continued to grow. In response to her arrival in Europe, *Punch*, the London satirical paper, published a seven-stanza mock-epic poem of praise under the title "An M.D. in a Gown." "Not always is the warrior male," it began, and though it hewed to the ponderous witticism that a medically trained woman saved her husband the expense of calling the doctor, it nevertheless concluded on a note that must have appealed to Elizabeth, despite its tortured rhymes.

> Young ladies all, of every clime,
> Especially of Britain
> Who wholly occupy your time
> In novels or in knitting,
> Whose highest skill is but to play,
> Sing, dance, or French to clack well,
> Reflect on the example, pray,
> Of excellent MISS BLACKWELL!

Confident that the English-speaking world, at least, would not forget her, she prepared to enter La Maternité, determined to see it not as a prison but as an opportunity.

～

On July 1, 1849, Elizabeth presented herself at a low door in a high wall and left Paris behind. Port-Royal Abbey, home of La Maternité for the last half century, consisted of a quadrangle of two-hundred-year-old buildings around a courtyard of flowerbeds and gravel paths, with a garden and a small wood adjacent. Those gazing up and out over its tiled roofs could glimpse only the highest domes of the city as proof that the wider world was still there: the Panthéon to the northeast, the Observatory directly south.

A colonnaded cloister surrounded the courtyard, but instead of the deliberate tread of contemplative nuns, the walkways now echoed with the hurried steps and birdlike chatter of dozens of young women swathed in aprons of coarse white toweling: the élèves, or midwives-in-training, among whom Elizabeth would live and study. Elizabeth followed an old woman up stairways and along corridors, all bare stone and plain wood, to the "funniest little cabinet of curiosities" as ornate as the rest of the building was austere: a small chamber overstuffed with chintz sofas and china figurines, embroidery and mosaic-topped tables. This was the parlor of Madame Madeleine-Edmée Clémentine Charrier, La Maternité's chief midwife, who had the curved spine of a crone and the twinkling blue eyes of a fairy godmother. Madame Charrier in turn conducted the new arrival to Madame Blockel, supervisor of the dormitories and the dining hall: red of face and squint of eye, with "tremendous projecting teeth" as well as "a tremendous vocal organ," which she put to constant use keeping the lively *élèves* in line.

Before Elizabeth had a chance to unpack, Madame Charrier was back with a crowd of students and a question: would the new arrival care to spend the night on duty in the *salle d'accouchements?* Someone handed over a clean apron ("with the injunction not to lose it, or I should have to pay three francs"), and Elizabeth plunged into her first shift on the labor and delivery ward.

Eight babies were born that night in a large room full of shadows, with a hearth at one end, candlelight winking off copper and tin implements, two rows of beds, and cabinets stacked with linen in the corners. In the center rose "a large wooden stand with sides, on which the little newcomers, tightly swathed and ticketed, are ranged side by side": wrinkled red faces peeking from beneath peaked caps bearing labels with name and gender, each infant wrapped like a mummy in black serge. Elizabeth's first letter home evokes an orderly scene of quiet competence—"very little crying" from the newborns, their student attendants "pretty and pleasant."

She left out the screaming pain of labor, not to mention the peril of giving birth in 1849. Even wealthy women, well attended in the comfort of their own bedrooms, died in childbirth. Only the most desperate—those rejected by their families or by society—gave birth in a hospital, where even if the wards were swept and scrubbed, no one washed hands, aprons, or instruments between patients. Puerperal fever was a permanent resident. So were rats. And while linens might be changed, mattresses that were repeatedly soaked in the fluids of childbirth stank, especially in July. The eight new mothers, exhausted, drenched in sweat, supine on blood-soaked sheets, appear nowhere in Elizabeth's account. "It was really very droll," she wrote.

Perhaps she meant to spare her family—mindful of her younger brothers—the pain and fear that preceded the tidy row of newborns. Perhaps she dismissed the new mothers—many of them beggars or prostitutes—as a category of nameless, faceless women rather than a collection of individuals. Perhaps she had already absorbed the French attitude toward patients as teaching tools. Or perhaps, after this shocking introduction, she was trying to reassure herself by projecting professional nonchalance. To her journal, she confided what was not for general consumption: watching the student midwives trying to turn a breech baby while the mother writhed and moaned in agony, "I almost fainted."

After such a beginning, it was no challenge to sink into sleep the following night, despite the close proximity of the fifteen young women with whom Elizabeth now shared a room. Her *dortoir*, up a twisting stairway with a massive, rough-hewn wooden banister, was a smaller echo of the labor ward she had just left, with rows of iron bedsteads and wooden chairs under facing walls of windows, a gilded crucifix at one end, and two small pendant oil lamps that radiated barely enough light to read by—if she had time or energy left for reading. There would be no privacy for the next three months, or however long Elizabeth could bear to stay.

The days were closely scheduled. The bell perched on the ridgepole clanged at five each morning, but Elizabeth kept her head on the pillow on principle. "Of course I lie ten minutes longer pretending to sleep," she wrote, "partly from anger at the noisy bell, partly to display to the angel, the remnant of independence that still remains to me." She was grateful for her Protestantism, which excused her from morning and evening prayers and the daily infant baptisms in the lofty stone chapel at one corner of the quadrangle. (What had once been the nuns' choir, separated from the rest of the chapel by an imposing iron grille, was now in constant use as a laundry.) After a quick wash and a hastily bolted bit of bread saved from the day before, Elizabeth rushed from infirmary rounds, to classes with Madame Charrier, to a lecture from the eminent Monsieur Dubois—"a little bald gray haired man, with a clear gentle voice, & very benevolent face." These were followed by study groups outside on the grass or at the heavy trestle tables in the *salle d'études*, once the nuns' chapter house. Elizabeth found these sessions far beneath her medical

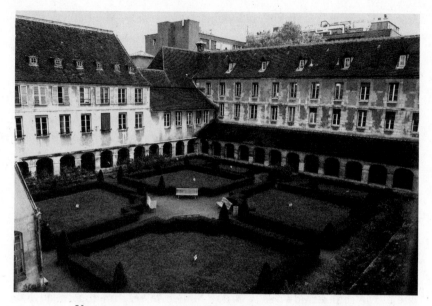

VIEW FROM THE STUDENTS' *DORTOIR* AT LA MATERNITÉ.
COURTESY DANIEL CLARKE

ability but excellent for French language practice, as each student in turn parroted the instruction of the leader. When the bell rang for the midday meal, the students repaired to the round tables of the refectory, where the plain hearty fare was always accompanied by something stronger than water. Elizabeth had left the temperance pledge far behind. "I am learning to take wine," she wrote. "Everyone advises me to do so, and I shall soon be able to drink my bottle a day."

After lunch there followed another lecture, slightly more soporific after the wine, and then the hour for receiving visitors in the students' parlor. Surrounded as she was by unseasoned girls with more enthusiasm than intellect—"we have every variety of temper," she wrote, "like dry & wet gunpowder"—Elizabeth thirsted for a draught of Blackwellian conversation. Anna visited occasionally but was easily deterred by bad weather or another magnetic séance. More often Elizabeth skipped the closely supervised visiting hour in favor of a self-prescribed course of hydropathy: she took a bath, though there was no more privacy to be had there than anywhere else. Six tubs stood side by side in a double row, presided over by a wrinkled old woman who scolded the bathers in an impenetrable patois. Elizabeth created her own solitude by closing her eyes, submerging her ears, and imagining herself "deliciously reposing on the heaving waters of some soft summer lake."

With each passing day, Elizabeth's level of active experience rose vertiginously—and in the absence of English-speakers with whom to discuss her new knowledge, she poured the details of her daily life into letters home. "I have been handling leeches for the first time," she wrote, "disgusting little things." France was a leader in the farming of medicinal leeches, which were particularly useful for bloodletting in inaccessible areas, like the vagina, where a lancet might do unnecessary harm. A leech could be introduced via a speculum and withdrawn when it had its fill of blood by pulling on a thread passed through its tail.*

Elizabeth's diligence left little room for the luxury of friendship, but one of the senior midwives, Clarisse Mallet, "a very intelligent ladylike young woman," took every opportunity to draw Elizabeth out of her reserve. "She cannot bear to see me alone," Elizabeth wrote. "It seems to the French a sign of deplorable melancholy." For once, Elizabeth found nothing to disparage, and began to take pleasure in her colleague's company. She appreciated Mademoiselle Mallet's observations on the wards and her cheerful tolerance of her own stilted French, though she did wish her new friend would stop touching her: "I have to welcome with a good grace, the pinches, shakes, & similar tokens of French affection." Intellectual communion was always more comfortable than an actual caress. Friendship was awkward, and writing about it was worse. "Shall I describe to you a little private dinner, given me by Mlle. Mallet?" she wrote to Henry. "I think it will suffice to say that it was very peculiar & very merry."

There was one other individual whose company Elizabeth enjoyed. This was Claude Philibert Hippolyte Blot, an attending physician a year younger than herself, slender and sleepy-eyed, with an elegant aquiline

---

* Though bloodletting has been discarded as a relic of the barbarous past, leeches are still in use. They secrete natural anticoagulants and are effective in draining congested blood from wounds to facilitate healing.

profile. She had the opportunity to sit by him every Tuesday while he supervised smallpox vaccinations—one of the few truly beneficial public health advances of the early nineteenth century—pressing his scalpel to each infant's arm. Elizabeth's awareness of Blot was mutual; when she ventured to ask him a question, she noticed, "he colours, or passes his hand through his hair and looks intently at the baby, in a very un-Frenchmanlike manner." Within a month of her arrival, Blot was sharing medical journals and pointing out unusual cases in the infirmary. Combining ambition with a lively wit, he earned from Elizabeth what was currently her highest compliment: "His sentiments seem to be good, but his character is certainly not French." After another month, he surprised her with a bashful request: would she help him with his English? "I think he must have been meditating this request for some time; it had

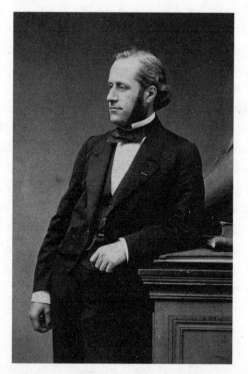

HIPPOLYTE BLOT.
COURTESY SCHLESINGER LIBRARY, RADCLIFFE INSTITUTE, HARVARD UNIVERSITY

hardly the air of spontaneous thought," she wrote in her journal. "I like him. I hope we may come a little more closely together."

These sympathetic colleagues aside, it was still a strain to spend every waking and sleeping hour among girls whom Elizabeth found at best picturesque and at worst simpleminded. As long as the *élèves* paid her the respect she felt was warranted, all was well, "and it sounded not a little droll to hear the scientific terms flowing so glibly from their laughing lips, which were busily employed in talking nonsense" whenever they were off duty. "Everything delights them," she wrote. "They are perfect children in their full, unthinking enjoyment of the present." In sunnier moods, Elizabeth endeared herself by phrenologizing them, or sharing a few English words with a giggling group.

It was just like her teaching days, only this time she had no authority over the students, and no room of her own. After a long day of strenuous medical effort—often preceded by a sleepless night on duty—their high spirits could drive her to distraction. Games of tag and wild dance parties broke out after the lamps were extinguished. Worst of all was something called "promenading the bedsteads." The heavy iron bed frames stood on casters, and the floor of polished tile was smooth enough that a gentle push turned each bed into a vehicle. A shove at the end of a row had a domino effect, and a bed launched down the center aisle with enough force could sail the length of the dormitory. Until the *élèves* ran out of energy and collapsed onto their pillows, sleep was impossible. But so was sustained irritation—not even dour Elizabeth could remain angry at these cheerful creatures for long, especially when, upon waking, "they begged me to excuse them because they were *so young!*"

The indignities of her accommodation were balanced by the undeniable value of the education she was receiving, as well as the gratifying recognition of her aptitude. Monsieur Dubois more than once lingered after a lecture to confer praise, which Elizabeth drank in like sunlight. "He wished I would stay a year and gain the gold medal," she crowed to her journal, "[and] said I should be the best obstetrician, male or female, in America!" A year at La Maternité, he insisted, would expose her to a volume of cases equal to what most physicians saw in a lifetime.

She believed him; she was feeling more like a real doctor and less like an impostor every day. "I am actually hand in hand with nature," Elizabeth told Marian. "I have had a dozen patients under my own care, I have aided in delivering more than a hundred—I have seen all that is remarkable in a thousand—I have bled & leeched & poulticed with my own hand, & watched disease daily." As the three-month mark approached, Elizabeth signed on for three more—personal discomforts could not outweigh the benefits of staying. And it would be easier now that she had established a definite finish line. "As I look forward to my departure the last of December," she reassured Marian, "I feel almost joyous."

A buoyant optimism gilded everything Elizabeth recorded. She was granted a precious day out with Anna, and for once gave herself up to "the pleasure of looking & moving & eating & everything that was natural, & nothing that was wise." She was proud to receive a visit from Charles Lee, the dean of faculty from Geneva College, though she was irritated that La Maternité's regulations forbade her from showing him around.

Madame Charrier, whom Elizabeth respected as "a woman of great experience," presented her with a lithograph of her historical namesake. The eighteenth-century Elizabeth Blackwell—a Scotswoman and no relation—was famed for her beautiful illustrations of medicinal plants, which had earned her enough to bail her doctor-husband out of a London debtors' prison. "I imagined a whole romance out of the picture," Elizabeth mused, "a romance of a beautiful, true spirit, struggling with a society too strong to be turned from its ancient habits of evil. But the pure spirit is not lost, it is working bravely still." She was beginning to feel like the engineer of her own journey, gathering momentum.

~(

CHAPTER 7

SETBACK

On the first Sunday in November 1849, Elizabeth was working upstairs in La Maternité's infirmary, trying to ignore what felt like "a little grain of sand, as it were, in one eye." She was too busy to attend to it, and her mind shied away from its probable cause.

In the predawn dimness that morning, she had been making the rounds of the newborns. One of them was suffering from purulent ophthalmia, an aggressive form of conjunctivitis contracted when an infant passes through the birth canal of a woman infected with gonorrhea. As she washed the tiny affected eye, the contaminated liquid splashed into Elizabeth's face. By evening her left eye was swollen, and when she woke the next morning, the lids were stuck together with gummy discharge.

Elizabeth requested leave to retreat to Anna's new rooms on the rue de Fleurus until the eye was better, but such coddling was beyond the rights of the élèves. She then sought the opinion of Hippolyte Blot, who wasted no time confining her to a bed in the students' infirmary. It was soon clear that both eyes were compromised. Today, though the danger of such an infection eating through the cornea is taken seriously, gonorrheal conjunctivitis is easily treated with antibiotics. In 1849 it was cause for profound concern. Though he kept his fears to himself, Blot knew that his friend was in real danger of losing her sight.

Hippolyte Blot and the faithful Clarisse Mallet made Elizabeth their highest priority, taking turns by her side for three days. It was fortunate that Elizabeth felt so warmly toward her attendants, because the treatments to which they subjected her were torture. They cauterized her eyelids. They syringed her eyes with the medicated eyewash known as collyrium; a pharmacopeia of the period mentions everything from rose-water to ammonia to sulfuric acid as possible ingredients. They applied leeches to her temples; they painted her forehead with mercury and hellebore; they administered mustard plasters, purgatives, ointments of belladonna and opium. Elizabeth lived on water and broth, her eyes enormously swollen, her sleep interrupted every two hours as Blot peeled away the opaque membrane forming over the more severely affected left cornea. It was all very far from the cold-water-and-fresh-air regimen Eliz-abeth preferred, which in this case was probably lucky. Had she been in any position to direct her own treatment, her future as a physician might have ended in Paris.

Anna received unprecedented permission to visit Elizabeth three times a day. The patient appreciated her sisterly attentions, but Anna was

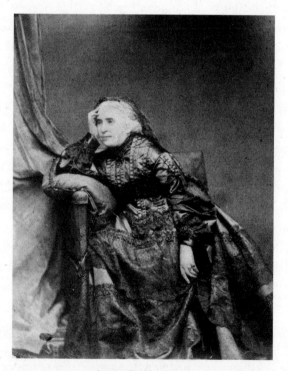

ANNA BLACKWELL.
COURTESY LIBRARY OF CONGRESS, MANUSCRIPT DIVISION, BLACKWELL FAMILY PAPERS

not a natural caregiver. "For the first few days after her illness began I wept almost the entire time," she wrote. "The next few days I spent in something very like swearing, & up to the present time have indulged in an equal amount of both." She informed the rest of the Blackwells, with a telling error, that Elizabeth had contracted "prurient" rather than "purulent" ophthalmia, and bemoaned "the great laws of solidarity that so sternly link us all in one, & so frequently make the noble & the good share in the penalties of the ignoble & the evil"—aggrieved that virtuous Elizabeth had been laid low by her degenerate patients.

Though she was grateful for the special care her sister was receiving, Anna flew straight to Baron du Potet for advice and was soon adding her own treatments to the regimen, giving the "magnetic influence" as much credit for Elizabeth's progress as the devoted efforts of the hospital staff. "I have frequently found her in such excruciating pain that speech was impossible, & a paroxysm of nervous distress & pent-up feelings forcing her from her fortitude & making her weep bitterly," Anna wrote. "*In five minutes*, setting my whole soul into the effort, I have had her sleeping quietly, unconscious of pain." Whether animal magnetism was imaginary or not, the comforting presence of an older sister, her soothing touch, and the cutlets and fruit pies that Anna brought to supplement the hospital fare were powerful positive forces—both for Elizabeth's health and for Anna's own sense of purpose, much as she might bemoan her own martyrdom. "I have, indeed, lost again almost all the flesh I had gained of late, in consequence of this outlay of vitality," Anna wrote. Thank goodness for du Potet, she insisted, "without whose constant aid I could not have borne a tithe of all this fatigue & anxiety, & the exhaustion which follows my constant action upon poor E's eye."

What she lacked in unflappability, Anna made up in journalistic gusto. Elizabeth's left eye looked nightmarish, and Anna did not spare the home folks. Much depended on the integrity of the cornea, for, Anna explained, "if the portion mortified should suddenly detach itself, the probability is that the eye would at once empty itself through the hole." She seemed at least as fascinated by Elizabeth's condition as she was horrified: "The pupil presents, just now, the appearance of one of those little misshapen blackberries of three granulations, & half-dried-up, that one sees so often on some scrubby little bush; if you can fancy such a one in dull-looking lead, you have just the appearance of this poor eye." Scar tissue on the surface of the cornea had to be cauterized repeatedly so as not to abrade the underside of the eyelid.

Throughout the ordeal Elizabeth maintained a superhuman degree of stoicism. For a woman who hid her own ailments, the situation was a particularly exquisite misery: not only was she in unimaginable pain, but her curtained sickbed stood in the middle of her own workplace, with her colleagues witness to every aspect of her helpless plight. Their tearful concern was not always easy to bear. "She is even sometimes almost tormented by the great number of little kindly-meant visits," Anna wrote of the midwives' attentions. "Great is the regret expressed on all sides that she should have missed such a *'jolie opération'*; such a *'cas interessant.'*" The enforced idleness was maddening, and beneath it lay the terrible fear that she would never be able to *see* an interesting case again.

Between agonizing treatments, Elizabeth remained relentlessly optimistic. "There never surely was a case of this disease round which such perfectly admirable conditions could have been united," she declared, grateful for Monsieur Blot's tireless attention and Mademoiselle Mallet's deft fingers. She insisted that she could feel her eye "working & pumping & setting things to rights." This confidence, however, was based at least partly on ignorance. "We do our utmost," Anna reported, "to keep her from suspecting the alarms & anxieties which any little change of symptoms creates."

After three weeks of darkness and pain, Elizabeth's less affected right eye began to clear, and her confinement to ease. One of her first acts was a gift for the tireless Blot, who would soon leave La Maternité to open his own practice. With Anna's help, she purchased a pair of lamps for his new consulting rooms, which sent Blot into an ecstasy of gratitude he could express only obliquely, as the institution frowned on personal interactions between an attending physician and a student, even when the student had a medical degree herself. "I do admire his delicate conscientiousness!" Elizabeth exclaimed. His solicitousness was a powerful medicine for Elizabeth's self-regard, if not her actual vision. "He admired my braid of long hair," she wrote, "[and] wondered how fingers without eyes could arrange anything so beautifully regular."

At the end of December, Elizabeth dressed for the first time since the injury, and with her eye bandaged and her head swathed in a veil, she slipped from the door of La Maternité into a waiting carriage. The hospital register records her departure *en congé illimité*: on unlimited leave, a designation that would keep her record free from the stain of failure, even as it closed this particular door firmly behind her. (In her memoir, Elizabeth made it seem as if she were ill in the hospital for only a few weeks when in fact it was closer to two months. She always hated to admit physical weakness.)

It was only a few minutes to Anna's rooms on the rue de Fleurus, opposite the western gate of the Jardin du Luxembourg, but even that was exhausting. Anna led Elizabeth upstairs, where she could no longer make out the details of the ceiling ornaments and the tasteful wallpaper, nor admire the view. "I felt very weak, and laughed hysterically the whole evening," Elizabeth confided to her journal, writing mostly by feel. She could discern the light of a lamp "as through thick mist," and tell when a hand was passed in front of her face but not much more—and that was with her good eye.

It would be the middle of January before she was able to venture outside on Anna's arm, heavily veiled in black lace and stepping carefully over a crust of frozen snow through the gates of the park. "I felt as if I could defy the cold of Siberia & rejoiced in every breath of the fresh sweet air," she exulted, her writing larger and looser than before. "I never smelt a summer nosegay of more soul rejoicing odour." Inactivity was taking a toll on her health. "I never was very fat you know, but now I am ridiculously thin," she wrote. "The anatomy of my neck is very unpleasantly displayed."

Elizabeth's conviction that God was her most faithful colleague never faltered. "I suffered according to a grand & beautiful law, that the highest must suffer for the sins of the lowest," she wrote, implying somewhat startlingly that her sufferings, Christ-like, would help to redeem humanity. Her belief that God was more powerful than anything medical science could offer was entirely explicit. "He fills me with a spirit of hope & confidence, that reacts continually against the disease & which will finally cure the eye." Given the limited pharmacopeia of 1849, belief in God's support remained a powerful drug.

The admiration of Elizabeth's mortal allies reinforced her sense of exalted suffering. Dubois, the obstetrics professor, put his praise in writing, affirming that Elizabeth had distinguished herself by *"son excellente conduite, son assiduité, son zèle, son intelligence et son instruction,"* and that her departure from La Maternité had taken place *"à mon grand regret."* His words were a comfort. "I am enabled by my sickness to go out in a halo of glorification," she wrote, insisting that she would be resuming her studies "as soon as I can go about without running into people" and celebrating the first anniversary of her medical school graduation with a glass of sweet Frontignan. Anna, who could be laid low by a passing cloud, marveled at her sister's optimism in the face of catastrophe, and brother Sam deemed her "a real sororal gem in the pinchbeck* family ring." Hippolyte Blot wrote a fulsome letter to the Blackwells extolling *"son noble caractère, sa résignation, sa fermeté, son courage."* Marian, clear-sighted as usual, was the only one to leaven her praise with candor. "I regard her course as a noble one, and I feel proud that woman should conquer so many obstacles and achieve what she has done," she wrote. But: "Elizabeth is a peculiar person. She does not please everyone."

~

Emily rejoiced with her family in the restoration of Elizabeth's health. Cozy as it was to gather hearthside for evenings of literary appreciation with her mother and siblings in Cincinnati—the family had just read Currer Bell's† *Shirley*, which they deemed superior to his *Jane Eyre*— Emily, now twenty-three, was ready to move forward. In the new year of 1850, she received a letter from Elizabeth's former employer in Henderson, Kentucky, inviting Emily to fill the same teaching position. If medical school was truly in her sights, she needed to earn some money.

---

* A copper-zinc alloy meant to look like gold and used in costume jewelry.

† In 1850 the world knew Charlotte, Emily, and Anne Brontë only by their pseudonyms: Currer, Ellis, and Acton Bell.

A month later she was on her way to Henderson, where she moved into the same room that had been Elizabeth's six years earlier. Elizabeth blessed the decision with a mixture of honest enthusiasm and older-sister superiority. "Everyone will be prepared to meet her pleasantly for my sake, & she will be more popular than I was, for I awed the people a little too much, I kept so strictly to myself & my books," she wrote. "I might have done more good, if I had opened to the kind feeling that every where awaited me." It was heartening to see Emily take her first step toward the partnership Elizabeth imagined. "Oh, I do hope Emily will succeed & begin to lay up a little fortune," she exclaimed. From her convalescence in Paris, she wrote letters of encouragement and advice—bossy but no less heartfelt—to Emily in Henderson.

Emily tackled her new surroundings with the same single-mindedness as her sister before her. Forewarned by Elizabeth's experience, she was more philosophical about Henderson's discomforts. Teaching took up six or seven hours each day, but otherwise her time was her own, to fill with study and walks in the woods. She brought home armfuls of cherry blossom and wished she had a book to help her identify the crimson songbirds that perched in the locust trees outside her window. The only real detractors were an aggressive mosquito population and too much solitude. "I think I never lived so entirely without talking in my life," she wrote, checking off another Sunday with some relief. Henry cheered her on with cheeky letters, signing off, "Farewell embryo Esculapius! & believe me yours ever, Phosphate of Lime coated with Gelatine & muscular tissue." A year older than Emily, he could tease her medical ambitions in a way he wouldn't dare with Elizabeth.

Like her sister before her, Emily found it unnerving to live among slave owners. But where Elizabeth—who had spent her teenage years steeped in the rhetoric of famous abolitionists—had felt called to act, Emily, only ten when she tagged along to the Anti-Slavery Convention of American Women, did not. She felt like a trespasser in the "infernal regions" when she entered the kitchen, full of Black people speaking "strange gibberish," and was equally alienated from the whites who benefited from their labor. "It seems to me the trouble the slaves give them is almost punishment enough for keeping them," Emily wrote, "but the people are so lazy that they must have someone to wait on them all the time, and so they think it would be impossible to have a free state." As judgmental as Elizabeth, but without the same adamantine idealism, she kept to herself and left the citizens of Henderson to their own opinions.

Writing from Paris, Elizabeth exhorted Emily to be careful. "I can imagine you well in my old room, with its half window," she wrote. "But you do wrong to study much at night, for your eyes have a tendency to inflame—& for pity's sake Emily, do not injure them." Elizabeth's impatience had intensified with the glorious news that, thanks to cousin Kenyon's efforts, she had been granted permission to study at St. Bartholomew's, the oldest hospital in London, under the aegis of James Paget, who was on his way to renown in surgery and pathology. This was thrilling, both for her own sake and for Emily's. "Now if I go & make a respectable common-sense impression upon the London M.D.s, I have a full persuasion that they will behave in a respectable common-sense way to my sister, & afford her the simple justice of a medical education," she wrote. "Here is another motive for getting my eye well—oh little organ, how much you are needed!"

～

For all Elizabeth's resolute optimism, however, the eye was not improving. The cornea had thickened and clouded, and whenever she used the healthy eye, the damaged one became swollen and painful. The hope that she might regain its use was receding. "I have been placed in a most difficult strait," she confided to Emily. "The thought of St. Bartholomew's hospital, & all the noble work that waits for me to do it, haunted me day & night." How to free herself from this depressing quandary? She did have one idea, which as usual made perfect sense to her and alarmed everyone else. "My intention is to study Hydropathy for a month or two this summer," she revealed to Emily. To study it intimately, that is, as a patient of Vincent Priessnitz.

Unlike every other medical mentor Elizabeth had hitherto consulted, Priessnitz had no training. A farmer from the Silesian village of Gräfenberg, near what is now the border of Poland and the Czech Republic, as a teenager he had been injured in a cart accident and told he had little chance of full recovery. Wrapping himself in wet bandages and drinking copious amounts of water, he restored himself to health, and word of his technique spread. He transformed his family's farmhouse into a water-cure sanatorium, treating his increasingly illustrious patients with plain food, exercise, and water—beverage, shower, bath, compress—and boasting enviable results. Regular medicine was getting Elizabeth nowhere, and cold water and fresh air had helped her in the past. It was time to put this alternative practice to the test.

Hippolyte Blot, who continued to take responsibility for Elizabeth's care, was appalled. "My kind young physician thinks I am a little crazy to take a long expensive journey & go all alone, to a half savage country, where a peasant takes the place of a physician—but I think I am very wise," she wrote. "Oh Milly Milly, if in a few months, I could regain my eye & find myself again strong & eager for work, wouldn't I bless those German mountains till my dying day?"

For this chance she was willing to leave her Paris friends behind—including Blot, whose attentions had expanded from the medical to the social. He often dropped by Anna's rooms in the evenings, ostensibly for English lessons, though he also enjoyed reading aloud to Elizabeth and Anna such improving texts as Ernest Legouvé's four-hundred-page *L'histoire morale des femmes*. "I shall miss him exceedingly when I leave, for there is a most affectionate sympathy between us," Elizabeth wrote. "But a reformer's life is not a garden of roses."

Elizabeth had always preferred to play the hero rather than the damsel in distress. Galloping off to continue her quest at Gräfenberg was vastly preferable to the possibility that Blot's admiration might twist into pity for her disfigurement. To her mother's brother Charles, a military man, she wrote, "I beg Uncle to feel quite sure that a brave soldier's niece will never disgrace the Colours she fights under, but will be proud of the wounds gained in a great Cause, and resolve more strongly than ever to 'conquer or die.'"

～

Few women in 1850, even if in perfect health, would have undertaken a solo journey of more than eight hundred miles via rail and carriage across the breadth of Europe. Elizabeth—gaunt, unsteady, half-blind, and alone—left Paris on June 16 and made the journey in six days, via Brussels, Cologne, Hanover, and Berlin. Her journal, scrawled in a jolting conveyance, is a triumph of will over discomfort: disjointed entries in an awkward, looping script written first in pencil and gone over later in ink; lines that weave out of horizontal; capital letters leaning drunkenly, their flourishes askew. In no mood to enjoy the view, she wrote her impressions in telegraphic bursts: "disappointed in the Rhine . . . country too flat . . . round Magdeburg duller & duller."

Ever in search of the ideal, she paused in her flight long enough to enjoy the work of old masters in Berlin, allowing herself a moment to indulge in pure feeling, not to mention gratitude at having preserved at least partial sight. In her rapturous descriptions of the paintings that held her gaze, she betrayed something of the yearnings she rarely allowed to surface. There was Titian's *Girl with a Platter of Fruit*, a portrait of the artist's daughter, full-figured, all creamy skin and rich brocade; and a more contemporary self-portrait by Angelica Kauffmann, looking directly at the viewer with self-possessed wit—both images of arresting, beautiful women, blooming with the kind of health Elizabeth had lost, attracting her in a way she could not articulate. But Elizabeth's favorite was perhaps the most telling: Correggio's *Io Embraced by Jupiter*.

> The most beautiful picture I ever saw—her head thrown back, the face expressive of divine bliss, ecstasy superhuman thrilling in every fibre, such ecstasy as only the embrace of a deity could give—the figure is exquisite in every way—the rounded limbs glow with soft light—his figure is dark & cloudy, veiled to the sight. . . . It is too beautiful to be called voluptuous—yet it is the most powerful representation of the love sentiment in a woman that I have ever seen.

In the painting, Io is a monumental nude, her lips parted in orgasmic passion, while Jupiter is barely discernible as a cloud of sooty vapor, divine love unburdened by threatening flesh. It is an image of sexual pleasure without carnality and without context, without submission or pain or disease or pregnancy; an otherworldly love, as idealized and impossible as Elizabeth's attraction to Hippolyte Blot would forever remain.

"I wrote to him," Elizabeth confided to her journal. "How strongly my life turns to him, & yet that terrible suffering has put a distance between us, that I fear nothing can remove." Both her pioneering ambition and her emotional awkwardness made any thought of intimacy impossible. When Blot announced his marriage less than a year later, she would send warm congratulations. For now, as she stood before Correggio's sensual masterpiece, it was consoling to imagine that such bliss was something "only the embrace of a deity could give."

Certainly bliss was not to be found at Gräfenberg. If Elizabeth had expected the wild sublime, she found only smooth-sided slopes, cultivated nearly to the peaks and dotted with tame white cottages. She had little money and even less German. At a loss, she took a hotel room, wrote a note to Vincent Priessnitz, and sat down to wait, "feeling decidedly blue."

In a gratifyingly short time, the door opened, and the fifty-year-old Priessnitz himself, "the High Priest of water," stood before her. With his pale blue eyes, weather-beaten features, wiry frame, and homespun clothing, he struck her immediately as "honest & good." He looked her up and down and declared that he could restore her vitality in six weeks, without doing her fragile eye any harm. She had heard that his establishment was full, but he reassured her. "You *can* come, child," he insisted. "Come this afternoon, and bring your things with you."

The plainness of the Gräfenberg sanatorium was part of its mystique. Priessnitz had expanded his farmhouse into an enormous five-storied white edifice with a stream rushing beneath, "something like one of our cotton manufactories," wrote Elizabeth, with room to accommodate and process, factory-like, hundreds of patients at a time. Though the ear might be charmed by the constant applause of rushing water, the nose wrinkled at the proximity of cows and the ubiquity of sodden wool blankets and linens stretched out to dry. Elizabeth was shown to the only available room, a sky-lit garret under the rafters with a straw-filled wooden bedstead and a green earthenware bowl atop the low bureau. "I must have looked rather dismayed," Elizabeth wrote, "for the girl hastened to inform me, that I had an Italian count & countess with their son & daughter for next-door neighbors." When the bell rang for the evening meal, Elizabeth found herself in a vast dining hall, surrounded by patients in formal dress, the ladies with their hair done up in flowers and curls, jewels sparkling on wide expanses of décolletage. Their daunting finery stood in odd contrast to the dismaying fare: a hard brown loaf "so sour that I could hardly swallow it." The fresh milk was some consolation. Exhausted and unable to comprehend the merry German chatter all around her, she retreated to her spartan room.

The cure began at six o'clock the next morning, with Priessnitz himself supervising the first treatment. To begin, there was "packing": a swaddling of the patient, first in a wet sheet, then in thick blankets and eiderdown, to induce sweating. This was followed by a series of cold-water baths, further wrapping in wet bandages, and glasses of water to drink. At noon the protocol featured an *abreibung,* a vigorous rubdown with wet sheets, followed by a sitz bath and more wet bandages; this process was repeated at four. In the hours between treatments, everyone took to the mountains.

Gräfenberg agreed with Elizabeth—at least according to her letters. "Everybody seems to have a good appetite—my own is ravenous," she wrote to the family. "Out all day in the open air, rambling over these wide hills, stimulated by the wind & the abundant cold water, I find myself suddenly in strong vigorous health, & the idea of sickness out here, seems a fable." Flowers and trickling springs and the call of the cuckoo made the landscape lovely, if not sublime, and she even made a friend: a handsome young American suffering from near-total blindness, who provided her efficiently with flattering male attention, a warm "home feeling," and the satisfaction of helping someone even more afflicted than herself. The only irritant she mentioned was her constant sense of sartorial inadequacy. "I find I have brought altogether too small a wardrobe for the demands of the place," a deficiency that exacerbated her tendency to shun the company of others.

To her journal, Elizabeth told a different tale. "The *abreibung* deadens my fingers, the sitz bath gives me colic, the wet bandages impede digestion," she wrote. "Tonight I went to bed with quite a feverish attack, which gave me unpleasant dreams the whole night." In her autobiography decades later, Elizabeth dispatched her final and devastating setback in a few lines: the rugged regimen proved "too stimulating," a "violent attack of inflammation supervened," and by the beginning of August, she had returned "with great difficulty" to Paris, in pain and largely unable to see. On August 15, 1850, the noted ophthalmologist Louis-Auguste Desmarres operated to remove what remained of her left eye and fitted her for a glass prosthetic. Ether had been used as an anesthetic for the first time in 1846; chloroform in 1847. Both were gaining in acceptance, but not all surgeons had adopted them. Dr. Desmarres might have used either one—or neither.

The loss of her eye ended any possibility that Elizabeth would become a surgeon, though her resolve to practice medicine remained undimmed. Alone in a Paris boardinghouse, she put her own surgery behind her and focused on the next chapter. "It is a sad business—she has suffered horribly," wrote Anna, who had herself fled the midsummer heat for the suburb of St. Cloud, sighing, "I am horribly tired just now, & suffering from the fatigue & excitement of other people's affairs." Elizabeth, her health rebounding rapidly, did not miss her sister's lugubrious company. It was time to return to London and claim the opportunity that had been waiting since May: continuing her studies at St. Bartholomew's Hospital.

From Cincinnati, brother Sam expressed his less self-absorbed support. "That poor only eye," he wrote. "Heaven preserve it, it is very valuable now."

CHAPTER 8

LONDON

Where Elizabeth had taken up science as a duty, Emily pursued natural history and astronomy with passion. "I must go to bed with my head full of comets," she wrote, reluctantly snuffing her candle. It would not do to squander her irreplaceable eyesight. After a lonely 1850 in Henderson, Kentucky—where excitement had taken the form of roast possum for supper, "served up with its legs pointing to the four points of the compass"—Emily was now teaching at home in Cincinnati, devoting her weekends to study with a sympathetic physician. Elizabeth's achievements seemed impossible, compared to Emily's daily failure to live up to her own high standards. "I wish I could acquire that kind of finished way of doing things that some people have," Emily confided to her journal. "I am exceedingly deficient in that. I have a something sprawling in my character. . . . I am all at loose ends and don't often act as I meant to act." Surely Elizabeth never wandered in such uncertainty. "I certainly have a great deal of a kind of proud scorn or scornful pride in my disposition which is no mark of a great character," Emily wrote. "I find friends nowhere, how grand it would be to have real friends, friends who raised one's emulation, who by their intellect, character, lives roused each other to noble action thought and feeling. I have never had, I believe I never shall have, a friend."

While Emily steeped herself in science, the rest of Cincinnati was afire with spiritualism, thanks to a visit from the touring Fox sisters, Margaretta and Catherine, of Rochester, New York. In the past year these celebrated teenagers had dazzled audiences with sensational public séances, during which mysterious rappings seemed to communicate messages from the spirit world. Henry had gone with his friends from the new Literary Club of Cincinnati, and one afternoon he sat discussing the phenomenon with one of them, Henry Warriner, in a voice loud enough to draw Emily away from her books. Warriner himself, it turned out, professed clairvoyant skill in divining people's characters by touching their writing.

Scientist or not, Emily could not resist this chance to peer into the future. She fetched a letter penned by Elizabeth and one she had written herself. Holding Elizabeth's to his forehead, Warriner focused his attention for several silent minutes. "If I get anything from this letter," he began, "the writer is a very superior person—there is an intense thirst for knowledge." He followed this generic opening with a string of words that did indeed seem to frame Elizabeth's unique force: enthusiasm, aspiration, perseverance, determination, ardor, ideality, "a great sweep and breadth of thought." Emily was riveted in spite of herself.

"I perceive great mental action," Warriner continued. "If it be a lady there is much more vigour and power than they generally possess."

"Do you perceive much benevolence?" asked Emily. Would her distant sister become the friend she craved?

"There is sincerity ... directness ... ," Warriner mused. "Benevolence does not strike me as prominent."

It was disappointing but not particularly surprising. "Do you perceive much ambition?" Emily wanted to know.

"There is no petty ambition but a high aspiration," came the reply, too close to the mark to dismiss. "There is great energy and firmness—a powerful will—it is a good nature—there is a good humor in it." That, at least, was heartening.

Taking up Emily's letter—unfortunately less substantial than Elizabeth's, but the only one Emily had to hand—Warriner meditated even longer than before.

"I perceive great intellectual activity," he said at last—again, a safe bet in the Blackwell household. But there was more. "There is something very luminous and lucid in the mind," he went on. "It is a less glorious, less glowing character—I do not see the same sweep of thought—there is more keenness and penetration."

"Which would succeed best practically," asked Henry, with a reassuring twinkle at Emily, "this individual or the last?"

"This one," answered Warriner, raising Emily's letter. "The other is too deep and enthusiastic, this one is more practical, more fit for business."

"Do you see any particular defect in this disposition?" Emily asked, seized by chronic self-doubt.

"No, it is well balanced," said Warriner. "There is more caution, more waiting for wind and tide—I should think his abilities might be beyond his success—but the intellect is very fine. . . . There is a sincerity and integrity that resembles the other."

"Would this person be a leader, or one who would like best to work alone?" asked Emily, striving for nonchalance.

"I do not think he would be inclined to take the position of leader," Warriner replied. "There is great self-reliance—does not ask or need the advice of others, but is inclined to let others go their own way."

This was flattering, but Emily dismissed it. "It appears to me like the description of the outside, and not of the inside," she complained to her journal that night. "It does not reach *me*." No one, not even a clairvoyant, could sense the turmoil she kept so deeply hidden. "He did not remark the intense longing for perfection, the passion for intellectual pursuits and the stormy restlessness of my disposition." Unless possessed of truly supernatural powers, Warriner could hardly have recognized what even Henry, so close to Emily in age and affection, failed to notice.

"You will be greatly pleased with Millie when you see her again," Henry wrote to Elizabeth. "She is possessed of a most admirable *balance* of physical & mental qualities—strong but not heavy, with clear definite common sense, quick, prompt, decided, quiet, cheerful & self possessed." He admired her unusual combination of imagination, capable shrewdness, and productive energy. "I don't think Emily knows what it is to be *blue*," he insisted, "for she is never idle & keeps up I have no doubt a steady active thinking even in her sleep."

Emily had recently completed her first practical experience at the bedside of her mother, who was suffering from a "terrible discharging tumour"—a pus-filled boil, or carbuncle—on her back. "I am surprised at my own powers," Emily wrote, though her clinical satisfaction was tempered with emotional unease. Pious Hannah inspired impatience in her scientific sixth child, and Emily was struck by the sad gap between duty and feeling. "Sickness would lose much of its horror if people were so noble that they attached their friends powerfully to them," she wrote, "but cold attendance during sickness must be painful and I pitied my mother when I felt how far apart we were." Attending diligently to Hannah's care, she kept her feelings, as always, to herself.

Emily's desperation to launch herself toward something larger grew daily, even as her own doubts held her back. By the summer of 1851, she had had enough. "I have been teaching for five years and my disgust and hatred of this most detestable occupation has risen to a pitch that is almost unendurable," she scrawled. "And life might be so glorious. Human nature so lofty and yet people go on potter potter in their little contemptible lives and seem to have no more conception of the mysteries around them, of their marvelous existence, than beetles."

～

Elizabeth, meanwhile, had found London a darker place than during her first eager visit eighteen months earlier. She arrived at the beginning of October 1850, as autumn began to take hold. Night fell early, daylight was dimmed by a blanket of smog, and her remaining eye burned and blurred. The city depressed her—"the dingy look of every building, the ugliness of the people, their rude unpleasing manners, their vulgar dress"—and the prospect of yet another search for respectable-yet-affordable lodgings, and yet another conservative medical community to confront at St. Bartholomew's Hospital, exhausted her. "I asked myself with astonishment, is this the same London?"

She was more alone this time, the sustaining sweetness of her acquaintance with Charles Plevins having curdled. "I will not speak of him, as I have nothing pleasant to say," she wrote. "I shall always feel grateful to him for his former kindness—but he is too bitter to suit me." She had no time for a disappointed admirer. Even her stalwart cousin Kenyon was less solicitous now. On a visit to Paris during Elizabeth's convalescence, Kenyon had met "a charming young Parisienne" named Marie de St. Simoncourt, and they had married at the end of the summer. "They are so perfectly enchanted with one another that really it is pleasant to think of two human creatures so perfectly happy," Anna wrote, professing herself *terribly* fatigued after having supervised the details of their Paris wedding. Elizabeth approved of Kenyon's choice, even as it diverted his attention from her.

To return to work was a tremendous relief. She found a large front room in Thavies Inn, a drab but respectable address a few steps from the bustle of Holborn, and rose at half past seven as the dome of St. Paul's, visible from her window, emerged from the morning mist. When the bells of St. Andrew and St. Sepulchre rang nine o'clock, she set out for St. Bartholomew's Hospital, an imposing quadrangle of pale Georgian facades darkened by decades of coal smoke. A hospital had stood on the site since the twelfth century; in the imposing Great Hall, gold leaf covered the ceiling, and epic murals by William Hogarth lined the grand staircase. Elizabeth had arrived at an ancient locus of British medicine, though the college itself had been formally established only five years since. "A little dark figure in doctorial sack with writing case under arm makes its way through assembling students, who politely step aside to let it pass," she wrote, denying herself even the luxury of the female pronoun.

A shortcut along Cock Lane allowed Elizabeth to avoid the teeming Smithfield meat market on her way, though the sounds, sights, and smells of the hospital were hardly better. Six hundred indigent patients filled the beds of St. Bartholomew's, and hundreds more crowded the benches of the waiting rooms, especially on Thursdays, when the most afflicted, fortunate in their misfortune, would be admitted to fill whatever beds had become vacant. Disease had its seasons: in winter the rooms were full of catarrhal coughing, replaced in summer with the moans of dysenteric cramp. Accident and injury were constants. Screams echoed from the operating theaters, and fumes poured from the apothecary's copper cauldrons of opiate syrup and "black draught," a laxative made from senna. The odor of putrefying flesh wafted from the dead house and the dissection rooms, and the distinctive roasted-almond smell of gangrene mingled with the reek of chamber pots. Inpatients did receive adequate meals, but the prevalence of sepsis, erysipelas, and other infections endemic to hospital wards meant they might pay the ultimate price for their porridge and potatoes. The use of antiseptic protocols was still decades away.

The terms of Elizabeth's admission allowed her to walk the wards, perform dissections if there was a private room available, and sit in on postmortems—as long as the deceased was female. She could attend lectures if the lecturer approved. Thankfully, her new mentor and the warden of the medical college, James Paget, led by example; Elizabeth held an unlimited ticket for his anatomy and physiology classes, and his colleague George Burrows followed suit in principles of medicine. She followed the stout and elderly Clement Hue on his rounds, taking careful notes on a young woman admitted with chest pains. "Auscultation shows a striking derangement of the heart action," she noted. "The heart appears to hesitate in contracting, then several violent contractions occur in rapid succession." With her sight compromised, she sharpened her hearing as a diagnostic tool.

ELIZABETH'S TICKET FOR JAMES PAGET'S ANATOMY LECTURES.
COURTESY LIBRARY OF CONGRESS, MANUSCRIPT DIVISION, BLACKWELL FAMILY PAPERS

As usual, Elizabeth's strategy for acceptance was to leave no opening for criticism. Paget's students gave her a round of applause when she joined them, and Lydia North Paget, who served as her husband's amanuensis, expressed bemused approval. "Well we have our 'Lady Doctor' here at last," she wrote. "The young men have behaved extremely well, and she really appears likely to go on her way quite unmolested." At the start of each term, Paget invited a dozen students at a time to come for breakfast. Elizabeth, happily included, was pleased with these "gentlemanly fellows," though they "looked with some curiosity at their new companion."

The women, in contrast, were disappointing. Invited to a dinner party at the Pagets', Elizabeth raised a critical eyebrow at the amount of bare skin on display, along with ballooning petticoats and endless frills. "Women so dressed out, don't look like rational beings," she complained, "& consequently they cannot expect to be treated as such." Scornful of the women she hoped to inspire, she nonetheless insisted that her male colleagues recognize and respect her womanhood. Paget himself, watching her from beneath a permanently furrowed brow, told her to expect more resistance from women than from men. "I am prepared for this," she insisted. "But a work of the ages cannot be hindered by individual feeling. A hundred years hence women will not be what they are now."

⁓

Elizabeth's blameless hard work masked a growing divergence from the orthodoxy of august St. Bartholomew's, which—after the investigative spirit of Paris medicine—she found somewhat dull. "Here there is no excitement," she wrote, "all moves steadily onward, constantly, but without enthusiasm." The stream of forlorn patients trudged past, accepting their doses of calomel and laudanum, emetics and purgatives. As Elizabeth's experience deepened, and as the shift from intern to practitioner approached, the question of what constituted legitimate and effective medicine remained hard to answer. At St. Bart's no one wanted to hear her opinions regarding cold water and fresh air, or her criticisms of the standard materia medica. "I must confess that this study of the old practice is both difficult & disgusting to me," she wrote, "but it is essential & I shall be diligent." She could not afford to alienate patrons like Paget.

Meanwhile, based on her own experiences as a patient, and despite her sincere hopes, "neither hydropathy nor mesmerism are what their enthusiastic votaries imagine them to be." The only way forward, she wrote to Emily, was to begin with "old-established custom"—the ineffective habits of the old guard—and try to establish an independent institution in which to introduce more enlightened approaches. That way "the very instant I feel sure of any improvement I shall adopt it in my practice, in spite of a whole legion of devils," she wrote. "Now E., future partner, what say you—is it not the only rational course?" Elizabeth's current approach to medicine was to observe, absorb, and obtain "that bedside knowledge of sickness, which will enable me to *commit heresy* with intelligence in the future."

More than ever, Elizabeth wanted Emily with her on her solitary path. "All the gentlemen I meet seem separated by an invincible invisible barrier, and the women who take up the subject are inferior," she lamented. "It will not always be so; when the novelty of the innovation is past, men & women will be valuable friends in medicine, but for a time that cannot be." For now, only a fellow Blackwell might merit her unconditional support. She would not risk her fledgling reputation by associating with any woman less dedicated than herself—and no hint of Emily's doubts or frustrations had reached her. Proud of the diagnostic skill she was acquiring with the stethoscope, Elizabeth instructed her "partner elect" to "auscultate Mother & the boys."

Though Elizabeth had met no woman in London with whom to share the practice of intelligent heresies, she was, for the first time, finding female friends to discuss them with. A few weeks after settling at Thavies Inn, she received a visit from a young woman who had been attracted to Elizabeth's reputation as a flower turns toward light. Bessie Rayner Parkes was twenty-one to Elizabeth's twenty-nine, a distant cousin by marriage, and the only child of "people whose position is so respectable," Elizabeth reported to Emily, "that the daughter dare not ride in an omnibus." Yet these same proper parents had given Parkes a liberal Unitarian education, with the result that "she will not wear corsets, she won't embroider, she reads every heretic book she can get hold of, talks of following a profession, & has been known to go to an evening party, without gloves!"

In Parkes, Elizabeth found a little sister to mentor in progressive ideas. "She is really a very noble girl, but chaotic & without definite aim," she wrote. "I shall be curious to know, if there are many girls like her, that is girls who think. I fear not." Parkes, in turn, was entranced by Elizabeth's history, which Elizabeth, warmed by her interest, related in vivid detail. "Such a tale!" Parkes wrote. "Of energy, & hope; of repulses from men, & scorn of her own countrywomen." She was particularly impressed by Elizabeth's illness and subsequent surgery, gazing at her new friend's face with horrified delight. "*I can't tell which eye it is*," she wrote. "Literally I looked & looked & thought it *wasn't* the one I thought last time." To Parkes, Elizabeth was part reformer, part gothic heroine. "Oh she is *such* a jolly brick," she gushed.

The recipient of this ardent account was Barbara Leigh Smith, eldest daughter of a wealthy member of Parliament who had never married her milliner mother, though he was unwavering in support of the five children she bore him. A man of radically progressive politics, Benjamin Leigh Smith might have justified this scandalous liaison with the argument that marriage would have made his mistress and their children his property. His eccentricity extended to his parenting: two years earlier, when his daughter turned twenty-one, he had settled upon her an income of £300 per year—an enviable sum from Elizabeth's impecunious perspective—and having the foresight to understand that illegitimacy might cause problems after his death, he took the unusual step of making sure she received access to her inheritance while he lived. Smith's financial independence made it possible for her to speak her mind, and she had already begun to publish her own ideas on the subject of reform. If Elizabeth was fond of the impulsive, disheveled Parkes, she was drawn to the statuesque Smith with something more like respect. Their friendship would be a lasting one.

Barbara Leigh Smith's nascent interests in public health and progressive education—and not, at this point, in woman suffrage—aligned with Elizabeth's own. Indeed, in Smith and Parkes, Elizabeth found spirits more kindred than their activist counterparts in America. That fall of

1850, Marian and Ellen, the youngest Blackwell sister at twenty-two, had attended the first National Woman's Rights Convention in Worcester, Massachusetts, and reported on it to Elizabeth with enormous enthusiasm. Elizabeth's response was lukewarm. "I have read through all the proceedings," she wrote to Marian. "They show great energy, much right feeling, but not a great amount of strong, clear thought."

As with Seneca Falls in 1848, Elizabeth could not agree with the convention's endorsement of woman suffrage. She felt, moreover, that the very term *woman's rights* was wrong-headed. "I cannot sympathise fully with an anti-man movement," she continued. "I have had too much kindness, aid, and full reception amongst men to make this attitude of women otherwise than painful to me." Her aim was toward a loftier, sexless ideal: "The great object of education has nothing to do with woman's rights, or man's rights, but with the development of the human soul and body." Elizabeth was stunned by the prostitutes she saw on every corner in London, "poor wretched sisters . . . decked out in their best, which best is generally a faded shawl and thin, even tattered dress, seeking their wretched living." She imagined a "grand moral army" of women mobilized in the pursuit of education and enlightened industry, with Queen Victoria herself at its head. Her new English friends seemed ideal comrades-in-arms. She loved their "vigorous thoughtful minds, that will not be contented with a selfish, frivolous life, and are struggling hard to change the senseless customs which fetter them."

Bessie Parkes and Barbara Smith, in turn, made Elizabeth their project, adorning her cheerless rooms with flowers and paintings and introducing her to their friends. When the hospital day was finished, she revived her idealism in the company of London's intellectual vanguard: people whose philosophical adventurousness she recognized as Blackwellian, whose ideas and pursuits, like her own, did not always align comfortably with English mores. "I have forgotten the smoke," Elizabeth told Marian, "I don't miss the sunshine, I have got beyond the external world of London."

There was the noted writer and art historian Anna Brownell Jameson, for example, whose analysis of Shakespeare's heroines the Blackwells had read to each other back in Cincinnati; the American abolitionist and children's author Eliza Lee Cabot Follen; the electrochemist Michael Faraday; the radical publisher John Chapman; and Chapman's live-in assistant editor Mary Ann Evans, better known to literary posterity as George Eliot. And there was Lady Anne Isabella Noel Byron, widow of the famous and infamous poet, whose memory, even a quarter century after his death, still cast an aura of glamour around her. As she approached sixty, Lady Byron focused her considerable intellectual and philanthropic resources on education, and Elizabeth hoped she might extend that generosity to the cause of women in medicine. After all, her daughter, Ada Lovelace, enjoyed considerable renown as a mathematician, a field in which Lady Byron had encouraged her. When, in the spring of 1851, an invitation arrived to visit the great lady at her home in Brighton, Elizabeth accepted immediately.

Elizabeth found everything in Brighton delightful: the elegant stone residences with their bow windows facing the spray off the Atlantic, the vast sunset view, and her delicate and distinguished hostess, whose air of quiet melancholy seemed deliciously entwined with her tragic past. The other guests were no less captivating. Fanny Kemble, the actress, swept into the parlor in rose satin and white fur, her dark eyes flashing as she declaimed a tragic passage in a thrillingly deep voice—the first time Elizabeth had heard Shakespeare delivered by a professional. At night, the wind howled around the house with appropriately poetic ferocity. Breakfast was a cozy tête-à-tête with Mrs. Jameson, who discussed fine art and female potential with fiery intelligence. When it was time to return to London, Lady Byron, swathed in purple velvet, escorted Elizabeth to the station in person and saw her onto her train "with the most hearty shake of the hand."

In Lady Byron, whose subdued voice belied a brilliant mind, Elizabeth found a sparring partner worthy of her respect; their correspondence would span years and continents and end only with the older woman's death a decade later. Elizabeth pushed back politely but firmly against Lady Byron's opinion that although a woman might become a doctor, she would always hold a secondary position in the field. "Dear Lady Byron," she wrote, "will you forgive, what almost seems to me presumption, in this free speech to one so much older and wiser than I am?"

Women were *not* more likely to be repelled by anatomy and physiology, Elizabeth insisted. "I can say most decidedly from my own experience, and from that of a younger sister," she wrote, "that what might seem the most repulsive parts of medical study, become profoundly interesting, when pursued scientifically." A woman's ability to study and practice was *not* threatened by her euphemistically "variable" health—though of course menstruation was "a subject I cannot discuss in a note," Elizabeth added. And though a female doctor might choose to specialize in women's health, "no one who has the true scientific spirit, when he has once obtained a glimpse of this magnificent land of knowledge, will ever be content to cultivate one little corner." Elizabeth begged Lady Byron not to make the fatal error of "ranking human beings according to *sex* instead of *character.*"

But Lady Byron had been shaped by different forces, in a different generation. "My earliest ideal of happiness was 'a life of devotedness to one,'" she wrote back, and hastened to correct Elizabeth's suggestion that such an attitude was idolatrous. Men and women, she reassured Elizabeth, should certainly be held to the same moral standards. "But I do not desire an equality of powers & privileges," she told her younger friend. "Where a Woman's capacity is such as to raise her to an equality with Men, I honor the Exception, but I would not make it the Rule." Much as she admired Elizabeth, she held to her conviction: "The oneness of dependency seems to me to constitute Woman's greatest happiness." They would agree to disagree.

～

The pain and loneliness of the previous year were receding memories. "Life opens to me in London," Elizabeth told Emily, "social life particularly." She could make the case that her social connections were more fruitful than her professional relationships. At St. Bartholomew's, she would always be a peculiar figure—"they would as soon think of making Queen Victoria an April fool, as venturing to joke with me, so fearful is the awe I inspire people with"—but outside the hospital, she was finding her true peers. One of these was Barbara Leigh Smith's first cousin, a woman named Florence Nightingale.

In 1851, just shy of her thirty-first birthday, Nightingale was wealthy, witty, well traveled, and monumentally impatient to shake off her family's conventional expectations and fulfill her calling as a humanitarian. She had recently dismissed her eminently suitable suitor Richard Monckton Milnes with a finality that dismayed her parents.* "To be nailed to a continuation and exaggeration of my present life, without hope of another, would be intolerable to me," she had written at the time. "Voluntarily to put it out of my power ever to be able to seize the chance of forming for myself a true and rich life would seem to me like suicide." Since then, she had journeyed through Egypt and Greece, and on her way home had visited the Deaconess's Institute at Kaiserswerth, near Düsseldorf, which trained laywomen in pastoral care and healing among the poor. Here, she thought, was a model of the kind of good she wanted to do in the world. Her family was appalled.

The arrival in London of a woman within a year of her own age and a fully qualified M.D. only fueled Nightingale's dreams of escape. Elizabeth was like no one she had ever met: a woman with ideals as lofty as her own, who had likewise turned her back on marriage and was actively in pursuit of her goals far from her family. In mid-April, Nightingale invited her new American acquaintance to visit her family's estate at Embley Park, a sprawling redbrick pile at the edge of the New Forest, with clouds of flowering azalea and rhododendron outside and lavish heaps of books within, overflowing the shelves onto tables and sills.

Elizabeth was equally taken with her swan-necked hostess, who kept in her pocket a diminutive pet owl named Athena, rescued during her visit to the Acropolis. "Walked much with Florence in the delicious air, amid a luxury of sights and sounds, conversing on the future," Eliza-

---

* Milnes was by all accounts a kind and generous man and was soon happily married to another; he was also a dedicated collector of homoerotic sadomasochistic pornography and led a double life to which his accommodating wife turned a carefully blind eye. Nightingale, who held exalted ideas regarding sexual purity, would not have made him a successful partner.

beth wrote. "A perfect day." Not only did Nightingale share her interest in health and hygiene, she also had similar thoughts about the unfulfilled potential of women. "Woman stands askew," Nightingale had written. "Her education for action has not kept pace with her education for acquirement." Nightingale's own education had likewise emphasized polish over pragmatism. That summer she would return to Kaiserswerth for three months as a nursing intern and begin to move in a new direction.

"Do you know what I always think when I look at that row of windows?" she asked Elizabeth now, gazing up at the monumental facade of her home with its ranks of stately gables and chimneys. "I think how I should turn it into a hospital ward, and just how I should place the beds!" In her vision, however, she was the matron in charge of the nurses, not the attending physician. Florence Nightingale, patron saint of nursing, and Elizabeth Blackwell, first woman doctor, would never agree about the role of women in health, but this first encounter was a passionate moment of recognition between two people whose choices most found baffling, if not horrifying. "She said she should be perfectly happy working with me, she should want no other husband," Elizabeth recorded. "As we crossed the fields, conversing on religious matters, it was a true communion."

Nourishing as it was to spend time with all these accomplished women, the stubborn question of making a living remained. Elizabeth had reluctantly accepted her cousin Kenyon's financial help, but after two years of study in Europe, she was impatient to support herself. And though London felt more like home than any American city ever had, it remained as rigid as ever, while in America there were signs that attitudes toward women in the medical profession were shifting. Medical colleges expressly for women had recently opened in Boston and Philadelphia. "My own mind is therefore made up to return, and that as speedily as possible," she told Emily. Her destination: not intellectual Boston or progressive Philadelphia but brash New York, her first American home, where no female medical institution yet existed.

As the weather warmed, Elizabeth made a final circuit of the London hospitals and drawing rooms in which she had found mentors and friends. At St. Bartholomew's, both Paget and Burrows offered written testimonials to her "zeal and assiduity" and told her that her example had prepared a path for women in the future. It was bittersweet: "They have learned to know and welcome me as I am going away, and are, as Mr. Paget said, sorry to lose me." Bessie Parkes was especially sad to part from her inspiring friend. "I very nearly astounded the opposite neighbors," she confessed, "by rushing in a dramatic way back again, which would have been exceedingly undignified & unsuitable to your respectable appearance."

CHAPTER 9

~

PRACTICE

New York had changed in the thirteen years since the Blackwells
lived there. The imaginary grid that city planners had laid over
rural hills and streams in 1811 was now built up as far as Fourteenth Street and beyond. Famine in Ireland and revolution in Germany
had pushed the city's population over the half-million mark. The spine
of Broadway connected a teeming spectrum all the way from the Battery,
past the throngs queuing at Barnum's American Museum, past the sim-
mering squalor of Five Points, and northward to the elegant environs of
Washington Square and the newly completed Grace Church—the length
of the thoroughfare choked by white-topped omnibuses, darting shop
boys, nervous pedestrians, and the carriages of the rich. Until recently
the gridlock would have included thousands of the city's roaming pigs,
but they had been rounded up and banished northward a few years earlier by the newly established police force. The completion of the Croton
Aqueduct in 1842 brought clean water to the manure-encrusted southern
end of Manhattan, drastically reducing the threat of epidemics, though
the mechanism of disease remained mysterious. New York was matur-
ing into a cosmopolitan capital. Surely there were enough open-minded
women—and sympathetic men—in this expanding hive of humanity to
support one female physician.

On September 12, 1851, a small item appeared in the *New-York Daily
Tribune*, the city's largest and most progressive newspaper. "Miss Elizabeth Blackwell, M.D., has recently returned to this City, from a two years'
residence abroad," it announced, generously exaggerating her experi-

ences at La Maternité, St. Bartholomew's, and Gräfenberg. "Miss Dr. B., we understand, has just opened an office at No. 44 University-place, and is prepared to practice in every department of her profession."

Two weeks after docking in New York harbor, Elizabeth had secured the endorsement of the *Tribune*'s founding editor, Horace Greeley, an intimate of Transcendentalist luminaries including Margaret Fuller, whom he had hired as his first literary editor. Hannah, Marian, and Ellen had come to New York as a welcoming party, and after some hunting, Elizabeth managed to rent part of a building within a few blocks of Washington Square, at the corner of Eleventh Street and University Place. Furnishing the empty rooms ate up much of her modest capital, and as it was not a boardinghouse—none of which would admit a woman who proposed, outrageously, to see patients in her rooms—she would be responsible for her own meals and housekeeping. But companionship was at hand: Marian planned to stay on with her in New York.

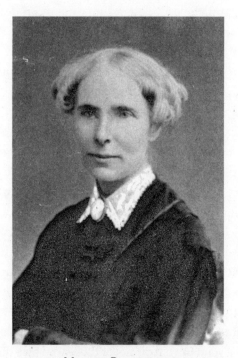

MARIAN BLACKWELL.
COURTESY LIBRARY OF CONGRESS, MANUSCRIPT DIVISION, BLACKWELL FAMILY PAPERS

If Elizabeth claimed Emily as a professional colleague, she had long imagined Marian as a kind of helpmeet, her calm encouragement an emotional bedrock for the life Elizabeth envisioned. "I think I have mentioned the comforting word you once spoke about my music, 'play on, people like to hear you, faults & all,'" she had written to Marian. "That little sentence has certainly given me courage a hundred times, & has helped me to conquer my nervousness . . . so you see you have laid the foundation of my fortune, & it will be absolutely necessary that you finish the good work, by taking care of it when it comes." It is unclear whether Marian's fragile health was the origin or the outcome of her circumscribed role as the family's caregiver, but Elizabeth was grateful for her presence, and kept a close eye on her headaches and dyspepsia.

Elizabeth's long and peripatetic apprenticeship was at last finished, her health restored, a permanent address established. She had letters of praise from some of the most prominent physicians in Europe, and allies on the American side of the Atlantic as well. From Paris, Anna sent confident congratulations. "I do not think there can be any doubt as to her success," she wrote. It was time to get to work. But in 1851 the term *female physician* meant something quite different from "woman with a medical degree." For most New Yorkers, it meant one person: Madame Restell.

Two decades earlier a woman of twenty named Ann Trow Summers had emigrated to New York from England with her husband and baby daughter. She found work as a seamstress but was soon widowed. Her second husband, the St. Petersburg–born Charles Lohman, was a printer and freethinker who admired his wife's independence. Surveying the opportunities for advancement, the couple settled on the thriving trade in patent medicines. Between her entrepreneurial spirit and his expertise in print advertising, they were soon in business, with a *nom de guerre* that became a household name. In March 1839 a substantial notice ran in the pages of the New York *Sun*, addressed "TO MARRIED WOMEN," and laying out the argument for birth control forty years before Margaret Sanger was born. "Is it not but too well known that the families of the married often increase beyond the happiness of those who give them birth would

dictate?" the writer asked. "Is it desirable, then, is it moral for parents
to increase their families, regardless of consequences to themselves, or
the well being of their offspring, when a simple, easy, healthy, and certain remedy is within our control?" Interested parties were directed to an
office on Greenwich Street and the services of a Mrs. Restell.

The debate on limiting family size had begun to appear in print in
the early 1830s, tracing its origins to the British Utilitarians and their
emphasis on the greatest good for the greatest number. This approach to
reproduction—that it was a virtuous act to avoid conception for the sake
of those already born—at first repelled most Americans, unaffected by
overcrowding and influenced by a Puritan tradition that saw procreation
as God's will and woman's holy purpose. But as advances in science and
engineering fueled American expansion and prosperity, the idea that
medical knowledge could enable a family to take control of its own future
had become easier to embrace. By the middle of the nineteenth century,
family size had begun a downward trend.

The Lohmans, however, promised not to prevent pregnancy but to end
it. Within a few months, their ads had moved from the theoretical to the
entirely specific:

> FEMALE PILLS.—MRS. RESTELL, Female Physician, informs the ladies
> that her pills are an infallible regulator of ******. They must not be
> used when ********. Prepared and sold only by herself.

The unprintable words were *menses* and *pregnant,* but the implication
was unmistakable. Business was brisk, and the clientele broad. For
the middle-class mother terrified of another dangerous delivery, no
less than the servant girl frantic to avoid the result of unwanted attentions, Mrs. Restell offered hope. Within the year, *Mrs.* became the more
fashionable *Madame.* And it wasn't just women who noted the address
at the bottom of the ads. Not infrequently, patients were delivered to
Madame Restell's door by gentlemen who hoped to erase the evidence
of their improprieties.

There was nothing infallible about those female pills, of course.

Madame Restell's remedies were herbal nostrums with active ingredients like tansy and ergot, used by midwives as abortifacients for centuries but hardly failsafe. When they did fail, there were other services she could offer. Women in a more advanced stage of pregnancy were invited behind a curtain, where, for a fee dependent on means, Madame Restell or her husband would rupture the amniotic sac with a pointed probe made of metal or whalebone. The patient was then sent home and instructed to seek the attention of a regular physician once the miscarriage began, a fabricated story of accident or illness preserving the ignorance of anyone who attended the woman during her recovery.

This approach was successful enough to produce a steady stream of grateful clients, but serious complications were also commonplace. When a patient died, the law placed the blame on the practitioner. Even when the procedure went smoothly, the idea of surgical abortion was unspeakable, and the power to end an unwanted pregnancy would surely encourage the weaker sex to transgress, if the shameful proof of sin could be so readily avoided. More and more states were codifying anti-abortion statutes. By 1849, Madame Restell had amassed a substantial fortune, as well as a criminal record.

It's difficult to say what offended New Yorkers more, Madame Restell's métier or her money. The mainstream press delicately refrained from discussing her practice, but condemnations circulated in medical journals not subject to such restrictions; one described her as "a monster who speculates with human life with as much coolness as if she were engaged in a game of chance." Pamphlets reporting on her trials—with their transcripts of graphic testimony—became best sellers. "Nature is appalled, that woman, the last and loveliest of her works, could so unsex herself, as to perpetrate such fiend-like enormities," declared one prosecutor in his opening statement. A whiff of sexual license clung permanently to this woman who helped the promiscuous hide their sins. But Madame Restell's earnings bought her skillful lawyers, and her clients included prominent names. Charges were often dropped, only to be followed by indignant editorials. "She has made enough money to drive a coach and six horses through the elastic meshes of the Law," complained the *New-York Tribune*. She did, in fact, take delight in driving her open carriage

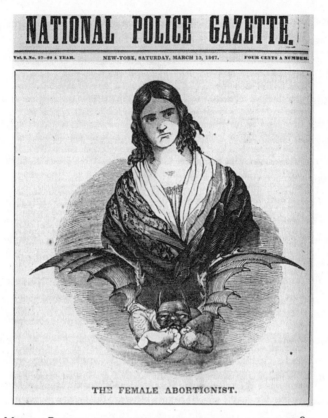

NATIONAL POLICE GAZETTE.

Vol. 9. No. 27—69 A YEAR.   NEW-YORK, SATURDAY, MARCH 13, 1847.   FOUR CENTS A NUMBER.

THE FEMALE ABORTIONIST.

MADAM RESTELL, AS PORTRAYED IN THE POPULAR PRESS, 1847.
COURTESY NATIONAL POLICE GAZETTE

up and down Broadway—a display of ostentation and confidence that seemed only to confirm her brazen wickedness. When another journal described her as "this noted 'Doctress,'" it was not a compliment.

Elizabeth was acutely aware of Madame Restell. The abortionist's emergence into New York notoriety had coincided with the dawn of Elizabeth's interest in medicine and perhaps helped to propel it—later, Elizabeth would remember her horror of abortion as formative. Restell's second criminal trial, in the fall of 1847, gripped the public just as Elizabeth left for Geneva College. Despite all of Madame Restell's powerful connections, she was sentenced to a year in prison. It could not have escaped Elizabeth's sense of irony that at the moment she accepted her

hard-won M.D. in 1849, the woman known as New York's most infamous "female physician" was incarcerated at the city penitentiary—and
on Blackwell's Island, no less.*

Where Margaret Fuller had provided Elizabeth with a positive argument for becoming a woman doctor, Madame Restell supplied the
negative. And while a modern feminist might cast Madame Restell as
a courageous practitioner of essential solutions for desperate women,
Elizabeth—who had never faced the fear of unwanted pregnancy and
never would—felt no such empathy. Even had she been tempted by Util-
itarian arguments about maximizing happiness, the Hippocratic Oath
she had sworn to uphold specifically prohibited abortion. "The gross perversion and destruction of motherhood by the abortionist filled me with
indignation, and awakened active antagonism," she later wrote. "That the
honorable term 'female physician' should be exclusively applied to those
women who carried on this shocking trade seemed to me a horror."

Loyal readers of the *New-York Daily Tribune,* upon seeing the
announcement of Dr. Blackwell's arrival in their city, might have remembered Greeley's thundering condemnation of Madame Restell's "horrible cupidity, depravity, and quackery" ten years earlier. He had always
pointedly refused to run the abortionist's lucrative advertisements. His
endorsement of this new lady doctor, therefore, concluded thus: "This
announcement is made without her knowledge or request, but in justice
to one whose past career and eminent qualifications entitle her to public
consideration and encouragement." The item carefully omitted any use
of the phrase *female physician.*

The *Directory of the City of New-York, for 1852–1853* lists Elizabeth for
the first time on page 63: "Blackwell Elizabeth, physician." Any pride she
might have taken in that entry, however, would have been diminished
by this one, in the Rs: "Restell Madam, physician." It would take more
than an endorsement from Horace Greeley to convince New York that Dr.

---

* Blackwell's Island, now Roosevelt Island, was named for its owner, Robert
Blackwell, in the late seventeenth century; there is no connection with Elizabeth
and Emily's family. It was the site of several grim municipal institutions, including a penitentiary, workhouse, and insane asylum.

Blackwell was something different. No one rang the bell at 44 University Place, though "insolent letters" occasionally appeared in the post. Without colleagues, without patients, and without an income, Elizabeth found herself suddenly becalmed, alone with her ideals.

༰

Elizabeth's return to New York, however anticlimactic, was the catalyst Emily needed. Her sister was waiting for her. It was time to shake off her tedious teaching routine in Cincinnati and decide where and when to begin formal medical study. "I imagine you sitting in your office day by day waiting for the patients who doubtless as yet don't come," Emily wrote to Elizabeth. She longed to sit down with her sister and discuss a thousand things, to find out at last if this calling for which Elizabeth had claimed her was really her true path.

Far from easing the way forward, however, Elizabeth's achievements had arguably made Emily's progress more difficult. Medical mandarins, appalled—and threatened—by Elizabeth's progress on both sides of the Atlantic, resolved ever more strongly to exclude women from established medical schools. Meanwhile Boston's New England Female Medical College and Philadelphia's Female Medical College of Pennsylvania, opened in 1848 and 1850 respectively, provided an obvious alternative. Why should women need to study alongside men if institutions for women now existed? In addition, Eclectic medical schools, like Syracuse's Central Medical College, had also begun to admit women; two of them, Lydia Folger Fowler and Sarah Dolley, had graduated in 1850 and 1851. The Blackwells dismissed both female and Eclectic institutions as unable to provide the level of rigor necessary to prove the legitimacy of female doctors, but the new schools made it all too easy for the gatekeepers of the medical establishment to reject applications from women. "I fear this stupid Philadelphia College may make it difficult for me to enter any college here," Emily mused. "But what has been done may be done again."

In the case of the Eclectic schools, with their emphasis on empirical observation and gentler methods, there was irony in this Blackwellian attitude. Both sisters held views on hygiene and medication that were more in line with Eclectic thought. "I am convinced that a new & nobler era is dawning, for Medicine," Elizabeth wrote, "when the low system of coarse & violent drugging shall give place to a more *spiritual practice,* better adapted to our delicate & wonderful *living* organism." But because the primary goal, to be acknowledged as physicians by the mainstream profession, was ideological rather than therapeutic, only a diploma from a regular—and male—institution would do.

The simplest plan, and the cheapest, would be for Emily to study at the Medical College of Ohio in Cincinnati. Though Emily craved a new identity in a different context, Elizabeth, having been a stranger and no less a target in Geneva, encouraged her to stay home. "Now though it might be very unpleasant to be gossiped about, I do not think in fact that you would be more annoyed there than elsewhere," she assured Emily. "You go so little into society, & I having been already fully discussed, you would probably come in for a smaller share."

Emily had grown up following her sister's instructions. To gauge the odds of being admitted at Cincinnati, she paid a visit to Dr. Reuben Mussey, a professor at the college who had discouraged her sister when she consulted him on the same question six years earlier. "I must tell you of my call for I think it will amuse you," Emily wrote to Elizabeth. Assuming she was a patient, Mussey had gruffly instructed her to sit down; pen in hand, he waited resignedly for her to relate "the details of some fearful disease" so that he could write her an even more fearful prescription. Once Emily conveyed her intent, his startled response was unequivocally negative, though when he realized whose sister sat before him, and heard the details of Elizabeth's European studies, he relented somewhat. "He said finally he did not think I could enter but he'd lay the matter before the faculty if I wished." Encouraged, Emily made the rounds of as many of the professors as she could, collecting several encouraging responses. "I came home tired and hopeful," she wrote in her journal, "full of the brightest anticipations of speedy study."

But when the faculty came to a vote, the answer was no. And so began a pattern of anticipation and rejection that would repeat for nearly a year: at one college after another—Cincinnati, Columbus, Buffalo—the passive support of many melted away before the active disapproval of a few. Even Geneva, which had granted Elizabeth her diploma, and Castleton, in Vermont, which had invited Elizabeth to enroll after she was already at Geneva, now turned their backs. At Cleveland Medical College, part of Western Reserve, Emily was told, "though the large majority of the profs and students wish to admit me, the minority were so decided in opposing that I am refused." And while the other rejections were dismaying, this one was particularly galling—because Cleveland Medical College currently had a woman enrolled among its medical students.

Her name was Nancy Talbot Clark. Having lost her husband and daughter to disease within three years of her wedding, she had turned to medicine and won the support of John Delamater, dean of the Cleveland college. She was now in the middle of her second term. She would receive her diploma two months later, in early 1852—the second woman, after Elizabeth, ever to do so—and listen to a commencement speech that praised her achievement even while announcing that "the Faculty deems it inexpedient, hereafter, to receive ladies as Medical Students." On the one hand, it was encouraging that another woman had managed to duplicate Elizabeth's feat—as Emily herself had said, what had been done before might be done again. But reaction against Clark's achievement at Cleveland had closed the door on Emily once more. It was hard to take the long view in the wake of such disappointment.

Even Emily's closest ally didn't always provide the encouragement she sorely needed. "I ask myself often if I do not expect too much sympathy and companionship from Elizabeth," Emily wrote. "Life sometimes appears cold and lonely in the future." Like Elizabeth, she had decided that practicing medicine was a way to inspire women "with higher objects—loftier aspirations—to teach them that there is a strength of woman as well as of man." But unlike Elizabeth, she wondered if it was presumptuous for one who knew herself to be full of flaws to aspire to such heights. "I think often my intense desire for greatness of nature and life is but a refined selfishness," she wrote in confusion. Her solace, as always, was the outdoors:

> It gives a wonderful zest to wood rambles when every new plant is
> a small scientific problem, every tree or herb the expounder of the

laws of the universe; when the banks and hollows are one extended college where Nature's every friendly voice pronounces the richest, most varied and suggestive instruction, of which I have now a series of concentrated notes in a bowl in my room awaiting further consideration.

Nature was the one school that would always admit her without question.

~

In New York, Elizabeth made the best use of her underemployed days. If no one yet trusted her with a stethoscope, she would use her pen instead. Drawing upon everything she had observed in her peripatetic training, she wrote a series of essays to be delivered as lectures on the subject of raising healthy children, girls in particular.

The lectures laid out Elizabeth's conviction that hygiene and exercise, rather than pharmacology, were the true guardians of good health and the pathways to a shining future. These ideas were not particularly novel or controversial—the eldest of the Beecher siblings, Catharine, had published similar thoughts in her best-selling *Treatise on Domestic Economy* a decade earlier—but Elizabeth's M.D. gave her opinions the imprimatur of science. Provide a child with warmth and cleanliness, simple food and fresh air, and the freedom to be active and useful, she instructed, and nature would restore the degraded human race to the glory of Adam and Eve, created in God's image. Deprived, in her current isolation and straitened finances, of access to a medical library, she deputized Emily as her research assistant and fired off requests for information to Cincinnati. "Send me a scrap from some old Chronicle about the beef & ale consumed by good Queen Bess," she wrote. "I speak in my introductory of the astonishing feats performed physically by oldentime women." She denounced a system of education that required children to sit confined indoors during their growing years, and extolled the ancient Greeks, who prized physical training for both sexes.

Girls should wait until twenty-five to choose a husband, Elizabeth insisted, by which age they would be better prepared both physically and emotionally for the challenges of marriage and motherhood. Despite her experience at La Maternité, she continued to romanticize childbirth:

> The mother, forgetful of weariness and suffering, lifts her pale face
> from the pillow, and listens with her whole soul. The physician,
> profoundly penetrated with the mystery of birth, bends in suspense
> over the little being hovering on the threshold of a new existence;
> for one moment they await the issue—life or death! But the feeble
> cry is the token of victory; the mother's face lights up with ineffable
> joy, as she sinks back exhausted, and the sentiment of sympathy, of
> reverence, thrills through the physician's heart.

Surely she had never witnessed a delivery so sweetly pure. But her writing
was consistent with the emerging "cult of domesticity" celebrating wom-
en's roles as mothers, teachers, and moral exemplars. Older and wiser
marriage choices made by robust and healthy individuals, she explained,
would provide the "physical conditions most favorable to the production
of a strong and beautiful race." As the middle-class trend toward smaller
families continued, it was becoming important to get it right with fewer
children. The best mother, increasingly, was not the one with the largest
family but the one who invested the most time and effort in her children's excellence.

The woman who had fought for the right to study the human body
alongside men was using her hard-won credential to help women within
the home, rather than exhorting them to follow her out of it. Elizabeth
continued to reject the overtures of the women's rights movement,
declining an invitation to take the stage at the third national convention
in Syracuse, even though she applauded its focus on women's education.
The convention's organizers might have breathed a private sigh of relief,
given the opinions expressed in Elizabeth's response to their invitation.
"I believe that the chief source of the false position of women is, the inefficiency of women themselves—the deplorable fact that they are so often
careless mothers, weak wives, poor housekeepers, ignorant nurses, and
frivolous human beings," she wrote. "In order to develop such women,
our method of educating girls, which is an injurious waste of time, must
be entirely remodeled, and I shall look forward with great interest to any
plan of action that may be suggested by your Convention."

Meanwhile, given the intimate nature of women's health issues and the necessity of winning influential individuals to her cause—not to mention her own discomfort with public speaking—Elizabeth preferred to educate a small number of women at a time, in a private setting. During the spring of 1852, she delivered her lectures to groups of like-minded ladies in a Sunday-school basement and began to build a small following among these freethinkers. Eliza Bellows, a woman of delicate health, took a particularly strong fancy to Dr. Elizabeth. Her grateful husband, the prominent Unitarian minister Henry Whitney Bellows, was happy to show the lectures to his friend George Palmer Putnam, a publisher whose list of authors included Washington Irving, James Fenimore Cooper, and Edgar Allan Poe. That June, Putnam printed them under the title *The Laws of Life, with Special Reference to the Physical Education of Girls*. The slim volume, bound in dark green leather, was satisfying proof of Elizabeth's progress as a public figure. "These lectures . . . are the first fruits of my medical studies," she announced in her introduction. "I would offer them as an earnest of future work."

Elizabeth's initiative impressed her reserved sister. "She certainly has some of the qualities of a really great woman," Emily wrote. "She has the power of making things succeed." Her eagerness to join Elizabeth in New York grew. "I want to see her to judge how far I can work with her and whether we can be really friends." For her part, Elizabeth was grateful for Emily's contribution to her writing and bemoaned the inefficiency of the distance between them. "Oh dear if my provoking fortune would only come to the amount of paying my way, how quickly I should say come on, Dr Emily this is the place for you!"

Though her practice still did not cover expenses, Elizabeth was beginning to see a trickle of private patients. It was clear to these women what Elizabeth had to offer: an authoritative intelligence; a good understanding of basic medicine; and best of all, the opportunity to confide the unspeakable details of gynecological trouble to a woman professionally qualified to help them. Their appreciation of her was evident and, for Elizabeth, sometimes embarrassing. "By the bye," she warned Emily, "one great annoyance in my practice that I really don't know how to meet—some of my patients will fall in love with me, do what I will—they absolutely haunt me—make the most enamored eyes, & three of them in unguarded moments, kissed me!" Even when she overcharged the demonstrative ones, they came back for more. These satisfied patients surely meant to convey nothing more than ardent gratitude, but Elizabeth had never liked to be touched and preferred to think of herself as above mawkish entanglements. Or perhaps it was a case of doth-protest-too-much. "I can assure you it's no small cross," she wrote. "I've no objection to kissing a healthy handsome man occasionally, but love passages with women are diabolical!"

If certain women were too enthusiastic, even the most open-minded men continued to feel a deep discomfort with a woman who attached M.D. to her name. As long as Elizabeth could practice alone, all was well—until she needed a second opinion. The first time she called in a male colleague for a consultation, unintentional comedy ensued. An elderly woman presented with severe pneumonia, and Elizabeth asked an old acquaintance—a kindly physician who had once treated her father—to confirm her diagnosis.

After his examination, he paced up and down nervously. "A most extraordinary case!" he exclaimed. "Such a one never happened to me before; I really do not know what to do!"

Elizabeth was baffled. Had she mistaken the symptoms of pneumonia? But the good doctor's agitation had nothing to do with the patient. He simply could not imagine a professional consultation with a female physician; the cognitive dissonance was too great. Elizabeth diplomatically suggested that perhaps he could think of it as a "friendly talk" rather than a clinical discussion. That did the trick: useful advice was conveyed, and the patient swiftly recovered.

～

Sharing Elizabeth's home in New York and watching her progress, observant Marian became a conduit between Elizabeth's daily experience and Emily's anticipation. "I think I will send you a few lines, & give you my advice about matters & things," Marian wrote to Emily in Cincinnati, "which of course, you after the manner of all our family, will take if it suits you & reject if it don't." Though Marian applauded her sisters' vocation wholeheartedly and even sometimes envied it, she believed a medical degree was useless. Elizabeth's diploma had done little to impress her colleagues and meant even less to her patients. "I am quite convinced that the position a woman will occupy as Dr will be according to her *real merit,* and the personal influence that she succeeds in exerting on others—not on a mere diploma," Marian wrote. "It is not so much study as *practical experience and tact."*

Legitimacy, Marian argued, was a matter of demonstrated skill, not credentials. If she were Emily, she would forget medical school, work with Elizabeth in New York for a while, and then go to Paris and enter La Maternité. "That experience has been of more real value to our sister than anything else," Marian insisted. "I can see that she takes hold of obstetric cases with perfect ease & self-confidence—secure of her own knowledge, & prepared for any emergency. . . . It is *general* knowledge of sickness that I think she lacks." Despite Elizabeth's leanings toward cold water and good hygiene, Marian thought she still put far too much store in "those old hateful mineral drugs" and trusted her professors and her textbooks more than her own common sense. Emily should learn from Elizabeth's example. "You are less conservative in your nature than E—& have seen more of heresies," Marian told Emily, perhaps alluding to the time Emily had spent with Anna's Brook Farm friends. "You must be eclectic—reformatory—universal—and I firmly believe you will do just as well." As for Elizabeth, Marian thought she would find her place "less as Dr than as teacher & professor & stimulator to others," proving, at this early stage, uncannily prescient. "I must say," Marian confided, swearing Emily to secrecy, "if I were taken sick . . . I would doctor myself & not call upon her for aid."

Though she appreciated Marian's candor, Emily had toiled too long to abandon her pursuit of a diploma—she wasn't going to fall short of the bar Elizabeth had set. And as spring advanced, there were hopeful signs that this goal might be attainable. Dr. Mussey, who had greeted Emily's original appeal with grudging caution, had since paid a visit to Elizabeth in New York and delighted her by mentioning "his clear perception," Elizabeth reported, "that [Emily] ought to be a doctor." Upon his return to Cincinnati, Mussey informed Emily that he thought her chances either at Dartmouth or at Chicago's Rush Medical College were promising. That was enough to make up her mind; waiting had become intolerable. She began to pack, planning to visit Elizabeth in New York before continuing on to New Hampshire, where Dartmouth College's fifty-year-old medical school attracted her more strongly than Rush, founded less than a decade earlier. The Dartmouth term would begin in early August. "I have marked out my course," she recorded in her journal.

"So Milly is actually setting out on her special life journey!" Elizabeth wrote to Sam upon receiving the news. "She must obtain admission somewhere, for the world wants her & must necessarily receive her."

~

CHAPTER 10

ADMISSION, AGAIN

On a sweltering evening at the end of July 1852, Emily Blackwell sat down to dinner with her sister Elizabeth for the first time in three years. An uncomfortable anticipation had grown with each passing mile from Cincinnati to New York. Elizabeth had traversed Europe, transcended prejudice and pain, and won the praise of famous physicians. The sister Emily thought she knew was bold, brilliant, and capable but also uncompromising, inflexible, and exacting. Her letters made it clear that she expected no less from Emily. Would she be able to live up to Elizabeth's formidable expectations? And even if she could, would she be able to live with her?

The woman who answered Emily's knock at 44 University Place had a face etched with new lines of age and illness. But Elizabeth's missing eye was hardly noticeable—except when the glass prosthetic glinted oddly in reflected light—and her eagerness to share her medical goals with Emily was obvious. "From Wednesday noon till Monday morning we talked almost without cessation," Emily wrote with relief. "I liked E.—she was not nearly as particular and fidgetty as I had the idea."

Elizabeth was equally happy with Emily. "Her visit gave me a feeling of deep joy," she reported to Lady Byron. "She has a noble intellect, clear and strong. . . . If she can obtain the needful impulse and direction from a superior mind, I think she will make a fine scientific physician." Whether that superior mind belonged to a medical mentor in Emily's future, or to Elizabeth herself, was unclear. But Elizabeth's respect for

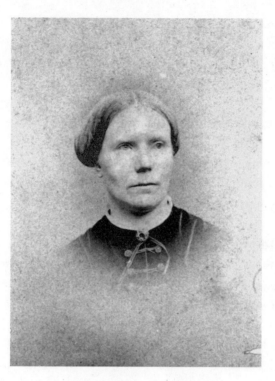

ELIZABETH, CIRCA 1855.
COURTESY SCHLESINGER LIBRARY, RADCLIFFE INSTITUTE, HARVARD UNIVERSITY

Emily was real. "I speak of her without hesitation—as a soldier of truth," she wrote, "rather than as my sister."

Galvanized by the brief reunion, Emily boarded the airless, creaking cars again for the long ride north to Hanover, New Hampshire. Its green and white New England charm enchanted her, as did the fresh faces of its forthright residents: "The men did not wear whiskers and the women seemed more able to take care of themselves." Blue hills, dry-stone walls, dark pine and hemlock among the spreading oaks and maples, the graceful elegance of the Dartmouth Green—it was "a different country from the west," a lovely setting for a new life. Surely the good news of her Dartmouth admission would follow without delay.

The professors, though courteous, remained unconvinced by this carefully dressed, well-spoken, accomplished young woman who had journeyed hundreds of solitary miles in order to make her appeal in person. She waited five days for their rejection, then packed her trunk once more. On the way south, she stopped at the Berkshire Medical Institution in Pittsfield, Massachusetts, for one more attempt. Berkshire had recently granted a medical degree to James Skivring Smith, a free Black man who went on to become the president of Liberia. But it wasn't ready to admit a woman.

Nine days after leaving for her glorious next chapter, Emily was back in her sister's stifling sitting room. "Why Milly, unfortunate child, so they've refused you," Elizabeth exclaimed as she walked in.

~

After years of wishing for each other's companionship, Emily and Elizabeth suddenly had more of it than either of them preferred. The dearth of patients had forced Elizabeth to a lower floor at 44 University Place, downsizing from two rooms into one. "I like the room," Elizabeth had written staunchly. "It has an air of pleasant gloom about it." Marian had gone to stay with a friend just in time for Emily's arrival, which was fortunate. Emily slept on the sofa, while Elizabeth had her bed in the six-foot-square dressing room.

The lack of space was an incentive for Emily to keep moving forward. Though Elizabeth was short of patients, she had made useful connections in the year since she arrived in New York, and now she got to work on her sister's behalf. Within the week Emily met Elizabeth's ally Horace Greeley, the newspaperman, who introduced her to the city commissioner in charge of Bellevue Hospital.

The oldest and largest public hospital in New York, staffed by the city's best-qualified and most public-spirited doctors, Bellevue served as pest house, lunatic asylum, and "warehouse for the destitute." Emily paid calls on its leading physicians, and by the first of September, the decision was unanimous: she would be allowed to attend lectures. This was unprecedented—though Elizabeth had gained access to St. Bartholomew's in London, no American hospital had yet welcomed a female student. John Wakefield Francis, consulting physician at Bellevue and co-founder of the New York Academy of Medicine, shook Emily's hand as he delivered the good news. "Now my dear," he instructed her, "if you have any difficulty up there come to me and I'll settle it for you." She was no closer to a diploma, but at least she would not be wasting her time. "Yesterday I had the satisfaction of taking out the first hospital ticket that has ever been taken by a woman in America," she wrote to her youngest brother George. It was good to have her own "first" at last.

The next day she was in the operating theater. A surgeon "in a long apron something like a butcher's," stiff with dried blood, explained to a ring of twenty students how to drain fluid from the chest as his shirt-less patient, "with a rather frightened look," shifted from foot to foot. Once the man was stretched on the narrow table, the surgeon selected an instrument and paused to invite Emily to move over where she would have a better view. "There was a great tumbling about directly, as if a cannon was about to go off there," Emily wrote wryly. "A small vacancy was left with students filed down each side, into which I stepped."

She watched as the scalpel opened an incision between the patient's ribs, and she did not look away until the wound was bandaged, "the students alternately watching the operation, & me." Emily ignored them. After so many years of gleaning on the edges of her chosen field, here she was right in the middle of it. "I shall certainly find the study of medicine interesting, however the practice may be," she wrote to her youngest brother. "Rather different kind of study than our botanical rambles, isn't it George?"

Emily soon became a familiar sight at Bellevue, walking the wards, attending postmortems in the dead house, and helping prepare prescriptions in the apothecary's shop. "The young Drs are used to my appearance and no longer stare at me nor laugh when I feel a pulse," she wrote at the end of her second week. She tried not to dwell on the moment when she had looked up at the blackboard to find a crude sketch of a woman wearing a Bloomer costume, the short skirt over loose pantaloons that had recently become a scandalizing symbol of women's rights. Above it, someone had chalked "Strongminded Woman."

Emily's intelligence and talent impressed her Bellevue instructors, and when she informed them that she would be leaving for Chicago to attempt enrollment at Rush Medical College, they were quick to offer letters of introduction as well as assurances that she would be welcome back at Bellevue between terms. Their gestures were genuine, but they were also likely relieved to see her go.

~

On October 29, 1852, almost exactly five years after Elizabeth arrived at Geneva in the rain, Emily reached Chicago under equally stormy skies. Within twenty-four hours she introduced herself to the president of Rush Medical College, Daniel Brainard, as well as his colleagues Nathan S. Davis and John Evans. The endorsement of the Bellevue brahmins made all the difference: it was easier for Rush's leaders to act boldly on Emily's behalf when they could point to men of large reputation who had already done so.

"They are all willing," Emily scribbled to Elizabeth that evening in incredulous haste. Brainard, Emily reported, was "a very reserved grave man—he says he neither favours nor disproves of women studying— they may do as they please." As far as the faculty was concerned, Brainard informed her, she was welcome. He cautioned her, however, that the decision to grant her a degree rested with the trustees, and he could not guarantee it.

At the end of her first lecture, Dr. Davis—voted favorite teacher by his students the previous year—motioned for silence. "I have introduced into the Lecture Room, with the cheerful consent of all the Faculty, a lady who proposes to spend the winter with us," he announced. Murmuring arose on all sides as he raised his voice. "To save all inquiry I will inform you that it is Miss Blackwell, sister of Miss Elizabeth Blackwell, who studied some years ago at Geneva and subsequently in Europe." Every face in the room was now turned toward Emily. "The Americans have the reputation of being a very gallant nation," Davis continued, his eyes sweeping the tiers of seats. "I need not tell you, you will be expected by your conduct this winter to maintain the national character." The students burst into gallant applause.

Emily's formal medical education was under way. "I have today completed one month's attendance at College," Emily wrote to George, "and therefore feel pretty sure that no interruption will now arise to drive me out—indeed I wouldn't go." As elsewhere, students paid their tuition by purchasing lecture tickets, which included a line for the student's name with a preprinted "Mr." In her writing case Emily now carried a stack of tickets: "all testifying, with a variety of flourishes, that Mr. Emily Black-well is entitled to attend the session of 1852–53," she noted with amuse-ment. Though she found "dirty little Chicago" not much to her taste, her professors pleased her enormously. James Van Zandt Blaney illustrated his chemistry lectures with elegant experiments that Emily wished her brother George could see. Joseph Warren Freer guided her dissections and deplored the dull state of her scalpels; he had turned to medicine after the death of his wife, which perhaps explained his unusual recep-tivity to the idea of a female doctor. John Evans, professor of obstetrics, insisted that Emily attend all his lectures on the "external generative organs," even though, unlike Elizabeth, she offered to sit them out. "I was glad to find my self-command sufficient to prevent even my colour from changing," she wrote afterward.

Like Elizabeth, Emily looked for allies at the top of the hierarchy. "I like Dr Brainard best," she wrote of the man who had founded Rush Med-ical College ten years earlier, "he is a man of decided talent and strong fearless character." The professor of surgery invited her to take a seat in the front row and asked her to tea with his wife. Encouraged, a few weeks into the term she followed him out of the lecture hall to ask a question as he was preparing to return to his office practice. Finding him receptive, she took a deep breath.

"Doctor, you don't want a student in your office, do you?" She could hardly believe she had dared to ask.

"I don't know but I should like a good one," he replied after a moment, hiding the quirk of a smile under his luxuriant mustache.

Emily met his gaze, outwardly calm but triumphant within. They talked for an hour about everything from surgery to her sister and walked together to his office, where he showed her around. "I went home how happy," she rejoiced in her journal. "I wrote to E., but could not sleep." Before dawn she was back at Brainard's office, organizing his library.

For the next fortnight, Emily spent all her free time at Brainard's office: reveling in his books, listening to his patients, meeting his colleagues, observing surgeries, and asking questions. Not only was the doctor will-ing to teach her, but his professional views were appealingly progressive:

He criticized the overuse of mercury-based calomel and condemned the proliferation of patent medicines and the scoundrels who profited from them. Most important, he seemed to place more value on Emily's abilities than on her gender. "The Dr has no other students, he will not take them," she reported proudly. "I regard this as almost as great an achievement as getting into college."

It didn't last. "And so two weeks have seen my office career commenced and finished," Emily wrote with a sigh. Although Brainard's patients were perfectly cordial, a handful of Chicago's more influential citizens apparently complained of her presence in his office, and he bowed to the pressure.

At the college, however, Brainard continued to be an attentive mentor. "I went yesterday with him to see him cut off a portion of a diseased eye," Emily recorded. "I held the patient, a young woman, who scratched away vigorously, though under the influence of ether—she said however she felt no pain, only alarm." Brainard called on Emily to assist him— in front of the class—during an operation to correct an infant's clubfoot, and praised her when it was over. She was pleased to discover that the actual experience of surgery—in 1852 still a dangerous, gruesome, messy endeavor, even with the introduction of anesthetics—was no more disturbing to her than it had been in the pages of her textbooks. While watching Brainard demonstrate amputation on a dog, she was happy to tell Elizabeth, "the blood affected me no more than so much warm water." But she did feel sorry for the poor creature later, when it came wagging up to her on three legs. Vivisection, a word coined by its opponents, was the dissection of living animals for experimental purposes— a practice endorsed by many physicians who believed either that animals felt no pain, or that their suffering was outweighed by the benefit to surgical knowledge.

In his lectures on syphilis, it was Brainard's custom to hand out graphic pictures of the ravages of the disease. With Emily present, he made a point of passing some to her first. "I examined them carefully with great composure, & then handed them on," she wrote. "It was nothing to me, & I don't think the class cared." The students respected their professor and president even if they didn't endorse Emily's presence.

Their hesitation, Emily realized, was a matter of collective ego more than individual chauvinism. "The reason many of the students dislike the idea of opening the college to women is that they have the idea that no other regular college would do it, but that the irregular colleges will," she wrote. "They think it would be rather derogatory to the honour of the institution in the opinion of the other colleges." They had little against Emily personally, but they shied from the risk that their own credentials might be devalued.

Daniel Brainard, Emily understood, felt much the same. She was a credit to him, certainly, but his institution came first. Brainard "would I believe admit any woman he had confidence in," Emily wrote to Elizabeth, "but he would not seriously injure the college to carry the point." And while he admired Emily, he doubted there were many women as committed as she. Emily, frankly, agreed with him: "When I saw the women who came to consult him at his office, I could hardly blame him for having no very high opinion of them."

Under Brainard's tutelage, Emily's attraction to medical practice, and her determination to pursue surgery, began to equal or even surpass her sense of medicine as moral mission. She enjoyed what she was doing and wanted to keep doing it for its own sake. Brainard, Emily told Elizabeth, "has liked me thoroughly ever since I told him if I could not study to my satisfaction here I would study in disguise at Paris"—a step Elizabeth had always refused, on principle, to consider. Heartened by Brainard's approval, Emily began to think of herself as a surgeon. "I would choose certain branches"—obstetrics and gynecology—"make myself the most skillful surgeon in America in that department, if possible—and I think it would be hard to keep me from succeeding," she wrote in her journal, with new confidence.

"I have come to the conclusion that operations though the showiest are by no means the most difficult part of Surgery," she wrote, with an acuity that belied her experience. The surgeon's true challenge, she saw, was not the bravura sawing of bone or the dramatic removal of a disfiguring tumor; it was deciding when and upon whom to operate, then managing the patient's recovery with meticulous attention—this more than a decade before Joseph Lister introduced the idea of antiseptic postoperative care. Her farsightedness extended to nonsurgical obstetric issues as well. "I feel convinced that some means might be found placing conception under the control of the individual," she mused in her journal. "Also of making the whole process of Gestation much more endurable—attended with fewer bad results to the health, strength and person than at present."

"Physicians have hitherto been men, who felt no special interest in the matter, the female side," she continued. "I have already planned a series of experiments with regard to it, some day I will carry them out." Where Elizabeth imagined a distant future of female achievement, Emily focused on the flawed present and what she could do to help women through the perils of pregnancy and childbirth. She confined these thoughts to her journal, however, and kept them out of her letters to Elizabeth.

A kind dinner invitation from the Brainards rescued Emily from her first solitary Christmas, but she preferred wind-whipped walks along the ice-piled shore of Lake Michigan to socializing. Soon she would be back in New York between terms, with no access to medical books or specimens. After dark one evening, she frightened the demonstrator of anatomy when he heard the sound of soft footsteps in the dissecting room. Leaving the premises as fast as dignity would permit, he returned with a light only to find "nothing more ghostly than Milly."

In quiet moments, Emily's thoughts turned toward Elizabeth, struggling to find professional traction in New York. "Her letters often make me sad—not from what she says but from a sort of unhappy atmosphere," she wrote. It was clear that Elizabeth was not getting anywhere by sitting and waiting in her consulting room, skimping on food and fuel. "I do hope you don't starve yourself," Emily admonished her. "I think you ought to burn a little more wood. It is excessively trying to be always shivering."

For years she had bobbed in Elizabeth's wake. Now she was gathering information and experience that matched Elizabeth's and in critical ways improved it. Having failed to attract a steady clientele among the wealthy, Elizabeth was thinking of offering her services gratis to the poor, to gain experience and win the sympathy of philanthropic New Yorkers. She outlined her idea for Emily, who discussed it at length with Daniel Brainard.

Brainard was unequivocal: advertising such services would make Elizabeth sound like another Madame Restell. "He said any young physician advertising that he would practice free on certain days at a certain place would be turned out of any society and stamped as a quack henceforth," Emily warned her sister urgently. A woman like Elizabeth—without a pedigree, an independent fortune, or any interest in making herself charming—could achieve her goal only by creating something larger than herself. Where the public would condemn an individual, it might endorse an institution. It was time to create one.

For the urban poor, private doctors were an undreamed-of luxury and public hospitals a nightmare of last resort. Those who needed something for a bad cut or a bad cold went to a dispensary: a free clinic for the poor. The idea had originated in London in the 1770s—as a way to serve those turned away from overcrowded St. Bartholomew's—and the first New York dispensary had opened in 1791. As the city spread northward and its population grew, more were added, each attending to its own neighborhood. By 1852 there were five major dispensaries and counting, funded by grants from the state and donations from the wealthy. They were important centers for the promotion of public health and had begun to serve an equally vital role in training young physicians. Establishing a small dispensary was an achievable goal. It would afford Elizabeth the medical autonomy she craved and perhaps become a place where other female medical graduates could learn.

Brainard was generous with his advice, and Emily conveyed his ideas to Elizabeth in fine detail. She would need a name ("say, the New York Institution for furnishing free med advice to indigent women & children, or any other title you pleased"), a board of influential trustees, a consulting physician and surgeon with impeccable reputations, and if she really wanted to make it stick, perhaps a charter from the state of New York. Given that the work involved matters of life and death, she needed to pick her people carefully. They must be true allies, such that "if ever a case should turn out ill and you should be criticized [they would] not come out & say they really didn't know anything about it."

Above all, Emily reported, Elizabeth needed to play by the rules, which were increasingly codified. The American Medical Association, founded in Philadelphia in 1847, had that same year published its *Code of Ethics*, which Emily exhorted Elizabeth to acquire and embrace; Emily's own professor, Nathan Davis, had been one of the sponsors of the document. The rules, of course, were part of a game created and controlled by men. Emily's letter concluded with a postscript. "Dr B thought it would be more imposing for you to have men's names for your officers than women," she wrote. "Alas poor women! But I believe it's true."

~

"I have often thought that if I followed solely my inclinations I should assume a man's dress and wander freely over the world," Emily wrote, once she was back in Elizabeth's cramped New York quarters. Where Elizabeth strove to stand alongside her male allies as an exceptional woman who had proved herself their equal, Emily yearned to shuck off her gender and make her way in anonymity.

Alone with her prickly sister and narrower opportunities for study, Emily found the productive momentum of her months in Chicago difficult to sustain. To her satisfaction, Daniel Brainard, visiting New York for a meeting of the American Medical Association, took the time to call upon his prize pupil. "He told me the trustees would make no difficulty about my graduation, so my way is clear," she wrote with relief. Elizabeth and Emily hosted the Brainards for an oyster supper—their living space so small, the guests had to file in and pull their chairs up to the tiny table one at a time—and Dr. Brainard regaled the party with tales of Emily's advent at Rush, and the stodgy opposition to her presence that he had handily dispatched. "We had quite a merry time," Emily wrote.

But as the New York summer grew sultry, doubts crept back. "I do not feel perfectly clear that I can establish myself in N.Y. and work in concert with E," Emily confided to her journal. Elizabeth's "nervous oppressive discomfort" was difficult to endure, and life in New York meant too much time shut up in places where she could not see the sky. To make things worse, her champion Daniel Brainard suddenly decided to spend the coming term in Europe. He reported that although Rush's board of trustees had, dismayingly, passed a resolution against admitting women henceforth, he assumed the decision was not meant to apply to *her*, as she was already midway through her studies.

Emily decided her way forward was clear enough to proceed—no other paths presented themselves. On her twenty-seventh birthday, October 8, 1853, she surveyed her position with stubborn conviction: "The future lies black with a golden glow beyond it."

~

She was right about both the darkness and the light. "I find I shall have more to contend with than I supposed," Emily wrote with impressive understatement from Chicago. The day after her return, and without her knowledge, the Rush trustees gathered for an emergency meeting and decided her fate. Rush Medical College would not allow her to finish her degree.

The decision was a case of moral cowardice that the *Chicago Tribune* was quick to call out, praising Emily's initiative and demanding an explanation for her shameful treatment. "It is too absurd," an editorial declared staunchly, "to suppose that any educated and reflecting female, who had the boldness to enter upon, and the perseverance to pursue this science, could not comprehend its truths, and administer its practice as well as a majority of the half-fledged youth who dabble in salts and soda." A letter from an anonymous Rush student appeared in response. "In behalf of the *medical class*, I wish it distinctly understood, by all concerned, that the young gentlemen composing that class are possessed of too much gallantry to repudiate the ladies in any shape," he wrote, with a roguishness that undermined the affirmation. This was followed by an editor's note: as far as the *Tribune* could ascertain, the trustees said they were acting at the request of the faculty, the faculty said the students had demanded it, and the students denied any such thing. "Now, it is very evident there is duplicity and double dealing somewhere," wrote the editors. "Who is guilty?"

Emily did not wait to find out. She had already left for Cleveland Medical College, Nancy Clark's alma mater. The school's dean, John Delamater, had once been Daniel Brainard's own mentor. Many of the Cleveland faculty members had been encouraging when Emily first sought admission two years earlier. And she was already halfway to her degree—surely Delamater could convince his faculty to admit her for a single term.

Her staccato journal entries attest to furious activity and flinty resolve, as well as a severe cold that left her shivering with fever and aching in every limb. But she was finished with uncertainty, and the Cleveland faculty seemed to recognize it. Within a few days of her arrival, she had taken her lecture tickets. "I am beginning to feel rested and settled," she wrote.

After that, finishing out the term was straightforward. Less than three months later, Emily sailed through her final examinations and was mightily amused, as she left the examiners' room, to overhear one curmudgeon mutter, "That is the only student you have passed whom I would introduce to practice in my family." Afterward, the school's co-founder, Jared Potter Kirtland, a copiously bearded old gentleman with kindly eyes behind his spectacles, presented her with a bouquet of flowers from his own hothouse—no small gift in the middle of February—and told her "it was not often that roses bloomed in winter, and it was not often professors had such a student," as Emily recorded proudly. "To which I of course replied that it was not often a student received flowers with so much pleasure."

Her graduation on February 22, 1854, was warmed by such expressions of solidarity on all sides. "Emily is now Dr. Emily Blackwell," Elizabeth wrote with satisfaction to Anna. "You have the honour of possessing two professional sisters!" On the day appointed for the graduating students to read their theses—Emily's was titled "The Principles Involved in the Study of Medicine"—she was surprised to see a woman enter the hall and sit down; after the readings, Delamater introduced her as none other than Nancy Clark herself, who had traveled from Boston to support Cleveland's second female medical alumna. The highest performance grade was 10, but the faculty awarded Emily 11 and, in addition to her diploma, presented her with a special commendation bearing all their signatures. Clark told her she had graduated "not only successfully but triumphantly."

The attention was gratifying, but Emily understood too well how ephemeral such enthusiasm could be. She had heard from allies in England, via Lady Byron, that the illustrious Scottish physician James Young Simpson would allow her to continue her training with him. She hoped her next mentor would be worth the journey to Edinburgh.

⤳

CHAPTER 11

EDINBURGH

E mily remained even-keeled even when seasick. "Judging from the fine flavor of carrot with which the operation ended, the greedy old ocean coveted even the soup I had eaten for dinner," she reported. "Probably when I am shut down in the cabin tonight I shall have another tussle with destiny, but if this weather continue I shall not know much of the horrors E was so troubled by." She had sailed from Boston at the end of March 1854, spending her last night with Nancy Clark, who saw her aboard with a bouquet of roses and a generous supply of biscuits.

The Royal Mail Steamship *Arabia*, built for the Cunard line only a year earlier, was magnificent: nearly a hundred yards from stem to stern, with two masts, two smokestacks between them, and two huge paddle-wheels on either beam. The main dining saloon, with seating for 160, was paneled in bird's-eye maple and ebony, hung with crimson drapes, and upholstered in velvet, with glowing stained-glass sconces depicting camel caravans "and other Oriental sketches" in keeping with the ship's name. Steam pipes beneath the floor warmed the staterooms, which were similarly done up with Brussels carpets and more red velvet.

Emily ignored its luxurious charms, perching contentedly in the lee of a smokestack, watching gulls tumbling in the sea-salted wind. Cresting waves foamed like spouting whales, and real whales spouted among them; icebergs resembled mountains or ruins or, in one case, "a little solitary watch tower." Even rough weather was gorgeous, and once she was safe in her berth, the crashing sea rocked her to sleep. Her young roommate—"an inoffensive Irish girl"—might wake her screaming that a ghost had invaded their cabin, and her fellow passengers might weary her with their "drinking smoking cardplaying & crowding," but these were passing irritations. The natural world continued to be Emily's solace.

Her solitary hours offered time to reflect on the three weeks she had just spent in New York. A month after Emily's graduation, Elizabeth had reached a milestone of her own: the opening of her dispensary. Following Daniel Brainard's instructions scrupulously, she had obtained a charter from the state and stacked her board of trustees with prominent men—many of them Quaker and several the husbands of satisfied patients. They included the *Tribune* editor Horace Greeley and his deputy Charles Dana; Henry J. Raymond, politician and recent founder of the *New-York Times;* and the jurist Theodore Sedgwick.

"The design of this institution is to give to poor women an opportunity of consulting physicians of their own sex," Elizabeth's carefully crafted mission statement began. "The existing charities of our city regard the employment of women as physicians as an experiment, the success of which has not yet been sufficiently proved to admit of cordial cooperation." At the end of a list of respected doctors who would serve as consultants, Elizabeth's name was tucked in discreetly as "attending physician." The minutes of an early board meeting suggest that even her trustees considered female physicians a hard sell. The original draft of their incorporation certificate softened the mission by stating that they would employ "medical practitioners of either sex," though it was "the design of this Institution to Secure the Services of well qualified female practitioners of Medicine for its patients."

The institution's name—the New York Dispensary for Poor Women and Children—was the grandest thing about it. Elizabeth had found a single small damp room on East Seventh Street, near Tompkins Square in the heart of Little Germany. She tacked a card to the door announcing the hours—Monday, Wednesday, and Friday, from three o'clock—until a more permanent tin sign could be painted. And three afternoons a week, instead of sitting in her room on University Place, she walked the mile to Seventh Street, and sat there.

The homely dispensary might not have matched what Elizabeth had imagined during her months of training in Europe, but it suited her approach as a physician. The tenement-dwelling seamstresses and cigar-makers who came for basic remedies also received guidance on household hygiene, ventilation, diet, child care—everything Elizabeth had described in *Laws of Life* for the wealthier women uptown. She dispensed job advice, recommended charities, and even handed out "pecuniary aid" to the most desperate. Sometimes she followed up with a visit to a patient's home. Elizabeth was practicing social work as much as medicine, and she was gratified to note that "in many cases the advice has been followed, at any rate for a time." The flow of patients wasn't more than a trickle, but that was beside the point: Elizabeth's institution existed at last, and it was a place to start.

Emily had passed through New York from Cleveland just as the dispensary opened. She spent nearly three weeks helping Elizabeth in her new venture, noting only that bare fact in her journal without further comment. Here was Dr. Brainard's advice in action, Elizabeth's newborn organization, awaiting Emily's more permanent help once her training was complete. But it was tiny, humbly situated, and had more to do with cough syrup and constipation than the newest advances in obstetric surgery. Emily was not sorry to be leaving for the operating theaters of Edinburgh and Paris. And perhaps Elizabeth felt a twinge of envy as she watched her go.

~

Upon her arrival in Liverpool, Emily gazed at her mother country with the eyes of a delighted tourist. Only six when the Blackwells emigrated, she thought of herself as American in a way Elizabeth never had; now back in Britain for the first time, "the people struck me as remarkably English." She paused at the edge of a crowd of children to watch a red-nosed Punch waving his pasteboard sword at a blue dragon with snapping jaws. Passing a baker's window full of "the most tempting plum buns, of course I went in and bought two." On the train to Birmingham, she gazed at the pastoral landscape: lambs, cottages, orchards. "It all had a sort of toyshop look," she wrote, "everything was so neat and finished, so green small & trim." Where Elizabeth had returned to the old country and saluted its superiority, Emily found it quaint.

The letter Emily had sent announcing her travel plans had taken a slower steamer than the *Arabia*, so she entertained herself by surprising the siblings she hadn't seen in nearly six years. Anna hadn't gotten up yet; her little sister's face peeping around the bed curtains produced, to Emily's delight, "a look of such bewildered amazement as is quite impossible to describe." Hearing Howard's voice in the parlor, Emily carried in the morning papers with a nonchalant "good morning." "If ever an apathetic youth opened his eyes," she wrote, "that young gentlemen did so then." Emily found her oldest sister and younger brother changed: Anna had gone gray, Howard was now bewhiskered, and both of them had erased Cincinnati from their accents and their dress. After lunch they went for "a real English walk, gathering kingcups and daisies from the hedgerow."

Emily wasted even less time than Elizabeth on family reunion, pushing on within days to London, where ever-helpful cousin Kenyon accompanied her on introductory visits to notable physicians. These included Elizabeth's mentor at St. Bartholomew's, James Paget, who was happy to see "another Dr. Blackwell" and heartily endorsed Emily's intention to study with James Young Simpson in Scotland. She met Elizabeth's friend Barbara Leigh Smith, who embraced her warmly and carried off a small stack of Emily's newly printed calling cards to share with well-connected friends. She toured St. Paul's and Regent Street and the British Museum with interest, but the works of artists and architects never touched her as deeply as the works of nature, and she was impatient to move on. Before she left for Edinburgh, Kenyon's wife, Marie, presented her with a gold brooch as a parting gift—an elegant French one rather than the gaudy enameled pins that were the current fashion. After all, Marie insisted, for Cousin Emily, "*il faut absolument quelque chose de sérieux.*"

The dramatic scenery on the journey to Edinburgh, as she rattled along in the cars of the Great Northern Railway, was much to Emily's liking. "The hills grew bold & bare," she wrote, opening into broad valleys cradling "little old villages of grey stone looking so solemn & antediluvian." Soon the hilltops glittered with lingering snow reflecting the last light of dusk; as they crossed the border at Gretna Green, Emily was lulled to sleep. Stumbling through a groggy arrival in the dark, she found her way to a bed at the Caledonian Hotel and awoke the next

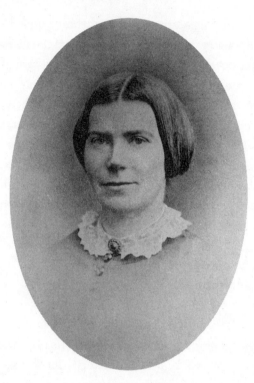

EMILY, CIRCA 1855.
COURTESY SCHLESINGER LIBRARY, RADCLIFFE INSTITUTE, HARVARD UNIVERSITY

morning to a view, framed in her window, of Edinburgh Castle high on its crag.

The University of Edinburgh had long been considered the best place to study medicine in the English-speaking world—the founding professors of America's first medical school, at the College of Philadelphia in 1765, had been Edinburgh graduates. Its population nearing two hundred thousand, the city had recently remade itself; in the New Town, north of Princes Street, rows of graceful terraced houses marched in stately contrast to the overflowing vertical squalor of the Old Town's ancient closes. Emily did not pause to consider the legacy of the Scottish Enlightenment, or her friendless arrival in an ancient city. As soon as she was dressed, she set out for 52 Queen Street, the home and headquarters of James Young Simpson.

In 1854 Simpson was a man in his exuberant prime, having held the University of Edinburgh's chair in midwifery and the diseases of women and children for nearly a decade and a half. He had been appointed physician to the queen in Scotland in 1847, the same year he became famous as the discoverer of chloroform as an effective anesthetic—a discovery he had made at his dining table in the company of several friends, each of whom inhaled a sample poured from Simpson's brandy decanter, felt a wave of giggling euphoria, and promptly crashed unconscious to the floor. His house, in the heart of the New Town, was—and still is—the only one in the row with a full fourth story, added to accommodate his seven children, his ever-expanding private practice, and the never-ending salon of writers, artists, statesmen, and physicians who joined him at breakfast, lunch, and dinner.

Emily presented herself at the pilastered front door of Number 52 and made the immediate acquaintance of Jarvis, Simpson's loyal butler and watchdog. "The servant who answered the bell was evidently well practiced in keeping people out," she wrote wryly. "He declined with the most inexorable politeness to take even the letter I had brought. . . . I should think a dozen ladies were sent off in the same satisfactory manner within five minutes." Emily waited several days, exploring the labyrinth of the Old Town. Simpson had been laid up with an attack of influenza, she learned—likely a cover for a bout of the depression that periodically halted his hectic schedule.

Her patience was rewarded. On her next visit to Queen Street, Jarvis escorted her through two long reception rooms full of patients to a sky-lit staircase at the rear of the house, where the great doctor's monogram was worked into the uprights of the wrought-iron banister. Emily ascended to Simpson's office. "I was received by a rather short stout man with a broad full rather flat face surrounded by a quantity of black wavy hair just touched with grey," she wrote. Barrel-chested and shaggy-maned, Simpson cut an unmistakable figure, with a shrewd gaze flashing from a somewhat porcine visage. William Makepeace Thackeray, part of the parade of guests at Simpson's table, described him as having the head of Zeus.

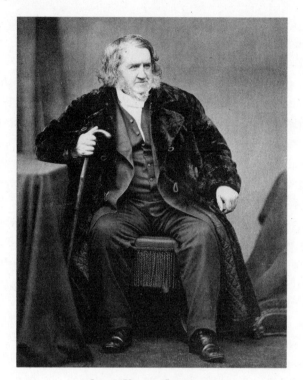

JAMES YOUNG SIMPSON.
COURTESY WELLCOME COLLECTION

Simpson shook Emily's hand and invited her to sit, clearly enjoying the effect on his startled patients when he addressed her—loudly and repeatedly—as "Dr. Blackwell." "There was one young English lady in particular," she recounted, "whose eyes really seemed as though they would never return to their ordinary size." That evening Emily accompanied Simpson and his wife and sister-in-law to their seaside retreat, Viewbank, near the fishing village of Newhaven on the Firth of Forth. After dinner they walked the rocky beach, peering into tide pools as Simpson pointed out limpets and jewel-toned anemones, hermit crabs and fossils—exactly the kind of ramble Emily liked best, in wondrous new surroundings. Mrs. Simpson and her sister dropped back discreetly, allowing the two doctors to talk. "I told him just what I wanted to do and he cordially offered to aid me in accomplishing [it]," Emily wrote. "It was past nine o'clock, but broad daylight, when, with very wet feet and very tired—but extremely satisfied with my first interview with Dr. S—I took leave, and they sent me home in their comfortable carriage."

Thus began Emily's transit in the crowded orbit of James Young Simpson. The next day she found the doctor at lunch, "surrounded by a perfect levee of friends who, any at least who were so inclined, sat down & took coffee &c with the most unceremonious freedom." All of them shifted their avid attention to this latest curiosity in Simpson's collection, talking to—and at—Emily until at last their host summoned his newest student to his busy consulting rooms.

Patients made their way to Queen Street starting at daybreak. The especially wealthy or notable were pointed straight up the front stairs by the ever-present Jarvis, and everyone else was directed to the waiting rooms at the back, to perch where they could after drawing a number in the order of their arrival. Most of these visitors were seen by Simpson's assistants, the man himself being out as much as he was in: lecturing at the university, making rounds at the Royal Maternity Hospital, or dashing between the grand homes of his wealthiest patients in his carriage. (His pocket pill case, with compartments for opium, morphine, and calomel, was labeled "Please return to 52 Queen Street" beneath the lid.) Any irritation at the endless waits and exorbitant fees, however, melted away in the presence of Simpson's equally outsized personality. He had the gift of attentiveness: every woman who came within range of his rosewood and ivory stethoscopes felt comforted and understood. "I believe I shall find my connexion with Dr S most fortunate," Emily wrote with cautious optimism. "He tells me to 'come about the house like one of the family' and see what he can show me."

Emily's work with Simpson proved to her that a patient's opinion of female doctors was usually in inverse proportion to her wealth. At Queen Street, even those who warmed to the idea of confiding their intimate troubles to a woman often balked at the impropriety of expanding the feminine sphere to include the medical profession. American women were a "fast set," they told each other, and women doctors clearly the "wild developments of an unreliable go-ahead nation."

Among the working class, Emily found no such issues. She took lodgings at Minto House, once an aristocratic residence, now converted to a small lying-in hospital in the crowded Old Town, with the steeple of Tron Kirk rising across the way. Minto House was a well-chosen address: it was cheap and respectable, and Emily could observe the half-dozen cases the hospital admitted each week and put her name on the list of students on call for "outcases." The indigent patients she saw there, and in the steep closes off the High Street and Canongate, cared not at all about the legitimacy or the propriety of her training.

Haring off down filthy passages and up narrow stone staircases in the wee hours to overcrowded rooms six or eight stories above the street could be unnerving, but the matron of the hospital pointed her toward the "most decent" patients. Emily became accustomed to her knock just as bedtime beckoned. "You wad'na be wanting another case tonight?" the matron would ask through the door. "There's an old body in haste for someone to her daughter—they live all alone in the house." In other words, there would be no degenerate males to threaten the lady doctor. Regretting the loss of sleep but grateful for these midnight opportunities,

EMILY'S TICKET FOR OBSERVATION AT EDINBURGH MATERNITY HOSPITAL, MINTO HOUSE, 1854.
COURTESY SCHLESINGER LIBRARY, RADCLIFFE INSTITUTE, HARVARD UNIVERSITY

Emily was sometimes out past three in the morning, though by then, in the Edinburgh summer, the sky was already growing light.

Her nocturnal experiences among the Old Town poor were an important complement to her daylight hours at Queen Street, where there was more watching than doing. Then again, James Young Simpson was worth watching. Now Jarvis waved her straight in and upstairs to Simpson's three connected consulting rooms, their walls covered in richly colored velvet. Simpson's own sanctum was the Red Room, while Emily generally stationed herself next door in the Green Room, waiting to be called upon to take a patient's history or even perform an examination—and keeping her lack of clinical experience carefully to herself. "I looked grave and did not tell him how very little I was able to detect during my first experiments," she confessed to Elizabeth. When Simpson sent her on a house call to a patient who needed to be bled for a gynecological complaint—requiring the application of leeches to her cervix—Emily was grateful no one from Simpson's practice was there to witness the clumsy job she made of it. "Today he has ordered leeches that I may apply them at his house," she worried. "How I shall succeed I don't know."

Most of Simpson's patients consulted him about ailments rather than pregnancy, and it was his innovation never to make a diagnosis without a pelvic examination. He took measurements of internal anatomy by means of a uterine sound—a curving metal probe engraved with calibrations—and felt for abnormalities of the uterus and cervix manually. "He makes a physical diagnosis of diseases of those organs just as he would of the chest, throat, &c," Emily wrote, surprised. "Nevertheless he is so skillful that in practice he conducts these examinations with little annoyance to his patients." Indeed, "his finger appears to have sight as well as feeling," she wrote with growing admiration. Simpson would have used his hands more than his eyes; though he was a pioneer in the use of the speculum, modesty dictated that much of the examination still happen out of sight, beneath the patient's skirts.

Emily had built up a degree of immunity toward charismatic medical men: from the start, she understood that Simpson's charm obscured the limits of his skill as a diagnostician and surgeon. "He has made in this way many remarkable cures—has killed a good many whom he says little about—has improved a very great many and has persuaded still more by his enthusiasm and firm conviction of the benefits of his treatment that they are much better when there was really not much difference," she wrote—an observer fully aware that the emperor was not always fully clothed. Emily had always chosen sincerity over glamour. Her professional reputation would be built on stronger science.

It did not escape her that Simpson performed his most daring experiments on charity patients. Mostly, however, his practice attracted the fashionable and the fortunate. "I have not seen a single case of syphilis or gonorrhea," Emily noted. "He seems not to have it among his patients." Some of their problems—various cancers, fibroid tumors—required surgical procedures with which Emily was familiar, but many were more ambiguous. "Through August & September he has a great many English patients," she wrote. "The gentlemen come north to shoot & their wives spend the time in Edinburgh being doctored!" Younger women presented with dysmenorrhea or amenorrhea: menstrual discomfort, or a failure to menstruate at all. Middle-aged matrons suffered from uterine prolapse—the toll of too many pregnancies, resulting in the displacement of the uterus into the vagina—or perimenopause, with its shooting pains and gushing periods.

Anna, similar to these vacationing patients in her concerns if not her cash flow, wrote to Emily seeking Simpson's advice. "Period generally about five weeks apart, but irregular; discharge always full of clots, some nearly black, like coagulated blood, some (smaller) bright red, like specks of raw meat," she reported with her usual graphic zeal. The list of symptoms went on for pages. "I should much like to know Dr. S's opinion of my case," she concluded. She did not ask for Emily's.

Popular gynecological remedies of the day ranged from hipbaths, prune juice, and leeches to the lower back, to mustard poultices, arsenic, suppositories, and fizzy lemonade. Simpson took a different approach. For many women, sometimes regardless of complaint, Simpson prescribed and inserted a "galvanic pessary" of his own invention: a copper disc with a stem of copper and zinc that he slid deftly into the cervix, and that patients professed not to feel at all. Pessaries were commonly used to support the internal organs of the pelvis and help keep them in

place; Simpson claimed his had additional electrochemical benefits. "I
have yet to be perfectly convinced that there is a real galvanic current at
work," wrote Emily. "I want to find some kind of galvanometer by which
to ascertain that fact."

One of the ladies who arrived to consult Simpson that summer was
Emily's own cousin-in-law Marie, Kenyon's wife. She was suffering from
a case of "stricture," a stenosis or narrowing of the cervix to which she
and Kenyon likely attributed their failure to conceive a child. Simpson
promised to cure her in a fortnight by surgically enlarging, or "dividing,"
the cervix, a procedure he performed frequently using an instrument
called a metrotome, an elongated switchblade with a hidden edge that
opened outward when the handles were squeezed. He inserted it into
the cervix, deployed the blade, and then swiftly pulled it out, scoring a
partial incision inside the length of the cervix. This was quickly repeated
on the opposite side. Sometimes it helped, and normal menstruation and
even conception followed. Sometimes, if the incisions were too deep, the
patient hemorrhaged.

Elizabeth, upon reading Emily's report of the situation, was dubious.
Wouldn't it be better to try dilation before surgery, stretching the cervix with a cylinder of waxed cotton, called a bougie, or a cone-shaped
piece of sponge, known as a sponge tent? Wouldn't surgical scarring only

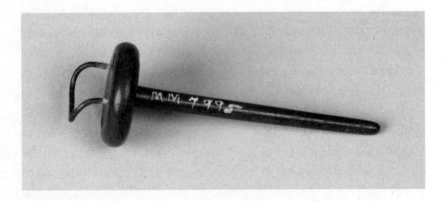

STEM PESSARY.
COURTESY NATIONAL MUSEUM OF HEALTH AND MEDICINE, PHOTO BY MATTHEW BREITBART

make the constriction worse? Elizabeth's concern was more professional than personal but no less correct; today cervical stenosis is not corrected with surgery.

The familial presence of Kenyon and Marie, and the rare opportunity to follow one of Simpson's patients over a longer term, made up for a disappointment that might otherwise have hastened Emily's departure from Edinburgh. Despite Simpson's support for her application to walk the female wards at Edinburgh's Royal Infirmary, permission was denied. Someone leaked the rejection to the press, and dozens of British newspapers reported on Emily's unprecedented request, some adding the patronizing untruth that Emily had "forthwith quitted the city in great chagrin at the ungallant reception she had experienced from her brother practitioners." Emily was irritated but undaunted. "I wish while they were about it they would have added the fact that I had been studying with Dr S for six months," she wrote. "Then I should think their notices might have done me a little good by making me known as the pupil of the first man in this department in Gt Britain."

Emily had intended to move on to London and Paris—to St. Bartholomew's and La Maternité—early in the fall, but although Marie endured her surgery without mishap, her recovery was difficult. Elizabeth encouraged Emily to remain in Edinburgh for Marie's convalescence, lest she provoke an "ineffaceable hostility" in Kenyon, after all his generosity to his doctor cousins. The repeated delays allowed Emily to accompany Simpson to the university for the graduation of the medical class. She watched the president touch each man's bowed head with an ancient flat black cap, murmuring *te medicinae doctorem creo*—"I create thee doctor of medicine"—as he handed him his diploma. Afterward, as Emily passed the platform on her way out, Simpson tapped her on the head with the ceremonial cap and recited the same invocation, "a joke which appeared much relished by his professional brethren," she wrote, unsure whether to laugh along.

She was coming to understand the limits of Simpson's esteem. "He rather likes the novelty of a woman Dr—has no objection to my being as far as possible indoctrinated into his view, and as I am sometimes useful does not dislike my being about his house and picking up what I can," she mused. "But he does not care about the matter—he will not in the least put himself to trouble to aid me."

The trouble Simpson had taken with Marie did not seem to aid her either—each treatment came with another setback. Inflammation, abscess, and ovaritis were compounded by the mouth sores caused by overuse of calomel, the mercury-based drug that Emily and other progressive practitioners had come to distrust. A frightening bout of peritonitis occurred while Simpson was out of town, and Emily spent a harrowing night at Marie's side, blistering her abdomen and soothing the pain with laudanum-infused poultices. "The whole case from beginning to end strikes me as a horrid barbarism," Elizabeth wrote from New York, voicing an opinion Emily refrained from stating explicitly. "I see every day that it is the 'heroic,' self reliant & actively self *imposing* practitioner, that excites a sensation & reputation; the rational and conscientious physician is not the famous one." Emily could not regret the extra months in Edinburgh—"I believe it has made the difference of life & death to Marie," she wrote, and acknowledged that taking responsibility for her cousin's care had "made a Dr of me"—but she was ready to learn from others.

The news that Elizabeth's friend Florence Nightingale was recruiting women to serve as nurses at Scutari in the Crimean War briefly piqued Emily's interest—not so much for the sake of clinical experience in the field, as in hopes of accessing new connections and opportunities within the medical establishment. Once she understood that Nightingale would hold the only position of authority, and that only in the sphere of nursing, she dropped the idea, "as I shall not of course accept a subordinate position." Elizabeth seconded this decision, unable to agree with Nightingale's conviction that women should be nurses and leave the doctoring to men. She was increasingly dismissive of the efforts that would soon make Florence Nightingale a household name. "She will probably thus sow her wild oats," Elizabeth wrote, "and come back and marry suitably to the immense comfort of her relations." An English correspondent of *The Una*, a new American monthly "devoted to the elevation of women," drew an explicit comparison between Nightingale's success and Emily's struggle. "It seems strange that it should be considered more unfeminine

for Miss Blackwell to visit sick women in the Infirmary of Edinburgh,"
the article pointed out, "than for Miss Nightingale to go to a foreign land,
and live among the horrors of war, for the purpose of attending to sick
men." The Blackwells were contributors to *The Una*, which was founded
by Elizabeth's friend Paulina Kellogg Wright. The anonymous correspondent might have been Anna.*

The days shortened in Edinburgh, its greens and grays cloaked occasionally in snow but more often in slush, the rotund Simpson swathed
always in a fur greatcoat, "in which article he is I verily believe broader
than he is long," Emily wrote. It was January 1855 before Marie was well
enough to travel, freeing Emily to leave for London. With her went a letter
from Simpson, proof that her extended stay had not been a waste of time.
"I do think you have assumed a position for which you are excellently
qualified and where you may, as a teacher, do a great amount of good,"
Simpson began.

> As this movement progresses, it is evidently a matter of the utmost
> importance that female physicians should be most fully and per-
> fectly educated, and I firmly believe that it would be difficult or
> impossible to find for that purpose anyone better qualified than
> yourself.
>
> I have had the fairest and best opportunity of testing the extent
> of your medical acquirements during the period of eight months
> when you studied with me, and I can have no hesitation in stating

---

* In the next issue of *The Una*, Elizabeth was quick to correct the aspersions
the anonymous correspondent cast, not on Nightingale, but on the leading physicians of Edinburgh. "Our English correspondent alluded to the injustice which Dr.
Emily Blackwell met with in Edinburgh," she wrote in an unsigned piece. After
pointing out that Emily had gone there to study not at the Royal Infirmary but with
James Young Simpson personally, she concluded, "It is therefore with feelings of
sincere gratitude that Dr. Emily Blackwell leaves the capital of true-hearted Scotland, and with the earnest hope that she may find elsewhere the same admirable
facilities in the pursuit of her chosen profession." Elizabeth was more interested
in elevating women than in criticizing men. And even with the Atlantic between
them, she could not resist quibbling with Anna.

to you—what I have often stated to others—that I have rarely met
with a young physician who was better acquainted with the ancient
and modern languages, or more learned in the literature, science,
and practical details of his profession.

Emily was pleased with this encomium, though its last line suggested
that Simpson, for all his ringing approbation, still found the idea of a
female physician uncomfortable. "Permit me to add that in your relation
to patients, and in your kindly care and treatment of them," he closed
reassuringly, "I have ever found you a most womanly woman."

⁓

CHAPTER 12

NEW FACES

"This medical solitude is really awful at times," Elizabeth confided to Emily in Edinburgh, in the spring of 1854. "I should thankfully turn to any decent woman to relieve it, if I could find one." Three days later she received a visit from a young woman with an austere severity about her dark hair and shadowed eyes, her strong jaw and wide mouth. By the end of the afternoon, Elizabeth knew she had found an ally.

Marie Zakrzewska was as ambitious and undaunted as Elizabeth herself. "With few talents and very moderate means for developing them," Zakrzewska would write in her memoir, "I have accomplished more than many women of genius and education would have done in my place, for the reason that confidence and faith in their own powers were wanting." Two years earlier she had achieved the impossible: appointment to the position of chief of midwifery at the University of Berlin. But her bad luck was as spectacular as her achievement, and on the day of her confirmation, her mentor and predecessor in the position died. Finding the politics and chauvinism of the medical community in Berlin untenable without his support, she emigrated.

She had spent the past year in New York trying and failing to continue her medical career. She spoke little English, but she would not consider nursing despite an invitation from a German doctor to serve as one. "I thanked him for his candor and kindness, but refused his offer," she wrote. "I could not condescend to be patronized in this way." After all, her mother had been a respected midwife, and her grandmother a veterinary

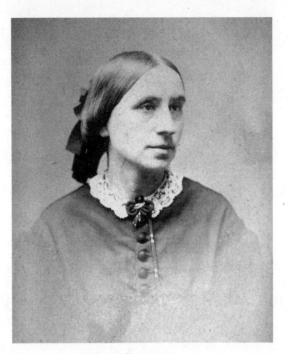

MARIE ZAKRZEWSKA.
COURTESY SCHLESINGER LIBRARY, RADCLIFFE INSTITUTE, HARVARD UNIVERSITY

surgeon. Her father was a scion of Polish nobility. Zakrzewska supported
herself and the siblings who had followed her to America with a shrewdly
managed business in knitted goods, and refused to concede her plans for
a medical future. Doubt was not something she suffered from.

Straining the limits of her German, Elizabeth listened to her visitor's
astonishing tale. Both as a physician and as an instructor, Marie Zakrzewska (pronounced Zak-SHEFF-ska and soon shortened, among the Blackwells, to "Dr. Zak") was better qualified than Elizabeth. "She knows far
more about syphilis than I do," Elizabeth noted, "and has performed version 4 times"—this last referring to the tricky process of turning a breech
baby in the womb before delivery. But penury and the language barrier
rendered Zakrzewska's credentials useless in America. Both her need for
Elizabeth's help and the depth of her experience ensured that she would
reflect well on her benefactor. Here, surely, was the perfect deputy. "There
is true stuff in her," Elizabeth wrote immediately to Emily, "and I am

going to do my best to bring it out." Perhaps Zakrzewska could obtain her M.D. at Cleveland Medical College, as Emily had. "My sister has just gone to Europe to finish what she began here," Elizabeth told her new protégée, "and you have come here to finish what you began in Europe."

Elizabeth's instant confidence in Zakrzewska stood in sharp contrast to her usual attitude toward women with medical ambitions, most notably Nancy Clark, currently the only female graduate of a regular medical college who wasn't a Blackwell. "Yesterday little Mrs. Clark called on me," she wrote to Emily. ("Little" Mrs. Clark was a year older than Emily. Neither Blackwell sister ever addressed her as "Dr.") "Hers is a good little nature, with some shrewdness too, but she wants independent strength." Elizabeth was unimpressed with Clark's narrow focus on obstetrics rather than the broader science of women's diseases and surgery. "This is evidently the natural tendency of present women," she tsked, "instinct and habit, not intelligent thought."

When Clark expressed her hope of joining Emily in Europe, both Blackwells were wary. "Would her companionship be unpleasant in any way?" Elizabeth asked her sister. "I don't want her to depend too entirely on me," Emily wrote back. "If she come and do at all well I will do all I can to help her." It was fine for Clark to pursue her vocation, in other words, as long as she did it somewhere else. "I find it as much as I can do to maintain a respectable standing medically among the physicians I meet at the Hospital & in Queen St," Emily told Elizabeth. "A more ignorant companion would certainly be no aid." The Blackwell sisters had no time or patience for any woman who might hinder their progress. And though neither mentioned it explicitly, it was not to Nancy Clark's advantage that, with her blue eyes and cupid's-bow mouth, she was undeniably attractive. She was also financially secure and had a doctor brother who planned to accompany her to Europe, further smoothing her path. In the Blackwells' opinion, Clark's seriousness—despite her diploma—was suspect. "I fancy she's a pretty little thing," Elizabeth wrote, "& that's about all."[*]

---

[*]   Clark studied successfully in Paris. On the voyage over, she made the acquaintance of Amos Binney, a recent widower. Within two years she married him and suspended her medical career; the couple had six children.

Yet since Clark's visit, Elizabeth had begun to question her own natural tendency toward solo superiority. In May she had attended a public lecture delivered by J. Marion Sims, a self-promoting surgeon known in his home state of Alabama for his experimental work repairing catastrophic vaginal and rectal fistula, the debilitating internal damage caused by prolonged obstructed labor. That he had practiced on enslaved women, without anesthesia, was something he downplayed to his contemporaries; later generations have condemned his ethics and questioned his legacy. Elizabeth knew him only as an ambitious outsider like herself, one who was rapidly drawing the attention of the New York medical establishment for a technique that could rescue afflicted women—prisoners in their homes, constantly leaking urine and feces—from a living death. (Sims's surgical technique is today of vital importance in restoring women to independence in the developing nations of East Asia and sub-Saharan Africa.)

Elizabeth was intrigued by Sims's stated goal of founding a hospital for the treatment of women—"much grander than anything I can hope to establish for many many years," she noted—and paid him a call, offering her support. "He is thoroughly in favor of women studying, and will treat them *justly*, which is all we want," she wrote to Emily, unaware of any irony. "He is a most fiery man, but with much sweetness nevertheless, honorable and a gentleman." His hospital, she hoped, would be an ideal place for female medical graduates to train.

Sims's apparent faith in medical women inspired Elizabeth to reexamine her own scornful attitudes toward her female peers. If exceptional women seemed scarce, it was Elizabeth's responsibility to find and cultivate more of them. "You must settle this matter, Miss Blackwell, for yourselves," Sims had told her: Women must elevate women and help each other "contribute to journals, get practice, show their force." His advice was dismissive—but also very much in line with Elizabeth's own thinking. She had never believed that the progress of women was the responsibility of men.

Connecting Zakrzewska to Emily's allies in Cleveland, Elizabeth smoothed her path to admission at Cleveland Medical College in the fall. Meanwhile the newcomer from Berlin was the ideal assistant at the dispensary in Little Germany, where her native language was an asset. Not to mention her company. Elizabeth felt the imperative of maintaining her tiny institution as at once credential, laboratory, and rallying point for women pursuing medicine, but the daily reality was a trial. "My Dispensary business is rather wearisome," she confided to Emily. "As it stands it seems to be of no special use except to give me a long hot walk." That summer indoor temperatures reached ninety degrees. From cooler Edinburgh, Emily sent encouragement: "I look on the little dispensary with interest as affording us the means of practice among the poor and then testing new methods and making improvements." The daily, steady effort of medical practice left Elizabeth unsatisfied and impatient. It attracted Emily profoundly.

~

Everything that Emily learned from James Young Simpson she reported faithfully in her letters to New York, filling the margins with sketches of instruments and techniques. She even sent a small pessary, which Elizabeth immediately tried out on a patient, unguided by anything other than Emily's description. It took a few attempts and a little improvisation. "She cried oh just as I judge it entered the cervix, & oh again as it passed the cervix—she said it was not pain, but like a *little electric shock* each time," Elizabeth reported. "It has been an immense satisfaction to have something rational that I could do." Rejoicing in Emily's famous mentor, she exhorted her sister to embrace her fortunate circumstances. "I do increasingly think that your position with the popular Dr Simpson, is a most rare chance for becoming known, both in America & Europe," she wrote. "I very much wish you could stay there a year, thoroughly recognized as his pupil."

But Elizabeth's insistence that Emily remain abroad meant her own isolation in New York would continue. Marie Zakrzewska left for Cleveland Medical College in the fall of 1854; in her absence, Elizabeth closed the dispensary. Its limited hours had made it difficult to connect with the women of the neighborhood; on some afternoons, Elizabeth waited alone and in vain. Rather than spend her modest resources on rent for both residential and underused professional space, she decided, with the help of a generous loan from sympathetic friends, to buy a house at 79

East Fifteenth Street, at that time located between Irving Place and Third Avenue. Without a disapproving landlord, she would be free to see private patients and carry on her dispensary work on her own terms. It surely did not escape Dr. Blackwell's notice that her new house backed onto the Fourteenth Street building that housed University Medical College, founded by New York University in 1841. For six years she would live within sight of its rear windows, even renting rooms to its students for extra cash. It would be another six and a half decades before New York University admitted a woman as a medical student.

Elizabeth was relieved to own a permanent home, and grateful for Marian's housekeeping in the three years since her arrival in New York. But whether as helpmeet or intellectual companion, mild Marian could not satisfy Elizabeth's craving for connection. Having eschewed marriage and motherhood for a career that existed more on paper than in practice, Elizabeth felt herself sliding toward depression. "I found my mind morbidly dwelling upon ideas in a way neither good for soul or body," she wrote.

Passive resignation, however, had never been her style. One day in late September, Elizabeth boarded a ferry bound for Randall's Island, northeast of Manhattan. Her destination was the juvenile department of the New York Almshouse, known as the Nurseries. She was going to pick out a child.

A five-minute walk from the ferry landing brought Elizabeth to a group of buildings built half a dozen years earlier, facing eastward into the salty breeze off Flushing Bay. Here lived more than a thousand children, ranging in age from three to fifteen. Some had been scooped from the streets, others deposited by desperate parents. Many were the children of recent immigrants: an "Infant Congress of many nations," as one observer recorded, noting—in the unsettling cultural shorthand of the day—the round faces of the Germans, the "dogged look" of the English, the "pleasure-loving lips" of the French, the "whimsically grinning" Irish. It was a "great depot of small humanities," Elizabeth wrote, "such forlorn children, assembled under harsh taskmasters, fast becoming idiots or criminals." Inmates of the Nurseries went to school, but their training in the sewing workshops and the vegetable gardens was more important. The best way off the island was through indentured labor.

"I must tell you of a little item that I've introduced into my own domestic economy in the shape of a small girl," Elizabeth announced to Emily, "whom I mean to train up into a valuable domestic, if she prove on sufficient trial to have the qualities I give her credit for." The transactional tone is startling, especially when juxtaposed with the rosy sentimentality of some of Elizabeth's writings on motherhood. But Elizabeth was less in search of a daughter than a useful companion. The small girl she chose—after several visits to look over the options—was Katharine Barry, a dark-haired, dark-eyed orphan of Irish parentage, thought to be about six years old. "She was a plain, and they said stupid child though good, and they all wondered at my choice," Elizabeth continued. "I gave a receipt for her, and the poor little thing trotted after me like a dog."

Removed from the institution, "Kitty" proved bright and diligent: "She is a sturdy little thing, affectionate and with a touch of obstinacy which will turn to good account later in life," Elizabeth wrote approvingly. It was cheerful to wake in the morning to a child singing "Oh Susanna" as she waited for permission to leave her bed. She was instructed to address her new guardian as "Dr. Elizabeth."

Elizabeth refreshed herself in the presence of Kitty's innocence. Introducing her charge to the idea of the divine one Sunday soon after her arrival, she was charmed by the child's response. "Oh nice God," Kitty chirped. "I like God, doctor, don't you?" Here was a stray soul to guide toward a better life, a tiny proof of all Elizabeth hoped to do for women. She liked to retell the story of Kitty's reaction the first time she was introduced to a male physician: "Doctor," she exclaimed, "how very odd it is to hear a *man* called Doctor!" Elizabeth enjoyed the challenge of this new experiment. "I have had, and I shall have a great deal of trouble with her, for she is full of intense vitality," she wrote after a year of Kitty's company, "but the results are worth the trouble."

Living with a child forced Elizabeth out of her single-mindedness. "Oh Doctor, wouldn't it be pleasant in the country today?" Kitty chirped one Sunday morning, and once she found her sunbonnet and filled her pockets with apples, off they set in the railcars that traveled up Second Avenue. A half hour's ride brought them to Jones Wood on the East River—bucolic fields of buttercups and groves of tall oaks that, in the next century, would become the massive medical complex of New York–Presbyterian Hospital, Memorial Sloan-Kettering Cancer Center, and Rockefeller University. Elizabeth settled herself in the shade to indulge in a long letter to her London friends, while Kitty floated woodchip "boats" in a pond nearby. "My friends here say they cannot imagine me, without this small shadow," Elizabeth told Barbara Leigh Smith and Bessie Parkes in London.

Kitty, in return, enjoyed a secure if circumscribed position within the Blackwell clan, appreciated and educated—Elizabeth sent her to the new and progressive Twelfth Street School for Girls—but never permitted to marry or pursue her own path. In a memoir dictated after Elizabeth's death in 1910, Kitty remembered her first encounter with the "very pleasant-voiced lady" who appeared on Randall's Island to claim her. "She came at the sunset-hour, and found me with my hands clasped behind me, gazing at the setting sun. She asked me, would I be her little girl?" For the next fifty years, Kitty would embrace the role of acolyte.

Elizabeth took comfort in these additions to her household: Zakrzewska, a sister doctor to stand in for Emily; Kitty, a daughter to compensate for her childlessness. She was less pleased with two new family members whose choice lay outside her control.

⁓

While their sisters were building medical reputations in New York and the capitals of Europe, Henry and Sam had been—quite literally—minding the store, their latest venture a Cincinnati hardware business. One day in the fall of 1850, a small woman with large eyes in a round face approached the counter. She introduced herself as Lucy Stone.

As a dedicated reader of the abolitionist press, Henry knew exactly who she was. The first woman in Massachusetts to earn a bachelor's degree, from Ohio's Oberlin College, Stone had been lecturing on slavery and women's rights for the last two years, sharing stages with Elizabeth Cady Stanton, Susan B. Anthony, and William Lloyd Garrison, whose radical views on abolition she heartily endorsed. Henry—who had been falling in and out of

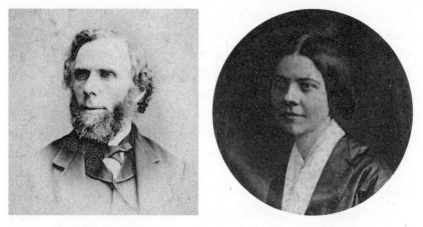

HENRY BLACKWELL. LUCY STONE.

COURTESY SCHLESINGER LIBRARY, RADCLIFFE INSTITUTE, HARVARD UNIVERSITY

love regularly since he was a teenager—liked Stone's politics, her famously bell-like voice, and her smile. But she was thirty-two and he was twenty-five. She might be a better match for his older brother Sam, he thought.

Three years later Henry watched Stone speak at antislavery meetings in New York and Boston, and though he balked at her Bloomer costume, he was smitten. "I decidedly prefer her to any lady I ever met," he told Sam. No matter that this lady saw the institution of marriage as another form of bondage, in which a woman's right to personhood and property was erased. In Lucy Stone, Henry had found a woman he could admire as profoundly as he admired his sisters.

A lifetime with those unbending sisters served him well in his ardent, dogged pursuit. His first step was a letter of recommendation from his father's old friend Garrison, proving his abolitionist bona fides. Then he set out for the town of West Brookfield, Massachusetts, where the itinerant activist had paused for a visit to her family. Arriving at the Stone farm unannounced, Henry found his beloved standing on the kitchen table, whitewashing the ceiling. She declined his offer of help. Undeterred, he waited for her to finish and spent the afternoon walking at her side.

On his way home to Cincinnati, he sent her two books: a volume of Plato and Elizabeth's *The Laws of Life,* the collection of lectures she had published a year earlier. How better to demonstrate his commitment to pioneering women? "I think you will like [Elizabeth's] lectures very much," he told Stone. Their courtship would continue for two years, while Henry tried to convince her that marriage need not be a prison. "If both parties cannot study more, think more, feel more, talk more & work more than they could alone," he declared, "I will remain an old bachelor & adopt a Newfoundland dog or a terrier as an object of affection."

Henry put himself at Stone's service, helping to arrange western speaking engagements and welcoming her to the Blackwell home in Walnut Hills every time she traveled within range of Cincinnati. He expanded his reforming energies to include women's rights and even made his first feminist speech, at the fourth National Woman's Rights Convention in Cleveland. But the turning point came in the fall of 1854. The Supreme Court of Ohio had ruled that any slave who entered the state—even if traveling with their master—had the right to freedom upon request. At an antislavery meeting just outside Cincinnati, Henry and the other attendees learned that a train would soon be passing through, carrying a Tennessee couple accompanied by an enslaved girl. Henry headed a party that boarded the train, asked the eight-year-old girl if she wanted to be free, and when she said yes, removed her forcibly from her owners.

For weeks afterward, Kentuckians stopped by Henry's store to stare at his face. A bounty of ten thousand dollars had been placed on his head across the river, and they wanted to make sure they recognized him if he crossed over. Gossip circulated that Henry had assaulted the white woman on the train. While he and his associates celebrated the girl's liberation, others saw it as an act of theft. Henry himself was somewhat startled at his own temerity and dismayed at the dent his activism put in his hardware business, none too robust to begin with.

But Lucy Stone was thrilled. "I am very glad and proud too, dear Harry of the part you took in that rescue," she wrote. "I exceedingly desire true relations for both of us." Perhaps this impulsive, devoted young man really could share her life without compromising her ideals. Within two months, they were engaged. Henry assured her that he would never dictate the disposition of her earnings, the location of their residence, or the nature of her role as his wife. He also assuaged qualms she would not discuss in a letter: "You shall choose when, where & how often you shall become a mother," he wrote.

Henry did not relax his astounding egalitarian ardor after his beloved said yes. "Lucy, I wish I could take the position of the wife under the law & give you that of a husband," he wrote. Even before their engagement was official, he had made her a second, more extraordinary proposal: at their wedding, he would read a public protest against the laws that deprived married women of their rights. "I wish, as a husband, to renounce all the privileges which the law confers upon me, which are not strictly mutual," he told her. "Help me to draw one up."

The reaction of his sisters to the engagement of their liveliest brother was mixed. Elizabeth, whose opinion Henry prized most, reserved judgment. Miss Stone came from the tribe of woman suffrage advocates she had always disdained. "We view life from such different sides," she hedged to Henry. "I thought discussion would be unavailing until personal affection had linked us together." To Emily, Elizabeth worried that Henry's adoration of this outspoken woman was a sign of his "morbid craving for distinction"—an ironic projection of her own hunger for recognition, compounded by the irritating sense that she was rapidly losing influence over her younger brother. "We must absolutely take the brightest view we can," she wrote with a sigh, "as it seems to be inevitable, and if Lucy will soften her heresies, it may be a very happy union." Emily was similarly cautious. "I hope that intercourse with our family may induce her to lay aside some of the ultra peculiarities that are so disagreeable to us," she wrote back, wary of Stone's exhibitionist extremism. "Certainly we will not allow it to break the strong feeling that has always existed among us if possible."

The nine Blackwell siblings now ranged in age from twenty-two to nearly forty; it was hard to imagine opening their circle to a stranger for the first time. Anna, having renounced America permanently, wrote a screed expressing shock that Henry planned to marry an American— which he, in a moment of Blackwellian blindness to his fiancée's feelings, blithely forwarded to Stone. But the family members still in Walnut Hills warmed to their future sister-in-law with each of her visits. "Sam says she is a most pleasant companion and very brilliant in conversation," Marian reported. "Ellen loves her heartily & says she belongs to us by nature. Mother cannot help liking her in spite of her dreadful heresies, and George in his cautious critical way remarks that his only objection is to her ultraism." Stone's feminism was fine, her abolitionist opinions all to the good, but the Blackwells had always stopped short of "ultra"-anything. They might have embraced ideas toward the radical end of the political spectrum, but they insisted upon a decorum that Stone, in their eyes, had abandoned the first time she wore bloomers in public.

Henry, guileless as always, sent a draft of his marriage protest to Elizabeth and asked for her comments. "She has very good taste," he assured Lucy, "& may make some suggestions of value." He had not shared a roof with his sister in nearly a decade; perhaps he had forgotten her horror of airing private matters in public, and her bluntness when she thought he was wrong. "I protest against a protest," she snapped in response, "and my short answer to 'Why?' would be, it's foolish, in bad taste." Henry's intention of making a political statement at his own wedding she condemned as "vulgar vanity." Marriage was an intimate act, she insisted. "Do not take the human nature out of it, by crushing it with platforms and principles." But even she could see that this time Henry would not be dissuaded. Having made her case against bad taste, she followed it with several paragraphs of detailed edits. The final draft of the protest incorporated most of them.

On May 1, 1855, with the sun barely up and the dew still wet on the Stone family's fields, Henry Blackwell and Lucy Stone stood before the Unitarian minister Thomas Wentworth Higginson and recited their marriage vows, which conspicuously omitted the word *obey*. A moment earlier Henry had read their protest, declaring that "this act on our part implies no sanction of, nor promise of voluntary obedience to such of the present laws of marriage, as refuse to recognize the wife as an independent, rational being, while they confer upon the husband an injurious and unnatural superiority." Newspapers across the country reprinted it.

The bride wore a silk dress in the dusky shade known as "ashes of roses." Though she would make history by continuing to use her maiden name after the wedding, in a letter to her closest friend she described

the event as "putting Lucy Stone to death." Her love for Henry was not
in question, but her continuing uncertainty about the institution of marriage gave her a migraine on her wedding day.

~

The friend to whom Lucy Stone had written of her wedding with such
black humor was a woman named Antoinette Brown. They had met a
decade earlier as students at Oberlin, where Brown—seven years
younger—had been warned upon arrival that Stone was "a young woman
of strange and dangerous opinions." Brown, possessed of opinions of her
own, immediately sought her out. The two became passionate allies,
often sharing a bed to continue their debates long into the night. Though
Brown held less militant views than Stone on abolition, religion, and
fashion, her belief in women's equality was just as bold. Her lifelong
ambition was to preach, and in the fall of 1853 she became the pastor of a
tiny Congregational church in South Butler, New York—the first woman

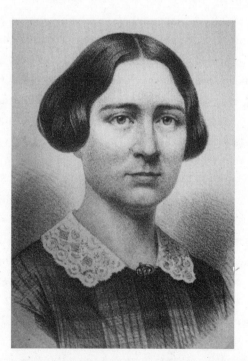

ANTOINETTE BROWN, LATER BLACKWELL.
COURTESY SCHLESINGER LIBRARY, RADCLIFFE INSTITUTE, HARVARD UNIVERSITY

in America to be ordained as a minister. Henry had tried to persuade her to officiate at his wedding to Lucy.

Henry embraced his Lucy's dearest friend as another sister, then strove to make her just that. When Sam passed near South Butler on a trip from Cincinnati to Boston, Henry encouraged his brother to pay a call. Sam did not regret the detour. "I forgot my drenched boots and the rain and wind without while busily talking with her for 3 hours," he recorded. "She seems to me to be a lady of judgment, very kind disposition and with the best principles and high aims," he continued. "I enjoyed the visit exceedingly."

Even as she won her own pulpit, Brown had begun to question the faith that required her to threaten the unconverted with hellfire, or condemn an unmarried woman who bore a child. Before a year was out, she left her congregation and joined her friend Lucy as a more secular kind of preacher. Like Lucy, when in Cincinnati she stayed with the Blackwells. And Sam, following Henry's example, began the patient process of convincing "Nettie" that marriage and women's equality were not incompatible. By Christmas 1855, Sam was able to write, "The love of her whom I love best on earth, though long withheld, is now wholly mine." Nettie, having learned from Lucy of the Blackwells' penchant for oversharing, gently cautioned her fiancé against forwarding her letters to his sisters. "They are for you, Sam dear, and full of haste, bad spelling, and confidences," she told him. "Elizabeth can easily get acquainted for herself."

Sam Blackwell and Antoinette Brown were married at her home in Henrietta, New York, on January 24, 1856. Sam borrowed Henry's white wedding vest, though he preferred his own sober black coat to Henry's dashing mulberry one. The wedding was less freighted with politics than Henry and Lucy's, though Sam and Nettie declared themselves joint owners of any property. The officiant was Nettie's magistrate father, and the event was sealed with "spirited miscellaneous kissing." Lucy sent her congratulations, joking that Sam "alone of all men in the world has a Divine wife."

The unmarried Blackwells were not the only ones ambivalent about these two weddings. Susan B. Anthony, who felt a sisterhood with both brides, scolded each of them for leaving her to work alone. Lucy, resolutely denying her own marriage misgivings, scolded her back. "You are a little wretch to even *intimate* that we are nothing now," she wrote to Anthony. "Let me tell you as a secret that if you are ever married, you will find that there is just as much of you, as before." Though both Lucy and Nettie would struggle to balance work with family, in Henry and Sam they had found men unusually well suited for the new role of feminist husband. The two brothers had been supporting professional women, emotionally and financially, since their teens. "I wish we had another brother for you, Susan," Lucy teased. "Would we not have a grand household then?" But Howard had moved to England, and George was only twenty-three.

~

Henry and Sam's marriages might have felt like a threat to the Blackwells' clannish bonds, but the addition of Lucy and Nettie actually brought the family closer, at least geographically. Neither sister-in-law considered Cincinnati a convenient base for a lecturing life. Meanwhile Elizabeth and Marian had more space in New York than they needed— even with the addition of Kitty and the return of Marie Zakrzewska with her medical degree. By the end of 1856, Henry and Sam had sold their business and packed up their mother, and nearly all the Blackwells currently on the American side of the Atlantic converged at the house on Fifteenth Street.

Kitty goggled in amazement one autumn evening as fifteen carts pulled up in front of the house, bringing all the Blackwell possessions from Walnut Hills, including the piano and a tin box containing Hannah Blackwell's precious wedding china. The house was suddenly filled to overflowing. Before long, Sam and Henry would establish new households across the Hudson in New Jersey; for now, though, Elizabeth's home was a perfect place for the arrival of the newest Blackwell of all.

Kitty was on her way to bed one chilly night when she met Dr. Zak coming downstairs. "Would you like to see a baby?" Zakrzewska asked.

"Yes!" Kitty gasped. "Where did it come from?"

"It came out of a cabbage," Zakrzewska told her, choosing to defer the start of Kitty's health education.

"Nothing so nice as a baby ever came out of a cabbage!" the child retorted, rushing upstairs. But there on a pillow in front of the fire was a tiny infant, and Sam was crying out "Don't you step on my baby!"

On November 7, 1856, Dr. Elizabeth and Dr. Zak had attended the birth of Nettie and Sam's daughter, a difficult breech delivery eased by the use of James Young Simpson's discovery, chloroform. "Thanks to our judicious doctors and to our Heavenly Father, all is well with both my Nettie and our tiny," Sam wrote with relief. Two days later the extended clan gathered at Nettie's bedside while Sam read out a list of girls' names. (Nettie was either too generous or too exhausted to object to this being a group decision.) "I was in favor of her being called Mary," Kitty remembered. But the Crimean War had just ended, and Florence Nightingale was now second only to Queen Victoria as the most famous woman in the world. Regardless of Aunt Elizabeth's philosophical differences with her illustrious namesake, the first Blackwell of the next generation would be Florence. Nettie and Sam went on to raise five daughters, two of whom—though not Florence—earned medical degrees.

Little Floy was barely two weeks old when one more Blackwell arrived at Fifteenth Street: Emily, home from Europe at last. After Edinburgh she had lingered for months in London, trapped by family drama: Marie's convalescence and Kenyon's ill health; cousin Sam's ill-fated love for Bessie Parkes; business troubles that forced her brother Howard to seek employment in India. All these unlucky Blackwells had looked to Emily for strength—a new and not unwelcome role for the even-tempered sixth sibling. "I have experienced for the first time the strange triumphant happiness there is in standing firm in a storm supporting those who are weaker," she wrote.

Meanwhile she had attracted respectful recognition in London—at St. Bartholomew's, Clement Hue had praised her "ardent love of knowledge, her indefatigable zeal in the examination of disease, her sound judgment and kind feeling"—and had finally reached Paris, where she walked in Elizabeth's footsteps, shadowing prominent surgeons, studying at La Maternité (without mishap) and even visiting Hippolyte Blot, now a father of two. She also came in for the same kind of snark Elizabeth had earlier endured. *Punch* had chuckled all over again, running a caricature of "Dr. Emily" as a mannish woman in bloomers, squinting diagnosti-

cally at a lapdog clutched by a wasp-waisted young maiden. "The surname of the lady is immaterial, and, moreover, it may be hoped, will
speedily be exchanged for another," the item read, "since if to be cherished in sickness is an important object in marriage, a wife who in her
own person combines the physician with the nurse must be a treasure
indeed." The joke was too stale to sting.

Confident in her work, Emily could ignore her critics. "The European
hospitals will never be closed to women again," she told Elizabeth. "My
studies here will do something to help others." She was tempted to establish herself in Britain but understood the basic paradox: she was welcome
precisely because the "old fogies" assumed that as soon as she completed
her studies, she would leave.

Emily reached New York in time for the merriest Christmas the
Blackwells had enjoyed in years. The oldest and youngest siblings were
absent: Anna was writing chatty dispatches for American newspapers
from Paris, Howard was on his way to Bombay, artistic Ellen was now

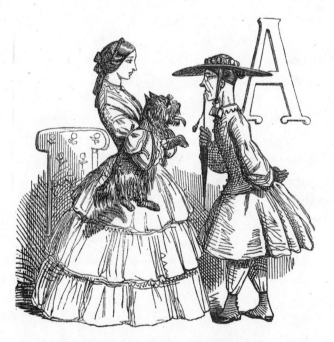

CARICATURE OF EMILY IN *PUNCH*, 1856.
COURTESY NEW YORK SOCIETY LIBRARY

studying painting in Europe with the likes of John Ruskin and Rosa Bon-heur, and George was lingering in Cincinnati. Lucy was on the road as usual. But crammed together at Fifteenth Street, the rest of the reunited and expanded clan indulged in roast beef and plum pudding. After din-ner, grandmother Hannah and steadfast Marian, Elizabeth and Dr. Zak and little Kitty, Sam and Nettie and baby Florence, Emily and Henry set-tled snugly in the parlor, singing favorite songs and reading aloud from Robert Browning's latest volume of poetry, *Men and Women*. There was a satisfying sense of return from western exile and European experiments to a base from which to launch larger plans.

Even from France, anti-American Anna could sense the consolidation. "As things have turned out, & the band being now increased by our very excellent and welcome new sisters, I can no longer even wish you all to return," she wrote with resignation, "but earnestly hope, on the contrary, that you may now really take root."

~

CHAPTER 13

INFIRMARY

"I have no turn for benevolencies," Elizabeth had written to Henry at the end of 1855. "I feel neither love nor pity for men, for individuals—they may starve, cut each other's throats or perform any other gentle diversion suitable to the age—without any attempt to stop them on my part, for their own sakes. But I have boundless love & faith in Man, and will work for the race day and night." Emily and Marie Zakrzewska were back in New York, each possessed of a diploma and substantial experience, and both of them were more interested in the practice of medicine than was Elizabeth herself. Let them manage the daily work of women's health. Elizabeth would focus on the grander goal of women's medical education, embracing the role she had always preferred: idealist.

There was still almost nowhere for a newly fledged female M.D. to acquire the practical experience that medical school did not provide. Elizabeth's hopes in J. Marion Sims and his Woman's Hospital had faded. "Dr. Sims has never called to see me, and is evidently striving to keep in with the conservatives," she wrote with disappointment to Emily. Sims had succeeded in establishing his Woman's Hospital in 1855, at Madison Avenue and Twenty-ninth Street, specializing in his signature fistula surgery; like Elizabeth, he understood that as an outsider he would be able to apply and refine his new ideas only in an institution of his own. It was now clear, however, that what Sims aimed to elevate was not the stature of women in medicine but the stature of J. Marion Sims. His Woman's Hospital was staffed entirely by men, and though he had recruited thirty prominent women as a board of managers, Elizabeth was not fooled. "Half are doctors' wives, the stiffest of the stiff," she complained, "the rest the richest & best known New Yorkers, but all of the fashionable unreformatory set." These society ladies were not going to solve the problem of practical training for female medical students. And thanks to the women's medical schools in Philadelphia and Boston, not to mention the Eclectic schools that now admitted women—however much the Blackwells might disdain the rigor of their programs—there were a growing number of female graduates to train.

Instead of cultivating more powerful men as trustees, Elizabeth now turned to their wives and sisters and daughters. Where Sims expected his lady managers to play a philanthropic and decoratively feminine role, Elizabeth asked her supporters to participate more actively. On Thursday evenings, they met at her house to discuss her educational mission for women and learn how best to promote it, as her disciples.

Elizabeth crystallized her thoughts in an address, "On the Medical Education of Women," that she published in December 1855 as a pamphlet that could serve both as a professional calling card and as a fundraising appeal. Her thesis, elegant in its simplicity, used the obvious example of obstetrics. "Women have always presided over the birth of children," she wrote—but in this enlightened age of forceps and chloroform, science had advanced beyond the unwritten wisdom of traditional midwifery. "The midwife must give place to the physician," Elizabeth declared. "Woman therefore must become physician."

Mindful of her audience—wives and mothers, not medical students—Elizabeth framed her project in terms they could embrace. "The grandest name of woman is mother—the noblest thought of womanhood is maternity," she assured them. However: "The woman who cares but for her own children, is a feeble caricature of womanhood, not its true representative." To realize the fullest grandeur of motherhood, women must extend their nurturing instincts beyond the fireside. Her vision neatly included both the female medical students who chose career over marriage and the society ladies whose generosity could support their training.

The benefits were obvious, Elizabeth explained. Medicine would be a broad new field of endeavor for unmarried ladies. As physicians, these women would in turn inspire and elevate a better class of nurses, a group Elizabeth continued to disparage: "their ignorance, faithlessness and inefficiency at present is proverbial." Women doctors would also, of course, rescue female patients from the "unnatural and monstrous" necessity of confessing intimate symptoms to men—or worse, in the case of inpatients, serving as case studies for male medical students, a terrible exposure that led to "bitter mortification" and "a deadening of sensibility." Even as she spoke on behalf of helpless hospital patients, however, Elizabeth seemed to fault the wealthier women who sought advice from doctor after doctor for their ailments, showing an "utter want of delicacy" in subjecting themselves to repeated examinations. And even as she feared for the "moral purity" of female patients both rich and poor, she laid no blame for this peril at the feet of her male colleagues, who had her "utmost confidence and respect." In aligning herself with the men, she implicated herself in their misogyny. Then again, she had never set out to *like* women—only to lead the way toward a world in which they were recognized.

It was not enough for women to earn medical degrees, she continued. Just as it was impossible to become a proficient musician by listening to someone discuss music theory, it was likewise impossible to emerge from the lecture hall a competent physician. All five senses must be tuned to the observation of disease, over months of repeated experience. "A system of medical education without continual practical instruction is an absurdity, or rather an impossibility," Elizabeth wrote. And while she had hoped her own example as a student—confirmed by Emily's repetition of her feat—would open the doors of all hospitals to women, she was wiser now.

"There is but one way of meeting the imperative need of our women for hospital instruction," she declared. "We must create a hospital to meet the want." Not a dispensary—a hospital, where female students could learn without restriction. "I know the difficulty of this undertaking," Elizabeth told the assembled ladies. It would require a huge effort of both publicity and fund-raising, guided by "sound judgment and good taste"—all of which she trusted her listeners to provide. She proposed the grand sum of ten thousand dollars and announced that the Thursday meetings would become sewing circles in preparation for a charity bazaar.

Marie Zakrzewska attended faithfully, though with growing impatience. The canny entrepreneurial spirit that had kept her afloat upon her arrival in New York recoiled from what she saw as Elizabeth's hopeless impracticality. "There was scarcely any life in these gatherings," she grumbled, "and when I saw ladies come week after week to resume the knitting of a baby's stocking (which was always laid aside again in an hour or two, without any marked progress), I began to doubt whether the sale of these articles would ever bring ten thousand cents." On Sundays, she and Elizabeth escaped for long walks on Staten Island or the Jersey side of the Hudson, refreshing themselves with sunsets and wildflowers. Their deepening friendship allowed Zakrzewska to suggest a more sensible plan: the foundation, for now, of a more modest "nucleus hospital."

Fund-raising began in earnest. Emily collected contributions from friends in Europe; Zakrzewska made trips to Boston and Philadelphia, explaining the project to progressive supporters of the female medical colleges in those cities. Even among allies, the idea of a woman practicing in a hospital was a hard sell. "If you must talk on hospitals, do not mention women doctors," one Fifth Avenue matron requested—though thanks to Florence Nightingale, it was perfectly fashionable to discuss nursing. A circular printed in June 1856 softened Elizabeth's pitch, insisting that while the new hospital would indeed be a place for women to receive medical training, it was also "designed to meet another want, not supplied by Hospitals generally, viz: an earnest religious influence on the patients." It would be a Christian charity above all, staffed by respectable nurses, in which "scientific instruction will always be subordinate to the welfare of the patient; each individual no matter how degraded, being regarded as a human soul as well as a body."

The house on Fifteenth Street filled with boxes and baskets of handiwork to sell at the bazaar. "I shall have an Art, Book, Fancy, Useful, and Refreshment table," Elizabeth decided—but the problem, as the ladies of Elizabeth's committee quickly discovered, was that no one would rent them a room in which to set up their tables, even if they paid in advance. At the last minute they secured a space at the Stuyvesant Institute, the very Broadway venue that had hosted J. Marion Sims's 1855 lecture announcing his women's hospital. This seemed auspicious—except that the ladies would not be permitted to use the lecture hall. They were welcome, however, to an attic loft three flights above, where nailheads stuck up from the floorboards and bare rafters ascended into the gloom.

Donated rugs and drapes and borrowed chandeliers soon dressed the space, and evergreen boughs hid the raw beams. For four days in December 1856, the Ladies' Fair charged ten cents admission for the privilege of shopping, and the *New-York Tribune* reported takings of more than $1,100 toward a projected $5,000, "the sum required to rent and furnish a suitable house for the accommodation and support of forty patients, with a dispensary for outside patients attached."

The paper also provided a satisfying clarification. "This enterprise must not be confounded with the Institution known as the Woman's Hospital, located on Madison avenue, which is now in operation, as that is a Woman's Hospital under the care, exclusively, of male practitioners," noted the reporter, referring to Sims's new establishment, "while this Institution is to be under the care and control of female physicians, with some of our eminent medical men attached as consulting advisers."

Sims had recently disappointed the Blackwells again. Despite Elizabeth's dim opinion of the women on his board, and perhaps due to her inspiring example, they had included in their bylaws a clause stipulating that Sims must hire a female assistant surgeon. The obvious candidate was Emily Blackwell, who upon her return from Europe was the best qualified—in fact, the only—female surgeon in New York. Sims ignored her, flouted his own board, and appointed Thomas Addis Emmet, a well-connected young surgeon whom Sims knew socially. The Blackwells' disillusionment with Sims was complete.

The *Tribune* was Horace Greeley's paper, and the bias of the article was clear. The Blackwells' project, it noted, had technically *predated* the founding of Sims's hospital, which was already receiving funds from the state; surely a similar level of support for the Blackwells would shortly follow. There it was, in print: affirmation that the Blackwells' goal was valid and should be realized, written by someone who seemed familiar with Elizabeth's "On the Medical Education of Women." Women, the *Tribune* declared, had always been healers—and now "manifested the capacity and the inclination to resume their old place in the modern profession."

⁊‍

The brick house on the corner of Bleecker and Crosby had been the home of the Roosevelt family, the branch whose most famous scion, later in the century, would be christened Franklin Delano. A remnant of privilege, it was built in the Dutch style with four chimneys and a dash of architectural elegance in its quoined corners. Its painted shutters and neatly swept stoop looked toward the fading elegance of Bond Street and the Corinthian flourishes of Colonnade Row, but the best addresses had already migrated farther north, to Washington Square and up Fifth Avenue. To the south and east, in the notorious slum of Five Points, wood-framed tenements sported broken windows like black eyes, and ramshackle stairways climbed crookedly up exterior walls from squalid cellars to airless attics, every square foot of living space claimed by too many of the city's most recent arrivals. On a visit a decade earlier, Charles Dickens had toured it with a police escort. "Debauchery," he wrote, "has made the very houses prematurely old." The Blackwells' New York Infirmary for Indigent Women and Children stood on the threshold between high and low, patron and patient.

Having raised just enough to secure the lease—from both private donors and the New York state legislature, which had allocated the same one thousand dollars it directed to all the city's dispensaries—the Blackwells planned to open on May 12, 1857. It was Anniversary Week, when progressive organizations like the Temperance Union and the Anti-Slavery Society held their national meetings in New York. The city would be full of sympathetic supporters.

It was also Florence Nightingale's thirty-seventh birthday. Though the "Lady with the Lamp" hewed firmly to nursing as the appropriate role for women in medicine, she had conferred a cautious blessing on the Blackwells' endeavor during her correspondence with Emily. The advent of women doctors was inevitable, Nightingale agreed; it was just a matter of the right woman leading the way. "She must have both natural talent and experience and undoubted superiority in her knowledge of

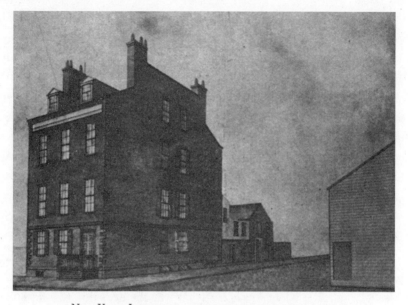

NEW YORK INFIRMARY BUILDING AT THE CORNER OF
BLEECKER AND CROSBY STREETS.
COURTESY NEW YORK ACADEMY OF MEDICINE

Medicine & Surgery," Nightingale wrote. "She must be entirely above all flirting or ever desiring to marry, recollecting that to her, the Apostle of the cause, her cause must be all in all." Both Blackwells could recognize themselves in those terms, even if they disagreed in theory with Nightingale's insistence that medical women must remain forever celibate. Whether the Blackwells were the right women Nightingale did not say, but she retained a deep respect for Elizabeth despite their divergent opinions. "Pray remember me most affectionately to your sister, whom I shall never forget," she had closed her letter to Emily. The Blackwell sisters were abundantly aware of the usefulness of Nightingale's fame, even if their opinions diverged. The date was not an accident.

Henry Ward Beecher, their keynote speaker, was another wise choice. Congregants and tourists flocked to his sermons at Brooklyn's Plymouth Church, familiarly known as "Beecher's theater"; on Sundays the Brooklyn ferries were dubbed "Beecher boats." For his exuberant homilies—encouraging seekers to pursue the truth of their individual natures—he was paid a salary of five thousand dollars a year, his success unmatched even by his best-selling sister, Harriet Beecher Stowe. The Blackwells understood the power of Beecher's rhetoric to propel their project. In its coverage of the infirmary's opening, the *New York Herald* devoted more column inches to Beecher's remarks than to any other aspect of the event.

If Nightingale and Beecher provided the sparkle of celebrity for the new undertaking, Elizabeth's steadfast ally, the Quaker doctor William Elder, supplied the heart. Elder had traveled from Philadelphia to witness the birth of an institution that would not only promote the progress of women in medicine but also, he predicted, correct the folly of current medical instruction. "All scientific medical works begin at the wrong end," Elder insisted, condemning the "fogyism and humbug" that infected the profession, and praising the Blackwells' intention to "educate the medical student in the Infirmary, by the bedside." He was sure they were standing in what would become not just a hospital but a female college. The Blackwells, he averred, were women of "broad faith," and the public could trust the virtue of their work. The abolitionist minister Dudley Atkins Tyng, another Philadelphian, arrived late, breathless and dusty from a delayed train, to confirm the spiritual fitness of the lady physicians. And lest anyone fail to mark the significance of the date, he cited Florence Nightingale, yet again, as proof of women's potential before offering a closing prayer.

The day was an undeniable success, but Elizabeth and Emily left the celebrating to others. Marie Zakrzewska found their restraint exasperating. "Elizabeth Blackwell seemed to feel some sort of gratification at the day of the opening," she wrote, "though she tried hard to conceal." Zakrzewska thought she could detect a more obvious flush of pleasure on Emily's face, though nothing like the triumph she felt was warranted. "It seems to me so strange that some natures always will be in opposition to themselves," she continued. "These two women for instance, have all right to be satisfied with their work and efforts . . . but still they won't acknowledge it either to others nor to themselves." Did they not realize that their supporters needed emotional satisfaction—good fellowship as well as good reform? "In spite of all I love them and feel sad that nothing

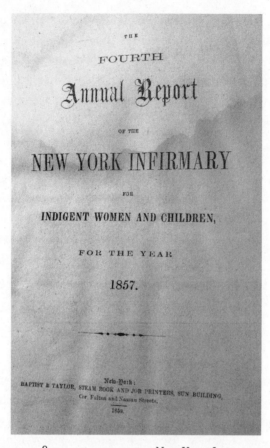

THE

FOURTH

𝕬nnual 𝕽eport

OF THE

NEW YORK INFIRMARY

FOR

INDIGENT WOMEN AND CHILDREN,

FOR THE YEAR

1857.

New-York:
BAPTIST & TAYLOR, STEAM BOOK AND JOB PRINTERS, SUN BUILDING,
Cor. Fulton and Nassau Streets,
1858.

ANNUAL REPORT OF 1857, THE YEAR OF THE NEW YORK INFIRMARY'S FOUNDING.
COURTESY NEW YORK ACADEMY OF MEDICINE

can cheer them up," Zakrzewska wrote. "Or do they perhaps show their joy in their bedroom where nobody sees them?"

〜

The infirmary building itself was an apt metaphor for an institution channeling middle-class largesse toward the needs of the poor, "fully respectable on the Bleecker Street side, and full of patients and misery on the other side and at the rear," as Zakrzewska described it. Around the corner on Crosby Street, the decorative touches of the facade vanished along with the middle-class complacency of the neighborhood. The dispensary was in the dining room on the ground floor—a luxurious space compared to its original incarnation on Seventh Street. There was a desk for the attending physician, an examination table behind a screen, and a workbench for preparing prescriptions. It was attended every morning by the lady physicians or one of their assistants: a series of new gradu- ates from the women's medical colleges in Philadelphia and Boston who paid for a practical opportunity that was as yet unavailable to them any- where else.

In the entrance hall, patients waited their turn on donated second- hand settees. The building was chilly in winter and airless in the hot weather, but it was spotless and well staffed, a paradise compared with the hellish conditions awaiting the sick poor at municipal institutions like Bellevue or Blackwell's Island. The second floor held two inpatient wards, with maternity cases on the third. The slant-ceilinged attic story was a warren of tiny rooms: sleeping quarters for students, nurses, ser- vants, and Marie Zakrzewska, who had moved in as resident physician. Though Blackwell was the name most closely associated with the infir- mary, it was Zakrzewska who devoted every waking hour to it during its first two years, tending not just to the patients but also to the build- ing, the larder, the linen closets, the medicine cabinets, and the staff. She was up before dawn to order provisions at the market, and after eve- ning rounds she gathered the students to review the day's patients while mending sheets. She made sure everyone was in bed by midnight, unless a crisis—or a baby—emerged. People might refer to the infirmary as the Blackwell hospital, but it was Zakrzewska who kept it going.

Elizabeth and Emily remained at Fifteenth Street, making the twenty- minute walk to staff the dispensary in the mornings and, in Emily's case, to treat surgical patients. At this early stage, the infirmary didn't actu- ally provide full-time employment for three physicians. Two-thirds of the beds remained empty. This was not for lack of patients but lack of funds; Elizabeth refused to spend money she didn't have. "It is a principle dis- tinctly laid down, that no debt shall be contracted by the Institution," read the annual report. Although the hospital's mission was to provide free care to the indigent, once it reached the limits of its meager resources, it accepted only those inpatients who could afford to pay four dollars per week. There weren't many of them. The Blackwells and Zakrzewska spent a substantial amount of time away from Bleecker Street, attending to private patients. It was their only source of medical income; the infirmary paid them nothing.

The *New-York Times* ran an enthusiastic notice of their efforts—"What the Lady Doctors Are Doing"—two months after the infirmary opened. The item cheered the infirmary's modest beginning, noting the founders' "ambitious plans for the future" and highlighting their "mortal horror of debt, quite unusual in similar enterprises." The "homelike" establishment was "as fresh and clean as if just swept by the proverbial new broom," and the nursing care was unusually good, "if one may judge from the physiognomy of the motherly-looking dames who have charge of that department." Surely the infirmary would prove to be the kernel of women's medical education in New York: "The plan is well laid, and only needs a refreshing shower of endowments and donations to hasten its growth materially."

All this was excellent publicity, but the article mentioned the Blackwell sisters only briefly before devoting a full paragraph to the credentials and merits of Dr. Marie Zakrzewska. "She is an enthusiast in her profession, and is of the timber from which good artists are made," the reporter enthused. "She is aided by the Drs. Blackwell." It is likely the reporter was Mary Louise Booth, a frequent visitor to Zakrzewska's attic quarters at the infirmary, and later the first editor of *Harper's Bazaar*. Dr. Zak had recognized the young reporter as a sister across disciplines: "I found that she also was a beginner in her career and had obstacles to overcome; as, for instance, hiding her sex by signing only her initials to whatever she wrote, or not signing at all." Their friendship had yielded exactly the kind of warm support Elizabeth and Emily found so hard to attract.

Policemen walking the night shift became accustomed to seeing the women of the infirmary coming and going at all hours. The doctors and their students spent significant time in "out-door practice," visiting patients and laboring mothers in the slums. Given the infirmary's limited finances, it was a good way to expand its reach and reputation without the extra expense of feeding and housing inpatients. Some nocturnal calls surely rattled the composure of even the bravest visitor, but those moments had their own value in plucking at the heartstrings of potential donors. "Night after night is spent by the young physician in these dens of misery," read one early annual report, "when the only bed is a heap of rags on the floor, and that heap is shared, perhaps, by a drunken husband, and here the newborn child is ushered into a world of woe." There is no record of either doctors or students coming to any harm beyond "unpleasant annoyances from unprincipled men." Though uptown ladies might draw in their breath and their skirts at the sight of a female with a doctor's bag, women of the tenements welcomed the unusual physicians into their private spaces. Women had always helped each other in sickness.

Their menfolk were not as sure. Who knew what really went on upstairs at Bleecker Street? When one woman died on the maternity ward, gossip flew: Weren't those lady doctors known to promote *hygiene* over calomel and leeches? What kind of doctoring was that? Though relatives had been present at the woman's bedside throughout her ordeal, by early afternoon members of her extended family—including men armed with axes and shovels—were pounding on the Bleecker Street door, condemning the infirmary for "killing women in childbirth with cold water." Their shouts drew a crowd that expanded to fill the sidewalk as far as Broadway; a few ran around and battered at the back door as well. The infirmary staff were trapped, their calls for help inaudible over the noise of the mob. At this point two policemen arrived, and the doctors had reason to be grateful for the reputation they had built in the neighborhood. Bellowing for silence, the officers ordered the rioters to disperse. Didn't they know the lady doctors did the best they could for their patients? After all, they scolded, "no doctor could keep everybody from dying some time."

This was not an isolated incident. On another occasion, a similar mob responded to the news that appendicitis had claimed a victim, though the patient had been attended repeatedly by Richard Sharpe Kissam, an eminent Bellevue surgeon who was one of the infirmary's consultants. This time Zakrzewska was able to send a note summoning Kissam, who told the angry gathering to fetch the coroner and have him examine the body in the presence of a "jury" of a dozen of them. "It was a sight to behold," Zakrzewska remembered. "These poor distraught men in overalls, with dirty hands, disheveled hair and grim faces, standing by during the autopsy, and at its close, declaring their satisfaction that death had been an unavoidable consequence of the disease." It was good to have champions like Kissam in a crisis, but the women he had just rescued must have wished they could do without his help.

By midsummer things were running smoothly enough that Elizabeth took a vacation, a solo weeklong ramble along the Connecticut shore near Lyme. Charmed by the blue and green and gold landscape, she filled her lungs with sea breezes, sometimes walking twenty miles in a single day. One afternoon an elderly gentleman driving a wagon in her direction offered her a ride, assuring her that he was a married man and she should feel no anxiety, despite the remote spot in which they found themselves. "I informed him that I had great faith in humanity," Elizabeth wrote, "& believed in men, not in tigers."

～

The infirmary's annual report for 1857 announced that nearly a thousand women and children had received care, though only forty-eight as inpatients. There had been thirty-six surgical cases, with Emily performing admirably as attending surgeon. "I have been delighted with the sound judgment and ability she showed, at every step," Elizabeth wrote after Emily's first successful operation. "I think a reputation in surgery will be sure to make her fortune in time, for it will be the very thing that will overcome the distrust women still feel in employing women Doctors." While a skeptic might insist that a feverish patient's recovery would have happened more rapidly under a male doctor's care, no one could question the skill of a woman who safely removed a tumor or corrected a clubfoot.

Word was spreading among the communities the infirmary served, and the trustees were happy to report that "the kindly, home-like way in which this charity is conducted, attaches the poor people to it, and they gladly return there." In fact, too many returned, and lack of funds forced the painful necessity of turning many of those patients away. But Elizabeth's adamant refusal to borrow money was prudent. The political turmoil that followed the Supreme Court's *Dred Scott* decision—which unexpectedly opened western territories to slavery—and the subsequent collapse of the market in western railroad securities led to a financial panic in the fall of 1857 that convulsed the country, closing New York banks for two months. Even as commercial credit evaporated, the infirmary proceeded with its work, unaffected. "Its funds have been managed with great economy," the *Times* wrote approvingly, "and, notwithstanding the commercial embarrassments of the past year, it is free from all debt, and has even increased the number of its beds."

Despite such proofs of success, Elizabeth, at least, remained unsatisfied. Though the Blackwells could claim staunch allies, most of New York's elite still looked at them askance. Remembering her enthralling encounter years earlier with Fanny Kemble in Lady Byron's parlor, Elizabeth brought Zakrzewska to pay a call when the actress visited New York, hoping she might offer her talent in support of the infirmary. Kemble listened attentively, but when she realized the attending physicians of this hospital for the poor were women, her reaction was immediate and thunderous. "She sprang up to her full height," Elizabeth wrote, "turned her flashing eyes upon us, and with the deepest tragic tones of her magnificent voice exclaimed: 'Trust a *woman*—as a *doctor*!—NEVER!'" Elizabeth and Zakrzewska left the hotel bemused and disappointed.

Elizabeth was increasingly unafraid to declare that America wronged its accomplished women. "When a woman has won herself an honorable position in any unusual line of life," she wrote in the *Philadelphia Press*, "she is still excluded from the companionship and privileges of the class to which she should belong, because her course is unusual." Her hard work had won her admirers, but she was still mostly unwelcome in the drawing rooms of the prominent people who could help her the most— people whose approval she craved more than she would admit. "Stop the sneer at any effort because it is unusual," she wrote with unguarded frustration. "Let us learn to regard women as human beings as well as women." She was weary of the gossips who wondered whether female doctors dressed like ordinary women, or cut their hair short like men.

It was good to have allies like Lady Byron, who had remained a flatteringly faithful correspondent in the years since Elizabeth had returned from Europe. "Your kind thought for our Hospital cheers me," Elizabeth wrote to her at Christmas 1857. To a woman as sophisticated and well respected as Lady Byron, Elizabeth felt no need to soften her sense of her own value.

Very few understand the soul of this work, or the absolute necessity
which lies upon me, to live out the ideal life to the utmost extent
of my power. My work is undoubtedly for the few, it is labor in the
interlinkings of humanity, and is necessarily difficult of appreciation to the mass, very slow in gaining their esteem. It has been
my most toilsome lesson, to translate my thought into the common
language of life, and I labour at this translation perpetually, and too
often remain still incomprehensible.

At least, she told her friend, she now had a loyal companion on her difficult path. "My sister is a noble helper, and we shall stand, I trust, shoulder to shoulder, through many years of active service." But even in her
gratitude, Elizabeth saw her younger sister as an aide, not a partner:
someone to hold the ground they had won, even if she herself was too
restless, and too ambitious, to settle there.

CHAPTER 14

RECOGNITION

"I am going to tell you my plans, which I have not yet mentioned to the family generally," Elizabeth wrote to her brother George in June 1858, "so keep it to yourself for a while."

The infirmary had been open for a year. Emily had attracted new interest with her own series of lectures for women, enlivened with anatomical illustrations borrowed from the city's medical schools. In Albany, she had successfully lobbied the New York state legislature for a grant that would place the infirmary on sounder footing. And she had overseen the care of one particularly important patient: Lucy Stone, who was expecting her first child at thirty-nine. "I should not object to its being a boy," Emily wrote, "but as the Blackwell family has always been distinguished by its women, I should be very well satisfied either way, and it may turn out a little Stone and no Blackwell after all." Lucy and Henry's only child, Alice Stone Blackwell, was born September 14, 1857, looking almost comically like her father. She would grow up to become a leader in the suffrage movement.

Emily's capable management allowed Elizabeth to look ahead—and to recognize the itch of her own dissatisfaction, despite the slow, steady growth of their practice. "Life in New York is monotonous," she wrote, "and it will continue so, for it arises partly from our position which is without money or connexions, partly from our nature which with the best endeavor, cannot enter into close relations with the society we meet." The wider approbation that Elizabeth craved remained elusive. Antoinette Brown Blackwell reported that few people on her lecture-tour travels had heard of the New York Infirmary for Indigent Women and Children—though mention of her own married name frequently elicited the question, "Whatever happened to that Elizabeth Blackwell, you know, the one with the medical degree?" Elizabeth might think of herself as a beacon of enlightenment, but her light was not shining as brightly as she had expected.

Barbara Leigh Smith had recently visited New York with her new French husband, Eugène Bodichon, an eccentric doctor sixteen years her senior, who spent most of his time in Algiers and affected a flowing white burnoose over his street clothes. Though the reform-minded Bodichons had planned their American wedding tour as an educative opportunity to observe southern slavery and northern liberalism at first hand, they paused for a pleasure trip to Niagara Falls, and Elizabeth brought Kitty along for the treat. Her friends urged Elizabeth to consider bringing her work "home" to England. Surely London was ready for women doctors, now that Florence Nightingale had become a household name?

Upon her return to England, Barbara Bodichon and Bessie Parkes founded a monthly magazine, the *English Woman's Journal*. The second issue, published in April 1858, included an extensive profile of Elizabeth and Emily, written with sororal pride by the Blackwell family journalist, Anna. Citing Queen Elizabeth I and the Huntress Diana as Elizabeth's models, Anna filled her account with the kind of hyperbole usually accorded a folk hero: how teenaged Elizabeth had proved her prodigious physical strength by hoisting a skeptical (and protesting) male visitor in her arms for three laps around the parlor; or how she had severely restricted her diet while at medical school, so as to remain pale of countenance no matter how trying the anatomy lesson. Anna mentioned neither the farcical circumstances of Elizabeth's acceptance at Geneva nor the tragic loss of her eye in Paris, and she was careful to correct the "very general misapprehension" that her sisters were American. As true daughters of Bristol, Anglophile Anna averred, Elizabeth and Emily had been "incapable of resorting to the system of puffing and self-vaunting so much in vogue among our transatlantic cousins." Their success, earned the hard way, Anna suggested, would be all the more lasting.

Though its circulation never exceeded a thousand, the *English*

Woman's Journal attracted an influential readership. One of these readers was Anna Maria Helena Coswell, Comtesse de Noailles, an eccentric and capricious young English widow whose brief and childless marriage to a French count had left her in a position to be extremely helpful to good causes. She was a shareholder in the *Journal* and let it be known that she was interested in supporting the Blackwells' work—in England.

It was this tantalizing possibility—a secure medical foothold in Britain, an aristocratic patron, and a chance to take her rightful place among a class of women she admired, including Florence Nightingale, whose fame had so outpaced Elizabeth's own—that Elizabeth now confided to George. "I think it very desirable to see England again," she told her brother, "and to test its possibilities." She had a perfect excuse for deserting the infirmary and indulging in a trip to Europe: her glass eye was giving her trouble, making a consultation with Auguste Boissonneau, the preeminent oculist who had originally fitted her, a necessity. Though Emily was skeptical of Madame de Noailles's overtures, Elizabeth ignored her. "I shall pursue the investigation as I think best," she wrote with autocratic confidence. "I am not sorry either to throw Emily for a while, upon her own resources, and force her into the responsibilities of practice—she has not yet braced herself to the work, as she must eventually, it being her only means of making money."

Elizabeth was correct that Emily's commitment to the infirmary was not as absolute as it could be. Beneath the competent composure of the thirty-one-year-old physician was the same frustrated uncertainty that had plagued Emily as a young teacher. Had she won her way to a medical degree, she wondered, only to face a life of lonely and uncredited labor, eternally eclipsed by the aggressive ambitions and prickly personalities of her sister and Marie Zakrzewska? Success as one of the world's first female physicians, she now understood, would involve more than good doctoring. It would require a constant active cultivation of public support—what the Blackwells referred to, with distaste, as "push." "An agony of doubt has burnt in my heart for months," she confided to her journal. Could it be "that this life of a Physician is so utterly not my life that I can not express myself through it—and worse—worse—that I might have done more in other ways?"

Elizabeth's departure, though it would mean more work for Emily, came at a perfect moment. In Elizabeth's absence, Emily could manage their project as partner rather than deputy and enjoy a respite from Elizabeth's brittle moods. "She needs change," Emily wrote of Elizabeth's European travel plans. "Her life in many respects would be a much happier one there than here." And Emily would now have a chance to deepen her own relationships with the patrons and private patients who had come to know Elizabeth first. By the time Elizabeth returned, Emily hoped, "I may have formed the commencement of a practice wh[ich] will enable me to remain here on better terms." For now, she recommitted herself to the infirmary—where, for the first time, she would be in charge.

~

On her last ocean voyage Elizabeth had been grateful for the presence of her cousin Kenyon; this time her companion was ten-year-old* Kitty— half ward, half servant—who continued to dispel the gloom of Elizabeth's habitual solitude. In fair weather the girl promenaded silently at Elizabeth's side, watching for porpoises and the dark silhouettes of storm petrels, which the sailors called "Mother Carey's chickens," while her guardian chatted with the captain and the first mate—who promised to "throw Kitty overboard" if she were seasick.

Elizabeth had sailed for Europe to secure her reputation, not to look after a little girl. Once in London she consigned Kitty to her brother Howard, on leave from India, and her sister Ellen, still abroad to study painting, with instructions to find the child some clothes and deposit her at a boarding school recommended by Barbara Bodichon at Ockham, in the Surrey countryside. "Dear Kittykin," Elizabeth wrote to her there, her handwriting and syntax enlarged and simplified for the child's benefit. "The weeks will soon slip away and Doctor will be back to see the progress Kitty has made." Progress, Elizabeth indicated, should be more practical than intellectual—the new generation of Blackwells, led by the toddlers Florence and Alice, needed looking after. "How nice it will be, when you can cut out little dresses for them, and sew them so fast, while

---

* Kitty's birthdate is obscure. In old age, she remembered celebrating her tenth birthday in the fall of 1859. Other sources place her birthdate in 1847.

they are playing around." She sent Kitty a birthday box containing a bonnet, a book, and a skipping rope, then left to visit Anna in Paris.

As an old woman, Kitty still remembered her bewilderment that fall, alone in a new country, surrounded by wary schoolmates who could not categorize this odd Irish-American orphan but were only too eager to eat her share of treacle pudding. Tardiness resulted in a day's banishment without meals, and as the fall deepened, chilblains bloomed on Kitty's feet. Her letters of distress to Elizabeth, she discovered with dismay, were never mailed. Finally, on a class excursion to the nearest town, she managed to slip one directly into the postbox, and Elizabeth responded with gratifying speed. That was the end of boarding school, but now Kitty would have to make her way to Elizabeth in Paris, alone.

Howard and Ellen left her at Waterloo Station in the predawn darkness, with a passport in one cloak pocket and a Paris address in the other. A child of means would never have made such a journey without a chaperone, and a girl of the working class would never have traveled at all. Kitty, always betwixt, traveled alone by train to Newhaven, by ferry to Dieppe (a crossing more than twice as long as the Dover-Calais route), and then by train again, arriving in Paris well after midnight. The French station officials, clucking with disapproval over the unsupervised child, tucked her into a carriage, and she rumbled off into the night.

"Having read, small as I was, too much about the Revolution," Kitty remembered, "I expected to be carried off to the Conciergerie"—the infamous prison that was Marie Antoinette's last stop before the guillotine. When the carriage halted unexpectedly, she feared the worst. Peeping white-faced out the window, she saw an oncoming cab and heard a familiar voice: "Is that you, child?" Elizabeth, informed that Kitty's train had arrived, had set out to meet her at the wrong station and caught up with her carriage at last, having recognized the child-sized trunk strapped to the roof. Kitty's memoir recorded fear and relief, but no blame. Certainly a true bond existed between the doctor and the grateful child she had rescued from the Nurseries on Randall's Island. But in the letters that survive from their yearlong stay in Europe—during which Kitty began to suffer from vision and hearing problems that would plague her for the rest of her life—Elizabeth makes almost no mention of her.

Her preoccupations were elsewhere. Barbara Bodichon had delivered a formal letter of "heartfelt welcome" signed by more than fifty of the influential Englishwomen in her circle, most notably Lady Byron, inviting Elizabeth to speak publicly on women's health and the importance of women doctors. Elizabeth was eager to accept, but the lectures she had delivered to Quaker ladies in New York church basements—and subsequently published as *The Laws of Life*—seemed inadequate for London's urbane elite. She remained in Paris to rewrite them and try them out on Anna, who, she told Emily, "represents an exaggeratedly English audience." She also needed to update her wardrobe: perhaps a black velvet hat "to give a little height & importance to the head." She hesitated at the expense but refused to allow wealthy patrons to underestimate her. "If it all falls through," she rationalized to Emily, "I shall bring back the clothes & we'll divide them between us."

A dignified appearance would also help put her audience at ease—an important consideration, given that her material was likely to make them uncomfortable. In a draft manuscript, she quoted a distinguished London matron who had once exclaimed to her, "You can hardly have an idea of the state of complete ignorance I was in, with regard to everything relating to the body, when I married!" Elizabeth's first lecture subject, therefore—approached with appropriately "reverential admiration" for an audience strictly limited to women—would be the reproductive organs.

Her explanation proceeded methodically from the almond-shaped ovaries, to the Fallopian tubes—lined with pulsing cilia "like a host of energetic little sweepers to be keeping their house constantly clean"—and onward to the uterus, which expanded from fist-sized quiescence to a "great industrial palace" of muscle and artery during pregnancy. To this point, the anatomy lesson was straightforward, full of domestic and mechanical imagery for these wives and daughters of capitalists. But as she turned to the external structures—vagina, labia, clitoris—Elizabeth's tone shifted.

"Let me here call your attention to a marked distinction which we observe in the functions of the Genital organs," she wrote. "We find that the Creator in his supreme goodness & wisdom, while endowing us with senses that place us in communication with the external world," she continued, "has connected the power of exquisite enjoyment with the proper exercise of those senses." She detoured into euphemistic metaphor—the flaming glory of the setting sun, the heart-piercing song of a bird, the slaking of a traveler's thirst with cold water—but soon returned to her point: "We find in the special organization which we are considering, a more abundant provision for exquisite sensation . . . than in any other part of the body." The clitoris, she pointed out, had no practical function except as a receptor of acute feeling. Her choice of image for female erectile tissue—"a spongy vascular body—in size and form, something like a great swollen leech"—was not unexpected for a woman raised in a culture that regarded sexual desire as a perilous temptation, but the fact that she was addressing physical pleasure at all, that she considered it an important part of a woman's physiological education, was startling. The women who attended this first lecture would surely return for its two sequels, when Elizabeth would make her larger point about the importance of training female doctors.

~

Before Elizabeth could take the stage in London, she needed to pay two important calls. The first was to Florence Nightingale, whom she found in January 1859 taking the water cure at Great Malvern. Nightingale had returned from the Crimean War in poor health, bedridden and complaining of chest pain—though she was still managing to churn out reams of cogent testimony on sanitary conditions in the army. Her friends and physicians feared the worst, but Elizabeth was not so sure. "I cannot help thinking that her condition is not understood, and that she is not going to die yet," she reported to Emily. "She converses with me, precisely as usual, her head clear, her enthusiasm alive, from two to three hours, twice a day." (Though Nightingale's invalidism would become part of her mystique, she would live another fifty years. Modern commentators attribute her symptoms to a combination of brucellosis—a bacterial infection acquired at the British camp in Turkey—and emotional health issues including post-traumatic stress disorder.) Public gratitude for Nightingale's work during the war had ballooned into the forty-five-thousand-pound Nightingale Fund, intended for the training of nurses. Three years after the war's end, it remained unspent.

All the Blackwells' fund-raising efforts were a molehill compared to the mountain of money Nightingale now controlled. Her hope, she told Elizabeth, was to establish new standards for nurses, eventually spreading her ideas regarding hygiene to mothers, teachers, and servants across Britain. Doctors, Nightingale felt, tended only to make things worse, interfering with nature's beneficence—but nurses, if properly taught, had the potential to restore vitality to humanity with attentive hygienic care. "She feels," Elizabeth wrote to Emily, "that I am the only person in the world that can help her, and she would be immensely relieved from the responsibility of the fund, which weighs heavily upon her, if I would throw [my] life into it."

Central to Nightingale's vision was the role of sanitary professor, to be installed in a major London hospital and placed in charge of training the nurses. "She thinks moreover that it ought always to be filled by a woman," Elizabeth wrote to Emily, "and that woman ought to be an M.D. She thinks I should fill it much better than she." It was an alluring prospect. The combination of Nightingale's influence and Elizabeth's credentials would be potent, and there was considerable overlap in their ideas; both women believed absolutely in the importance of hygiene and education, and Elizabeth frankly preferred the role of professor to that of clinician. But Nightingale's plan was to improve public health, not to elevate women. "She does not think that England is prepared to educate women Doctors," Elizabeth wrote. "She would really take me as a valuable exception."

Elizabeth could not reconcile their divergent perspectives. "She wishes, I see, to absorb me in the nursing plan, which would simply kill me," Elizabeth confided to Barbara Bodichon. The practice of medicine was Elizabeth's answer to Margaret Fuller's call to arms; it made her a model to others, living proof of woman's true potential, and she refused to give it up. Nightingale, meanwhile, saw the promotion of female physicians as an indulgence. "I remember my impression of your character—that you & I were on different roads (altho' to the same object)," Nightingale wrote to Elizabeth after her visit. "You to educate a few highly cultivated ones— I to diffuse as much knowledge as possible." They might have renewed their personal friendship, but on the professional level each would always conclude that the other was missing the point. From New York, Emily summed things up succinctly: "FN's idea evidently is not to aid you in yr work, but to engage you in hers," she wrote. "Keep quietly clear of her."

Elizabeth made her way back across the Channel and southward to the Italian Riviera for her first encounter with Madame de Noailles, another woman who spent most of her time supine—though any similarity to Miss Nightingale ended there. The indolent countess moved through the Mediterranean countryside lounging full-length in an oversized carriage; she retired early, slept late, and enjoyed three extravagant meals during her limited waking hours, with a chamomile-infused bath before dinner. She had exasperatingly little sense of the value of either money or time. "The most characteristic adjective for her is scatterbrain," Elizabeth wrote to Emily, "impulsive almost to insanity, full of whim." Elizabeth had intended to give her a private reading of her lectures, but over the course of her five-day visit, she found it impossible to capture the countess's attention long enough to get through them.

"I can hardly tell you how disgusted I felt by the luxurious self-indulgent objectless life of the wealthy English abroad," Elizabeth declared[*]—but Madame de Noailles spoke of giving the Blackwells a small fortune, and for that Elizabeth was willing to look past her excesses. "She has true instincts and certain aspirations which may be relied on," Elizabeth insisted to Emily—among them "great faith in women, & the desire to help them, and a great interest in the question of health." Her impulsiveness, in fact, might work to the Blackwells' advantage. "She told me frankly, she could not bear being bored," Elizabeth wrote. Regular annual donations were boring, so instead the countess gave Elizabeth a thousand pounds on the spot and the promise of five thousand more, with the expectation that Elizabeth would open a women's hospital in the

---

[*] Frances Hodgson Burnett—author of the beloved children's novels *The Secret Garden* and *A Little Princess*—would caricature Madame de Noailles's notorious excesses in "Piccino" (1894), the story of an English noblewoman abroad who, captivated by a peasant child, decides to buy him for her amusement. De Noailles actually did exchange money for a young Italian girl when she saw a painting of her in a Paris salon; the painting was not for sale, so she bought the original.

English countryside. Buoyed by this windfall, Elizabeth returned to London, ready to win more allies with her newly revised lectures.

Their frank content alarmed even her closest friends. Bessie Parkes thought the ladies would recoil with a "shriek of horror," but Elizabeth was undeterred: "I simply laugh, and disbelieve her." On March 2, 1859, she faced her first audience—"about 150 people, of considerable influence"—and even the popular press seemed to approve. "Now, let us for a moment imagine a person intrusted with a complicated and delicate piece of machinery," noted the popular monthly *Chambers's Journal*. "Imagine that person to be ignorant of the principles of the construction of that machine," it continued—such was the plight of women expected to guard their families' health in ignorance of physiology. Of course, "in a journal of this character, we can only allude to the more purely medical portion of Dr. Blackwell's discourse," the article concluded delicately— but its sympathetic tone was clear: intimate knowledge of physical health, imparted to women by fully trained female doctors, was "subject for much earnest thought."

One member of Elizabeth's audience responded with particular earnestness. Elizabeth Garrett, the twenty-two-year-old daughter of a prosperous Suffolk businessman, had read Anna's profile of the medical Blackwell sisters in the *English Woman's Journal*. Inspired by the thought of "something definite & worthy to do," Garrett attended each of the three lectures with growing interest, attention that was reciprocated once Barbara Bodichon introduced the two Elizabeths. "Last night I saw a Miss Garrett who very much pleased me—a young lady who is quietly forming her determination to study medicine," Elizabeth reported to Emily. "I think she has the pluck to take it up." Garrett was not nearly as decided as Elizabeth assumed—"I remember feeling very much confounded & as if I had been suddenly thrust into work that was too big for me," the younger woman wrote—but to her own surprise, the study of medicine suited her. Six years later she would become the first woman in Britain to qualify as a doctor.

As she prepared to repeat her lectures in Birmingham, Manchester, and Liverpool, Elizabeth allowed herself a moment of delighted optimism. "There is an immense charm in this fresh field, where solid

English heads receive the highest view of truth, where generosity and largeness of idea meet you at every turn," she exulted to Emily. "I like working and living in England, immeasurably better than in America, and there is no limit to what we might accomplish here." Surely the material support she and Emily needed to establish themselves in this far more congenial setting would soon present itself. For the moment, she resolutely ignored a recent warning from Florence Nightingale. "I do not think you know how little your audience represents the public opinion of England," Nightingale wrote. "I do not draw discouragement from this— but neither should I draw encouragement from them as you do."

In Elizabeth's absence, meanwhile, Emily was starting to believe in a future for the institution they had founded in New York. But she had no one to discuss her thoughts with, and visiting her brothers—now decamped to more spacious suburban quarters in New Jersey—was not restorative. "They have got so completely to look upon me as a Dr that I can't go near them without being pounced upon with regard to the baby's bowels," she complained. With the Fifteenth Street house now filled with boarders to cover expenses, Emily spent most evenings alone in her attic room, reading Elizabeth's rose-colored reports on establishing a new future in the old country, and writing two worried pages back for every one she received.

Emily understood the seductive allure of London, but there were good reasons to resist. The New York Infirmary had one advantage over anything England could offer: it existed. It would not be easy to create a similar institution in England. The graduates of the American women's medical colleges who arrived at Bleecker Street fed its purpose as a training hospital for female physicians; in England, women were not yet allowed to study medicine at all. And as Emily became more comfortable with leadership, it was hard for her to imagine trotting off in Elizabeth's wake once again, "a younger, less well known partner, to make my position by extraneous efforts upon the outskirts of yours." How could they abandon what they had struggled so hard to create in New York? "My liking is for Europe—if circumstances were favourable," Emily told

Elizabeth. But: "My judgment is for America, and for completing our work here."

Uncertainty complicated the decisions Emily faced in Elizabeth's absence. Should she search for a building that could serve more effi- ciently as both hospital and residence in one? What should she tell their patients and donors, now that rumors had begun to fly that Elizabeth wasn't coming back? Impetuous Bessie Parkes had published a line in the *English Woman's Journal* expressing the assumption that Elizabeth would now establish herself in London, "as her sister, Dr. Emily Black- well, is well fitted to supply her place across the Atlantic." And then there was the question of Marie Zakrzewska.

Elizabeth had been right in her original estimation of Dr. Zak: she brought enormous energy and skill to her work. Perhaps too much. Her role as the infirmary's resident physician meant that hers was the face its patients and staff saw most, and her talent as a practitioner, her knack for self-promotion, and her easy openness won her enviable popularity. "In looking over the book I see she has at least twice as many patients every week as I have," Emily complained to Elizabeth. "She is evidently desir- ous to get a position which we can not let her occupy—the superintend- ing woman influence in the Hospital."

Dr. Zak had begun to upstage the Blackwells in their own institu- tion, yet she did not hold herself to Blackwellian standards, whether in terms of her housekeeping ("Z doesn't even make her bed," Emily tutted) or her clinical practice. On one occasion, Zakrzewska—herself recover- ing from illness, probably from overwork—called in reinforcements for a difficult delivery. Emily and her consulting surgeon, Richard Sharpe Kissam, found the mother's vagina lacerated and the infant's scalp cut and bruised by Zakrzewska's clumsy use of forceps—an error she at first denied. Mother and child survived, but Emily was incensed: not only had Zakrzewska shown poor judgment and sloppy technique, she had made an unfavorable impression on their male colleague, something a woman doctor must avoid at all costs. "The whole affair has greatly shaken my confidence in her as an intelligent authority in difficult obstetric cases," Emily wrote.

At this fraught moment, a providential offer arrived from Boston: would Dr. Zakrzewska consider taking a newly created clinical professorship at the New England Female Medical College? "I felt that a larger field for my efforts might be opened there in connection with a medical school," Zakrzewska wrote pointedly, "rather than in New York where the two Drs. Blackwell controlled the direction of efforts toward what seemed to them wisest and best." Emily heartily agreed. "We can not make the hospital what it should be while she is living in it," she told Elizabeth. Sending Zakrzewska off with their blessings to a prestigious new position in Boston was a happy ending for everyone. "The Lady Doctors in Bleecker Street" were at last winning the approval both of their patients and the male physicians whose respect they craved. As Zakrzewska prepared to leave, Emily laid out her vision for the future.

First they needed to consolidate home and work in a single larger building, one plain enough not to intimidate the patients, elegant enough to make their genteel patrons feel at home, and substantial enough to attract the female medical students who would become the next cohort of women doctors. For that, Emily reminded Elizabeth, was the point: to be not the first female M.D.s but the first of legions. "If ever I come to the conclusion that this is not to be hoped—that our success is only exceptional," Emily wrote, "then as far as I am concerned the life is an utter & miserable failure even if I made a fortune by it." This was the best argument for staying in New York: despite England's charms, Emily had seen little sign there of prospective medical women "as hopeful as these young green independent Americans."

Once everything was properly arranged in one building—perhaps "one of those old fashioned 2nd Avenue houses," Emily suggested—they would need to adjust the public perception of their own relationship. "I have had our names put as a firm in the Directory this year," Emily announced: where the previous city directory had listed "Blackwell Elizabeth, physician" just above "Blackwell Emily, physician," the new edition had "Blackwell Elizabeth & Emily, physicians"—a small thing, perhaps, but not to Emily. It was inefficient, not to mention demoralizing, when private patients insisted they would see only the elder Dr. Blackwell. If

Elizabeth returned, she and Emily must "get people to regard us as medically on the same footing."

It was increasingly clear that Elizabeth *was* going to return. The
applause in Britain was not translating itself into cash, and "half crazy"
Madame de Noailles had proved a difficult patron, insisting on terms
that Elizabeth could not grant. "I confess I've had a good cry about it,"
Elizabeth wrote to Emily. "I find that my feelings were beginning to take
strong root in England, and it will be somewhat of a struggle to give all
this new life up." But she would not return empty-handed. She had a
thousand pounds, earmarked by Madame de Noailles for the creation of a
small sanatorium outside New York City, which could double as a country
retreat for herself and Emily. She had new allies in London, who promised to send over young Englishwomen for training at the infirmary—if
the English were not ready to educate female medical students, the Blackwells would teach them in New York. And she had realized a historic and
symbolic goal.

"I have only one piece of information viz that the Medical Council has
registered me as Physician!" Elizabeth scrawled to Emily just before her
departure. Britain's Medical Act of 1858 had required the registration of
all medical practitioners, and Elizabeth's foreign degree, and the fact that
she had treated a few private patients while in London, allowed her to slip
through. She was now the only woman included in Britain's first Medical Register. The loopholes that had enabled her admission were swiftly
closed, but when the medical profession at last opened to women in Britain, Elizabeth would be ready.

"Your registration is a good thing," Emily wrote with understated
approval in August 1859. "I am glad the old fellows got so far." But the
recognition seemed to her less important than getting on with the work.
She closed this last letter before Elizabeth's return with a pragmatic
reminder of her original errand: "Mind you are well provided with eyes."

~

CHAPTER 15

WAR

The American Civil War broke out in the middle of a letter to Barbara Bodichon. "I wrote the above 10 days ago—very different is the state of things now," Elizabeth told her friend on April 23, 1861. She had started writing just hours after the Confederate attack on Fort Sumter; now she resumed in a new reality. "Rebellion of the most formidable character threatens the subversion of the government and invasion of our very homes—everyone is up & doing."

As far back as 1856, Elizabeth had been describing "the overbearing insolence & outrages of the pro-slavery party," which called forth an equally fiery spirit in the North: "never were evil & good more strongly presented face to face for deadly strife." Five years later she was more cynical. "I think it is much more of a fight for the tariff, than for principles," she told Barbara. "I think the great majority of the country are perfectly willing to accept almost any compromise with slavery, if they could ensure safe commercial relations." Her take betrayed a strengthening bias. There were more obvious causes for the war—the divisive election of Abraham Lincoln, disagreement over states' rights, the widening cultural gap between the industrialized North and the plantation society of the South—but Elizabeth felt more than ever like an expatriate in America. In writing to her closest London friend, it was easy to slip into an attitude that cast Americans as boors driven by money. "Nevertheless this is a great country and I cannot but feel an interest in it," she wrote, "although the people are strange to me, and their souls very shallow."

The national emergency realigned the Blackwell sisters toward a single larger purpose, just as they had begun to diverge. In the year and a half since Elizabeth's return from England—and despite a move to a new house at 126 Second Avenue spacious enough to hold both the infirmary and the Blackwell residence, exactly as Emily had recommended—Emily had lost her optimism about their joint venture. Elizabeth wanted to teach women the principles of both medicine and hygiene, but she hastened to place those subjects in "their true position, in which I believe the latter stands much higher than the former." Women physicians, as Elizabeth now defined them, should be teachers armed with science. "I do not look on a good medical training as having power to make men of women," she wrote, "but as a most valuable educator of their own natures." Emily, increasingly skilled and confident both in the operating theater and in the labor ward, wanted to train women as surgeons and clinicians on a par with men—and when she considered the callow, untested medical graduates arriving at the infirmary for training, she despaired. "Doubt is disease," Elizabeth had written, but when it came to the future of women in medicine, Emily had her doubts.

For Emily, the work had become toil rather than triumph. "She has taken an extreme dislike to it," Elizabeth wrote to Barbara, "and though she performs her duties conscientiously, she only does in medicine what is unavoidable & no longer studies with any future object." As soon as she saved enough to live on, Emily had announced, she would leave the profession. "Though I was bitterly disappointed," Elizabeth wrote, "I have now accepted it as inevitable. I used what influence I could at first, but the subject is now never discussed by us."

The war erased all thoughts of the future—there was only now. Emily's crisis of confidence would have to wait. "We are compelled to direct the women who in a frantic state of excitement are committing absurdities in nursing talk," Elizabeth scrawled hastily to Barbara. "I hurry this off, for a thousand engagements press."

The wave of Union enthusiasm threatened to crash chaotically unless channeled and focused. Americans had only the dimmest understanding of the realities of war—the last large-scale conflicts on American soil had occurred long before most of the population had come of age. Already railcars bursting with poorly packed supplies were heading south. Wilting vegetables and fermenting preserves spilled over bales of unsuitable clothing, including thousands of unwieldy Havelock hats, meant to keep the sun off the neck, but mostly used by the men as coffee filters or cut into pieces to make the oiled patches used in muzzle-loading rifles. Eager, untrained would-be nurses were rushing to Washington to volunteer.

On April 25, Elizabeth and Emily called an informal meeting to discuss how best to help. They were astonished when more than fifty women and several sympathetic men crowded into the infirmary. The result was an appeal that ran in New York newspapers on April 28. "To the Women of New York and especially to those already engaged in preparing against the time of Wounds and Sickness in the Army," ran the heading. Right-minded women were invited to the Cooper Institute, a short walk from the infirmary, in order to help "organize the benevolent purposes of all into a common movement."

The next evening between two and three thousand women thronged the vaulted space of the Cooper Institute's Great Hall, its fluted columns rising from a sea of bonnets and its floorboards invisible beneath jostling hoopskirts. Just a year earlier, Lincoln himself had stood at the same podium to deliver a speech—rejecting the expansion of slavery into the western territories—that propelled him toward the Republican nomination for president. Now cheers erupted as Lincoln's vice president, Hannibal Hamlin, made an unexpected appearance: a testament to the well-connectedness of the infirmary's allies, and also to the current administration's need for help from any quarter. "God bless the women!" Hamlin finished, to tumultuous applause.

A stream of illustrious speakers, all of them men, followed: ministers and physicians and even a surgeon who had witnessed the attack on Fort Sumter. Among them was Henry Whitney Bellows, the influential Unitarian—and husband of one of Elizabeth's first patients—who had helped shepherd *The Laws of Life* into print a decade earlier. He attended the infirmary meeting and emerged from the massive Cooper Institute gathering as one of the leaders of a new organization: the Women's Central Association for Relief. Led by a board of twelve men and twelve women, it was charged with collecting aid and comfort for the soldiers, managing a central depot of supplies for distribution, and selecting women to serve as nurses.

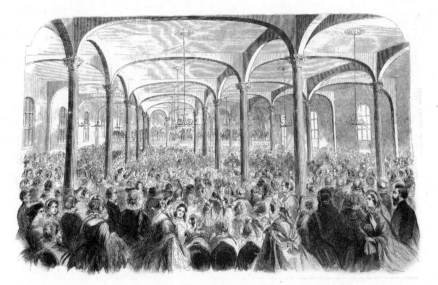

FIRST MEETING OF THE WOMEN'S CENTRAL ASSOCIATION OF RELIEF,
COOPER INSTITUTE, AS REPORTED IN *FRANK LESLIE'S ILLUSTRATED
NEWSPAPER,* MAY 11, 1861. *COURTESY NEW YORK SOCIETY LIBRARY*

This last item, of course, was the chief preoccupation of the Blackwells.
Elizabeth was named chair of the registration committee—the only female
officer in the organization—charged with identifying and training the
most promising individuals among the flood of women eager to do more
than knit socks and roll bandages at home. Many of them had read Florence Nightingale's recently published *Notes on Nursing,* with its thrilling
exhortation: "Every woman is a nurse." "There has been a perfect mania
amongst the women, to 'act Florence Nightingale!'" Elizabeth wrote with
some exasperation. But the scope of opportunity for women to work as
professionals in the field of health had suddenly widened dramatically—it
was a powerful moment for the Blackwells to put their ideas into practice.
Emily even traveled to Washington to meet with General Winfield Scott,
the "Grand Old Man" of the Union Army, who at first opposed the very
idea of women nursing the soldiers. He changed his mind.

The sisters quickly drafted a report, "On the Selection and Preparation of Nurses for the Army," which became the template for the recruiting effort—a template modeled explicitly on "the printed records of Miss

Nightingale's invaluable experience in army-nursing." Their first priority was to discourage frivolous interest; once the grim challenges of wartime nursing were made clear, they hoped, "much of the noble enthusiasm of women, whose sole desire is to serve their country in this momentous crisis, will be directed into other channels." Likely candidates would be between thirty and forty-five years of age, possessed of a strong constitution, good references, and restrained manners, and amenable to taking orders. They would dress soberly, as dictated by the committee—no hoop-skirts. Once chosen, they would submit to a course of medical training at approved New York hospitals and await the call to the front. Interested parties should come to the registration committee's offices on the fourth floor of the Cooper Institute between two and four in the afternoon. Kitty liked to come and watch as Elizabeth and Emily interviewed prospective nurses. "Girls of eighteen came and swore themselves black and blue that they were thirty," she remembered, "in order to get into the service."

Through the late spring and early summer of 1861, Elizabeth and Emily poured themselves into war work. Women and men, working alongside each other for the collective good: it was a gratifying realization of Elizabeth's youthful hopes. But in order to fulfill its mission, the Women's Central needed to open a clearer line of communication with the architects of the war. In May, Henry Whitney Bellows took a delegation of board members to Washington, a city that was unfamiliar to him. In need of a savvy guide, he found his way to Dorothea Dix.

A generation older than the Blackwell sisters, Dix had built an international reputation on advocacy for the insane, working for asylum reform on both sides of the Atlantic as a lobbyist, not a medical practitioner. She was a passionate admirer of Florence Nightingale and her work with the British Sanitary Commission. When the war began, Dix made a beeline for Washington and was soon overwhelmed with inquiries from women eager to volunteer. She was a logical liaison for the Women's Central: nurses trained in New York could be sent to her for deployment.

Touring military camps and hospitals at Dix's side, Bellows and his colleagues began to envision a Washington-based entity that could not only oversee women's relief efforts but also advise the military on sanitary issues. In mid-May they submitted a proposal to Simon Cameron,

the secretary of war, outlining their ideas for a commission of philanthropists, military experts, and physicians to receive the goodwill of the
people and direct it toward the health and comfort of the soldiers, as dictated by the latest scientific information. In England, this kind of effort
had followed only after the Crimean War, its purpose to analyze past
mistakes and recommend improvements. In forward-thinking America, Bellows's proposal insisted, such measures must be taken immediately. The proposal was swiftly approved, and in June 1861 the United
States Sanitary Commission was born, with Bellows as its president in
Washington and the Women's Central as its auxiliary in New York.

The informal April meeting at the Blackwells' infirmary had led
directly to the creation of the most important civilian organization of the
Civil War. But as Bellows and Dix rose in prominence, the Blackwells
retreated in frustration. "We shall do much good, but you will probably
not see our names," Elizabeth wrote to Barbara Bodichon, "for we soon
found that jealousies were too intense for us to assume our true place."
The Sanitary Commission was happy to enlist the efforts of females and
physicians, but not of female physicians.

The Blackwells' infirmary was pointedly excluded from the list of New
York hospitals approved to train nurses, those hospitals having made it
clear that they would refuse "to have anything to do with the nurse education plan if 'the Miss Blackwells were going to engineer the matter,'"
Elizabeth quoted with disgust. These were the same hospitals that continued to prohibit female medical students on their wards—they were
not about to partner with female physicians now. And it wasn't just the
male medical establishment that objected; several lady managers of the
Women's Central, Emily noted, expressed concern "lest our name should
make the work unpopular." With casualty figures growing daily, it was
unpatriotic for the Blackwells to argue. "Of course as it is essential to
open the hospitals to nurses, we kept in the background," Elizabeth
wrote in resignation. "Had there been any power to support us, we would
have fought for our true place, but there was none."

To compound the insult, the most prominent role in the nursing
effort—Matron General and Superintendent of Women Nurses—had
gone to Dorothea Dix. "Miss Dix, though in many respects an estimable

& sensible woman, is deficient in the power of organization, and has no idea of the details of Hospital management & the requisitions for this peculiar service," Emily wrote. "I think there cannot fail to be much confusion." Elizabeth was less restrained. "The government has given Miss Dix a semi official recognition as meddler general," she spat. "A showy false thing has more success than an unpretending truth and it is very difficult to make truth pretentious, it does not puff up nearly as readily as falsehood." Emily might have been accustomed to following another woman's lead, but Elizabeth was incensed by Dix's appointment, especially when her own medical qualifications were so much stronger.

Elizabeth and Emily continued to work long hours for the Women's Central during the first year of the war. But a year was as much as they were willing to give. In June 1862, Elizabeth told her brother George, "We completed the 100 nurses that we have sent on to the war—wrote up the annual report, made up the treasurers accounts, and then resigned our place in the Registration Committee." Not only had their male colleagues left them behind as the Sanitary Commission in Washington grew, but the ladies of the Women's Central Association for Relief had disappointed them as well. "They were inclined as summer came on to do as they did last year," Emily wrote in exasperation, "all go out of town and leave the whole work of the Committee on our shoulders." Wartime philanthropy was no match for the swampy heat of a New York summer, at least for those wealthy enough to escape it.

Elizabeth and Emily had diverted enough energy from their own work, especially given the implacable chauvinism with which their tireless efforts had been received. From this point, they let the war go on without them. Intermittent and incomplete engagement was not unusual on the Union home front. Sam, Henry, and George, now in their thirties and a decade older than the average Union soldier, stayed home; Henry was among those who opted for "commutation," the practice of paying cash— about $300—to avoid military service. Older men with wives, children, and professional responsibilities tended to see enlistment bounties as a form of patriotic contribution. "I have given up reading the newspapers and following politics, for it all seems such an unsatisfactory muddle," Emily confessed to George. "I see no issue and as I can't do anything

I don't allow myself to be so absorbed in public affairs as people are generally."

The sisters turned their attention to the project of building a small cottage on a wooded ridge in Bloomfield, New Jersey, using the money Madame de Noailles had earmarked for a sanatorium. The retreat would provide therapeutic fresh air and greenery for the infirmary's patients, and much-needed relief for their exhausted doctors. The house was still under construction in January 1863, when President Lincoln issued the Emancipation Proclamation—followed in March by a national draft to replenish the Union forces. "Our carpenter & mason will put no heart in their work till drafting day is over, they are so afraid of it," Emily wrote.

In New York City, white working-class resentment—sparked both by the draft and by the fear that emancipated Black workers would soon flood the labor market—resulted in several days of lethal violence in 1863, known to history as the Draft Riots but quickly devolving into white-on-Black terrorism. Kitty and Elizabeth were in New Jersey when they heard news of the violence, and immediately headed for the city: Elizabeth to protect her patients, and Kitty to protect Elizabeth. Leaving the ferry at Cortlandt Street and unable to find a carriage, they walked the two miles to the infirmary in the July heat, warily skirting a muttering mob on Broadway.

At the infirmary, they found the patients in a state of panic, clamoring to turn out the single Black woman on the ward lest she draw the attention of the rioters. As Kitty remembered it, the white patients were tersely informed that they were free to leave; the Black patient would be staying. No one left.*

---

* In her old age, Kitty dictated her memories to various family members. An earlier version of this story is slightly different: upon reaching the infirmary, Elizabeth and Kitty found the wards empty except for the Black woman. When the staff refused to turn her out, the white patients had fled. In both versions the infirmary staff is honorably protective of the woman in peril. In the earlier one, they are unable to influence their racist patients, who leave en masse; in the revision, their principled stance inspires their patients to swallow their prejudice and stay. Elizabeth pledged her life to raising humanity to a nobler plane, and Kitty was her most devoted acolyte. It seems in keeping that Kitty might have revised her memory to show the Blackwell example in the noblest and most successful light.

Once the Bloomfield house was ready, Elizabeth spent every weekend there, gazing over the hills and picking out the ships in New York harbor with her telescope. "The green flickering light, the rustling leaves, and moss & flowers, charm all my senses," she wrote. "If I am anxious they soothe me, if sad they cheer, if worried they calm." Though she brought ailing patients along to recuperate, the cottage's salutary properties were most enjoyed by Elizabeth herself. (Despite Emily's love of the natural world, there is less evidence that she spent much time there. For her, its most salutary property might have been that it provided a break from Elizabeth's company.) "You will wonder at my hopes & plans, while the country is in such a state," Elizabeth acknowledged to Barbara. "But strange to say, business never seemed more flourishing, and every sort of undertaking seems to go on as usual. I think [this] a hopeless war, which I trust Providence will bring good ends out of—I cannot approve of either side—so I work on."

Three years into the war, Elizabeth at last traveled to Washington herself—as a tourist. Though her train rolled through "villages of tents & shanties & baggage waggons" on the outskirts of the capital, she described what she saw with a blithe cheer that belied the bloodshed just a hundred miles to the south; more than ten thousand Union soldiers were dying at the Battle of Cold Harbor, and no one could yet know that this Confederate victory would be General Lee's last. "We have had charming weather," Elizabeth wrote gaily to Kitty. "I am certainly seeing Washington under the best possible auspices." Her upbeat observations were likely intended to spare her ward's tender teenaged sensibilities, but they may also have reflected her own detachment from the conflict.

Escorted by her old Philadelphia friend William Elder, who now held a position in the Treasury Department, Elizabeth took in government buildings and monuments, the city's avenues and squares, the wonders of the Library of Congress, and the lavish fare at her hotel, from mock turtle soup to strawberries and cream. She paid a call on Dorothea Dix, "making acquaintance with the lady, and watching her style of working." But Dix was hardly the most notable of her encounters.

Dr. Elder had brought Elizabeth to see the public reception room at the

President's House, and she was admiring the view of the Potomac from its windows when Judge William Darrah Kelley, a congressman from Philadelphia and close friend of Lincoln's, happened upon them. "Why don't you go up and see the President?" he asked them. "He is all alone, it is a good chance for you." The visitors were startled, but as Elizabeth told Kitty, "Dr. Elder & I are always ready for any deed of daring." Shepherding them upstairs, Kelley "swept aside the usher & opened the door of a large comfortable square room on the second floor."

Elizabeth was surprised at the sight of the "tall ungainly loose jointed man" who stood before her. "I should not have recognized him at all from the photographs—he is much uglier than any I have seen," she wrote. "His brain must be much better in quality than quantity, for his head is small for the great lank body, and the forehead very retreating." Phrenologically speaking, Lincoln was underwhelming—an impression that was reinforced when he perched himself on a corner of his worktable and "caught up one knee, looking for all the world like a Kentucky loafer on some old tavern steps." It was hard to credit this gangling character as the brilliant writer and thinker she knew him to be.

A more gregarious or aggressive woman—Marie Zakrzewska, say— might have seized this rare opportunity to engage the president of the United States on health policy and the future of women in medicine. But Elizabeth's disappointment in the Sanitary Commission was still fresh, and face-to-face confrontation had never been her style. After a brief exchange of pleasantries with the president, she excused herself. "Altogether it was a most characteristic little peep, immeasurably better than any parade glimpse," she wrote, "so I considered myself quite in luck." In her memoir, the chronicle of her own campaign, she neglected to mention the meeting at all.

Elizabeth's account of her visit to Washington did not edit out the war entirely, but even when confronting the brutal reality—some of the wounded were quartered at her hotel—she sounded more like a sightseer. She was disappointed in the Department of the Navy—no model warships or rebel flags to see—but perked up at an invitation from a young army doctor to tour the four-hundred-bed Douglas Hospital, a few blocks from the Capitol. In one ward full of wounded men, she paused by the bed of a "handsome dark eyed young man" who, with his elderly father by his side, seemed "comfortable though weak"—a peacefully poignant tableau that was unfortunately ruined by a sudden "torrent of red blood pouring from a hole in the middle of his thigh."

Elizabeth soon took her leave, with "a very cordial greeting from the excellent young Doctor," who gave her a souvenir photograph of the hospital. She had always been more interested in institutions than in individuals. And though the national crisis was not yet over, she and Emily had a new institution in mind.

~(

CHAPTER 16

COLLEGE

The last thing the Blackwells had intended was to found a women's medical college. Their goal had always been to open existing colleges and hospitals to women, not to segregate women in separate, second-class institutions. They had watched in irritation as the female medical colleges in Philadelphia and Boston grew and prospered, attracting patrons and publicity with apparent ease. "They have each quite a large number of superficial people engaged in pushing what each year I think a sillier & sillier scheme," Elizabeth complained to Barbara Bodichon. "The products are as worthless as you can well imagine & I have yet to see the first decent doctor come from either of those schools."

The Blackwells had founded their New York Infirmary as a place for newly fledged female M.D.s to train, but the graduates who joined them over the next decade were less than impressive. Young women had weaker educational backgrounds than their male counterparts, and at the women's medical colleges they studied with professors who were often mediocre—by definition, or else why would they be teaching at a women's medical college? "I am sick of the farce of bestowing degrees upon these half educated school girls," Emily wrote. The Blackwells' disdain might be legitimate—they had worked harder in pursuit of their own credentials—but it confused their allies when these two pioneers of women's medical education heaped scorn on women's medical colleges. "It is the old difference between me & the woman's rights party," Elizabeth wrote, "too conservative for the reformers, too progressive for the conservatives."

Compounding the problem was the old-world formality Elizabeth and Emily projected. New Yorkers might hold up the Blackwells as examples, but they didn't particularly enjoy their chilly company. It was much easier to embrace women like Ann Preston, alumna and soon to be dean of the Female Medical College of Pennsylvania, a woman whose "sentimental air of martyrdom" the Blackwells abhorred. Preston had received a warm (and lucrative) reception when she came to lecture on physiology and hygiene at the invitation of the New York Infirmary's trustees; when asked why they had overlooked the infirmary's own founding physicians, these ladies protested, "Oh we couldn't go to [the Drs.] Blackwell as we do to Ann Preston—we are almost afraid of them." Unwilling to unbend, Elizabeth and Emily struggled to connect with the very women they inspired. "Somehow they always seemed to feel that it was not their place to come & help us," Emily wrote, "but to stand by & see what we were doing."

The situation came to a head with the establishment of a third women's medical college, this time in New York City itself, not far from the infirmary. Its founder, Clemence Sophia Lozier, had received her degree from the Central Medical College in Syracuse, one of the Eclectic schools that Elizabeth and Emily dismissed. "If we could have joined with these persons we should have done so," Elizabeth insisted, "but we found their ideas of medical education so low, their hostility to the profession so rooted, and their distrust of us, so marked, that it was impossible to join forces. . . . The whole thing is a repetition of the Boston and Philadelphia attempts on a still poorer scale."

Incorporated in April 1863, Lozier's New York Medical College for Women trumpeted its own founding in a way the Blackwells found galling. "Being the first in this city," its annual report proclaimed, "it may be regarded as an index of advancing civilization, as well as in its character marking the progressive era in medical science." All of its trustees were women, and Lozier announced her intention to strive eventually for a faculty that was likewise entirely female. Elizabeth thought this was ridiculous. How could an aspiring woman doctor hope to succeed if her professors were themselves relatively inexperienced women? "The true plan is for women to use men for their own objects," she wrote, "not exclusively of course, but just as far as they can better accomplish their object by so doing." She dismissed Lozier's students as "a vulgar little class of women, led by one of the commonest type of woman's rights women."

So: the superior medical education available to men was—despite Elizabeth and Emily's successful examples—still off-limits, and the institutions that did offer medical education to women were, at least in the Blackwells' opinion, woefully inferior. How should they proceed? By changing their minds, though not their standards.

~

"We believe that the time has come to form a really good school of medicine for women," Elizabeth announced to a meeting at the infirmary. It was a week before Christmas 1863; Abraham Lincoln had delivered his address at Gettysburg a month earlier. Though the war dragged on, the Blackwells drafted a speech that both summed up their criticisms of the state of women's medical education and pointed a way forward. The "blank wall of social and professional antagonism" faced by aspiring women doctors may have begun to crumble, but they still suffered from a disabling lack of access: not just to schools and hospitals but also to prizes, professorships, medical societies, and the stimulating companionship of colleagues. And then there were the more fundamental handicaps. "Women have no business habits," the address declared, "girls are seldom drilled thoroughly in anything; they are not trained to use their minds any more than their muscles; they seldom apply themselves with a will and a grip to master any subject." Combine this lack of discipline with the pecuniary instability that propelled most women toward a profession in the first place, and it became clear that what women needed was, if anything, a medical education superior to that available from any existing medical school, male or female.

For a combined total of thirty years, Elizabeth and Emily had immersed themselves in the question of what comprised legitimate, rigorous medical education. They had studied all branches of medicine, not just obstetrics and gynecology. They had experimented with leeches and mercury, blisters and sitz baths, botanical remedies and magnetism and surgery. They had examined specimens under the microscope and lectured on diet and hygiene. They were more eclectic than the Eclectics in their openness to the broadest spectrum of useful approaches to healing, and they could quote from the traditional medical texts by heart. Now they envisioned a program that took all their experience into account—one that would have daunted most of the young men they had once studied with.

Examinations would be held in the laboratory and by the bedside, and students would have to demonstrate their skills, not just parrot back their lessons. They would be expected to speak up in class and work individually with their professors rather than listening and watching in a passive herd. A woman's traditional caregiving role might endow her with natural instincts as a physician, but instincts were insufficient: "It is knowledge, not sympathy, which can administer the right medicine; it is observation and comprehension, not sympathy, which will discover the kind of disease." The Blackwells' college might be for women, but it would command respect from the male establishment.

The speech was a statement not just of intention but of action already underway. The infirmary's trustees had applied to the New York state legislature, which had duly responded with an act "to enable the corporation entitled 'The New York Infirmary for Indigent Women and Children,' to grant and confer the title of Doctor of Medicine." (In keeping with its new, larger mission, the term *Indigent* was at this point officially dropped from the infirmary's name.) As firmly as she had once opposed the founding of a women's medical college, Elizabeth now embraced it. This, she proclaimed to Barbara Bodichon in the fall of 1864, was now "the San Greal* of my life, the deep unchangeable undying interest." Emily certainly shared her sister's views on adding rigor to the medical curriculum. For the moment, they could agree.

Robert E. Lee surrendered on April 9, 1865, and five days later Abraham Lincoln was assassinated. His death inspired Elizabeth in a way his living presence had not. "The great secret of our dead leader's popularity was the wonderful instinct with which he felt and acted the wishes and judgements of the great mass of the people," she wrote. Populist instinct was something Elizabeth had always lacked; now, for the first time, she was admiring rather than disparaging it. "I never was thoroughly repub-

* Holy Grail

lican before; there was always a shade of conservative aristocratic tendency," she mused. "But I am so thoroughly now, heart and soul." She felt ready to lead again.

༞

On March 5, 1866, Emily turned to her journal for the first time in years. "The circle is broken," she wrote. "Ah dear Howard! Poor Anna!" After a second sojourn in India, thirty-five-year-old Howard had returned to England in shaky health. In February he died, alone.

Anna was devastated. Howard, fifteen years younger than she, had been not just brother but also son and soulmate, the only sibling to have joined her in leaving America behind. "I had built on that beloved life as on a rock," she wrote in anguish. "Whether I shall really be able to outlive this loss I have no idea." Knowing Anna's histrionic tendencies, no one was seriously worried, but her grief created a compelling reason for another trip to England, which Elizabeth was only too happy to seize. She spent the summer and early fall of 1866 in Paris and London, enjoying a series of encounters that confirmed and intensified her eagerness to complete her work in America.

The first encounter, in London, was with Elizabeth Garrett, the young Englishwoman who had attended Elizabeth's 1859 lectures and with whom she had been corresponding ever since. Garrett had pursued her medical education doggedly wherever she could, ignoring female peers who saw her as "a kind of 'social evil' they don't wish to know" and a male medical establishment that dismissed her. "Science, at best, seems to sit upon a woman like the helmet on the temples of Minerva," read a florid editorial in *The Lancet*, "an incongruous adjunct, conceived by Poetry, not earned by stern experience and actual prowess in war." But the comparison to the classical goddess of wisdom and strategy was unintentionally apt. Garrett's determination grew with each obstacle, and she eventually exploited a loophole in the charter of the Society of Apothecaries that enabled her to sit its examinations and receive certification to practice. In July 1866, a month after her thirtieth birthday, she founded her own dispensary for women and children, St. Mary's, in Marylebone.

Elizabeth arrived in London in time to attend the opening ceremony. "In Miss Garrett we have the first legally qualified female practitioner which England can boast,"* proclaimed Dr. Archibald Billing, a fellow of the Royal Society. "In America, where they move faster than we do, I am assured that women doctors are establishing themselves fairly in the good opinion of the public." Perhaps he was aware that one of them was listening.

The second encounter lifted Elizabeth into an unfamiliar state that felt suspiciously like happiness. "I have had an unexpected pleasure in the renewal of friendship with an old comrade," she wrote to Marian. Hippolyte Blot had invited Elizabeth to spend a Sunday with his family at their country retreat while she was in Paris. It had been seventeen years since Blot saved Elizabeth from total blindness at La Maternité. "The intimate friendship of a man of one's own age, with whom a great deal of chum feeling exists, and of whom you are very fond, has a very great charm," she wrote with unaccustomed warmth. "[It] is giving to the last part of my stay, an intensity of life, that is very refreshing to a half starved soul." Within her own family, Elizabeth's relationships were often fraught; outside the Blackwell clan, they were almost entirely professional. It was a balm to relax with an old friend, a rare example of a man who considered her a peer. Elizabeth had never endorsed Florence Nightingale's rule that medicine demanded celibacy of its female practitioners, even if in practice she had never broken it. It was satisfying to recall the frisson of personal attraction she had once felt.

Also in Paris, Elizabeth caught up with a woman whose history had been entwined with the Blackwells' since the beginning of their medical presence in New York. Mary Putnam had been a girl of ten when her father, George P. Putnam, published Elizabeth's first book, *The Laws of Life*. At seventeen, just as the Blackwells moved the infirmary to Second Avenue, she had joined them as a student: "a very talented girl," Elizabeth had noted approvingly. Later, Putnam became the first woman accred-

---

* The first acknowledged female practitioner, that is. Half a century earlier, in 1812, the University of Edinburgh had conferred a medical degree on James Barry, a slim, smooth-cheeked young man who went on to spectacular success as a high-ranking military physician. Not until his death in 1865—the same year Garrett qualified to practice—was it discovered that Barry was originally female.

ited by the New York College of Pharmacy, and in 1864 she received her diploma from the Female Medical College of Pennsylvania. She continued her education in Boston at the New England Hospital for Women and Children, with Marie Zakrzewska. But Putnam's unusual ambition remained unsatisfied, so she pursued it across the Atlantic.

"Little Miss Putnam, who is gaining her first experience of Europe, is quite intoxicated with Paris," Elizabeth reported. It was gratifying, a generation after her own studies in Paris, to mentor a stellar student whose medical education she had initiated. Elizabeth helped Putnam find lodgings in the Latin Quarter and even unbent enough to complain to her about Anna: "a great Spiritualist much to the Dr.'s distress," Putnam noted, who "thinks she is continually receiving communications from the brother who has recently died." Venting to Putnam apparently did Elizabeth good. "When she went away," Putnam wrote, "she actually kissed me for the first time during the period of our long and friendly acquaintance!" Putnam was the first woman admitted to the medical school of the Sorbonne; her success drew Elizabeth Garrett away from her dispensary in England to join her in pursuit of more advanced medical education. Garrett would be the first woman to receive a degree in Paris. And Putnam, once she had hers, would become one of the Blackwells' most important allies in New York.

～

The ranks of accomplished women doctors were growing, and the Blackwells could take much of the credit for showing them the way. They were not, however, ready to be overtaken. Even sharing the path remained difficult for them. Clemence Lozier and Sarah Dolley, who had earned a degree from the Eclectic college in Syracuse in 1851, invited the Blackwells to join them in an effort to establish a much-needed national association of medical women. The sisters swatted away this gesture of solidarity. "They will, as always, parody a good idea," Emily fumed to Elizabeth, "pretend falsely to meet a real want, and lay hold of the work in so shallow & vulgar a way as to make it impossible for us to work with them, and yet cut ground from under our feet, and place us at the disadvantage of standing aside & in the background, while they noisily assume the centre of public notice & action."

Elizabeth and Emily preferred a quieter kind of progress. In 1866 they created the position of "sanitary visitor," sending their interns to attend patients in their homes not only when they were ill or in labor, but also to teach preventive hygiene. One resident assistant who filled this innovative role was Rebecca J. Cole, the daughter of free Black laborers in Philadelphia. Born in 1848, Cole received a classical education at the Institute for Colored Youth, the oldest African-American secondary school in the country, and went on to become the first Black graduate of the Female Medical College of Pennsylvania. After finishing her thesis on "The Eye and its Appendages" in 1867—with a thorough explanation of purulent ophthalmia—Cole had arrived at the infirmary, where she "carried on this work with tact and care," Elizabeth wrote approvingly.

Cole would return to Philadelphia and become an early voice against racial bias in public health, asserting that "the respectability of a household ought to be measured by the condition of the cellar," not by the complexion of its members. There is little surviving material related to her time at the infirmary, but her position—and the lack of comment upon it in the Blackwells' correspondence—is evidence of their unusual open-mindedness regarding race. Some of the infirmary's more conservative supporters—and plenty of its white patients—must have reacted to Cole's presence with less equanimity. Rebecca Lee Crumpler, in 1864 the first Black woman to earn a medical degree, from the New England Female Medical College, immediately moved to Virginia to work among the newly emancipated. Susan McKinney Steward, who received her degree in 1869 from Clemence Lozier's New York Medical College for Women, practiced in Brooklyn's Black community. The number of Black women doctors would slowly grow in the decades following the Civil War, but most of them studied in the South at schools founded to educate the formerly enslaved, and practiced exclusively among Black women. Cole's presence at the New York Infirmary was a noteworthy exception.

The opening of their own college would mark the end of the Blackwells' shared journey toward the moral high ground. Though her own name remained permanently associated with the New York Infirmary, Elizabeth knew that her sister was outgrowing the role of deputy. "Emily . . . does grandly at the centre of this movement," she confided to Barbara, "and exercises a certain imperiousness as head of the establishment which is not unbecoming." Emily was ready to lead, and Elizabeth was ready to leave. They could see the point ahead where their paths diverged, and both looked forward to it with some relief. (A postscript in a letter to George, who had begun to prosper in real estate, betrays Emily's state of mind. "When you write on money matters direct me personally," she instructed, "otherwise Eliz always opens the letter.") On November 2, 1868, trustees, friends, physicians, and a small group of students gathered at Second Avenue for the opening of the Woman's Medical College of the New York Infirmary.

"True growth is slow (as we measure time) and silent," Elizabeth began her inaugural address. Then, in case the implied rebuke to the "noisy," "pushing" leaders of the other women's colleges wasn't clear, she went a step further: "It is an easy thing to found a poor college." Their school would surpass its predecessors with a program even more stringent than Elizabeth and Emily had outlined in their address five years earlier. They would offer an unprecedented three years of study instead of two. Their course of lectures would build progressively year to year, rather than simply repeating the same material twice. And theirs would be the first medical school of any kind to feature a professor— Elizabeth herself—devoted to the subject of hygiene. Emily would take the chair of obstetrics and diseases of women; otherwise, the faculty was male. Students would be tested yearly by a board of examiners that included Elizabeth's earliest allies: Austin Flint, who had published her 1849 thesis in the *Buffalo Medical Journal*, and Stephen Smith, her classmate from Geneva, who had gone on to help found New York City's board of health.

"This school is the only one that the profession has confidence in, the only one it has sanctioned," Elizabeth concluded, somewhat inaccurately. Graduates of the Philadelphia and Boston women's medical colleges were gaining recognition, some of them as the Blackwells' own deputies, and students at Clemence Lozier's school—which had since moved to within a few of blocks of the infirmary on Second Avenue— had the same right to observe at Bellevue and other New York hospitals as the Blackwells' students did. But the Woman's Medical College of the New York Infirmary—embodying everything the Blackwell sisters had learned about effective medicine and public health—insisted upon a level of excellence at least as high as any to be found in American medical education and indisputably higher than that of the existing women's colleges.

Henry J. Raymond, the founder of the *New-York Times* and trustee of Elizabeth's original dispensary, spoke next—though, he was quick to point out, Dr. Blackwell's remarks had left him with little to add. Echoing Henry Ward Beecher at the infirmary's opening ceremony in 1857, Raymond declared that women's "keen intuition of the nature of complaints, and ready perception of the best remedies; their large sympathy for the suffering and their gentle solicitude during convalescence rendered them far more acceptable to patients than were men." Twelve years later

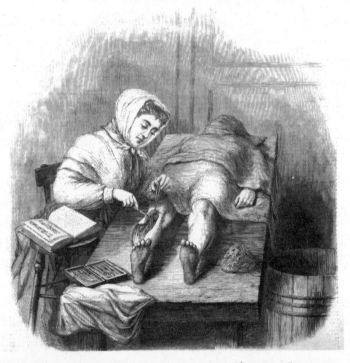

DISSECTION AT CLEMENCE LOZIER'S NEW YORK MEDICAL COLLEGE FOR
WOMEN, IN *FRANK LESLIE'S ILLUSTRATED NEWSPAPER*, APRIL 16, 1870.
COURTESY NEW YORK SOCIETY LIBRARY

the sisters had become only too skilled at keeping their impatience with sexual stereotypes to themselves. Raymond's words would resonate usefully with his readers.

After a tour of the infirmary's modest wards, the gathering dispersed, and seventeen students began their first term. One of them was a twenty-eight-year-old Englishwoman named Sophia Jex-Blake. The darling of a wealthy and well-connected family, possessed of strong opinions and high spirits, Jex-Blake had set her sights on admission to Harvard. Rebuffed, she found her way to the Blackwells, who promised an equally exacting course of study. Elizabeth reserved judgment on this rather forward young woman—"I'm afraid she won't be very amenable to discipline"—but here at last was their first English student, and she seemed to be made of the right stuff. "If I am to be a doctor at all," Jex-Blake declared, "I mean to be a thoroughly good one." She wrote happily to her mother of lectures and dissections and petitioning Emily for five minutes of fresh air between classes ("to which she instantly assented as desirable"), but only two weeks into the term Jex-Blake received word that her father was dying, and rushed home. She would go on to become a pioneer of women's medical education in England.

Elizabeth herself would not remain in New York much longer. Eight months after delivering the opening address at the Woman's Medical College, and long before its first diplomas were granted, she returned to England forever.

～

In her memoir nearly three decades later, Elizabeth skated briskly over her decision to leave. "In 1869 the early pioneer work in America was ended," she wrote. "Throughout the Northern States the free and equal entrance of women into the profession of medicine was secured." This wasn't true even at the time her memoir was published, let alone in 1869, but she framed her departure as a logical next step.

> Our New York centre was well organized under able guidance, and I determined to return to England for a temporary though prolonged residence, both to renew physical strength, which had been severely tried, and to enlarge my experience of life, as well as to assist in

the pioneer work so bravely commencing in London, and which extended later to Edinburgh.

This was accurate. Also accurate, though unsuitable for the valedictory conclusion of a memoir, were several other motives. For a woman who thrived on new challenges, running a hospital and a medical college was exhausting, exacting, repetitive work. The pressure to raise funds—often from people who failed to pay her the personal respect her symbolic achievement warranted—was relentless. Elizabeth was tired of exile in America, tired of striving for an ideal future in a state of chronic dissatisfaction with the present. And as Emily came into her own as a practitioner and professor, she was both better equipped to sustain the institutions they had founded and more difficult to share them with.

Though Elizabeth's crisp summary leaves out these tensions, a hastily penciled sheet in what seems to be Emily's hand preserves them. Emily may have welcomed the prospect of Elizabeth's departure, but the manner of it was important to her. "Partnership (of 10 years with identical names and initials and practice so intimately associated if terminated at all, ought) *not* to be terminated without *at least* six months' notice—say July 1 1869, or Jany 1 1870," she scribbled. The infirmary and the college were indelibly associated with the name Elizabeth Blackwell; her exit would shake the faith of the institutions' trustees and donors and deter prospective students and patients. In order to remain effectively at the helm, Emily would need to reassure the public of her own competence and sincere intention to stay put. The notes outline the idea of Elizabeth first moving her own private practice to an office uptown as an interim step, leaving Emily in sole charge. The pattern held true to the end: Elizabeth was thinking of her own future, gazing at the horizon and eager to set sail, while Emily wrestled with the practical details.

Though she may have framed her trip to England as exploratory, the family could tell that Elizabeth's move was for the long term. "If you would take a peep at Aunt Elizabeth's room, I think you would be rather astonished at its appearance," Kitty wrote to her favorite "cousin," Alice Stone Blackwell, now nearly twelve. "Trunks, boxes, books, clothes and papers, cover the floor in every direction; so that our room is in a con-

stant and uncomfortable state of litter." Elizabeth was leaving her ward
behind for now—the extended family had come to depend on Kitty's
help both with Grandmother Hannah and with the grandchildren. But
before she left, Elizabeth wrote a will, naming Emily and George as her
executors and Kitty's guardians. (Never mind that Kitty was by now in
her early twenties—Elizabeth still addressed her as "child.") Elizabeth's
modest assets were to be divided among her sisters, and her possessions
shared between Emily and Kitty, with a stipulation that Kitty should have
a piano. It was the tidying-up act of a woman who expected to be out of
reach for the foreseeable future.

Elizabeth sailed in July 1869 and took up residence with Barbara
Bodichon in London. Though her plans for the future were unclear, she
remained the only female on the British Medical Register, and she had
personal ties to the young women now attempting to storm the gates of
medicine in Britain. In September in her native Bristol, her attendance
at the congress of the National Association for the Promotion of Social
Science—where "many admirable people of large ideas" greeted her
warmly—bolstered her confidence.

She was soon writing a carefully diplomatic letter to the New York
Infirmary's board of trustees. "They claim me, on all hands, to remain
here this winter, and give an impulse in the right direction, to the medical
movement which is going on here," she announced, stretching the truth.
For the sake of the movement—not on her own whim, she insisted—she
would remain in London, at least for the time being. By midwinter, at
least privately, her mind was made up. "I am settled in England," she
wrote to Kitty. "I have not the slightest intention of returning to America
and DV* will never cross the ocean again. . . . I belong here, and here I
shall stay." The infirmary and college annuals would continue to list her
on the faculty and the board of trustees; it would be fifteen years before
the title "Dean of Faculty" appeared by Emily's name.

Emily had no time to dwell on the manner of Elizabeth's departure or
the duration of her absence. The college's second year was upon her. Lectures began in October 1869 with fourteen students, fewer than expected,

* *Deo volente,* "God willing."

though "I did not indulge in as sanguine expectations as some," she was quick to point out. The college was in many ways the embodiment of its founders: admirable, impressive, and somewhat forbidding. Its term began earlier in the fall than that of other schools, its academic standards were higher, and three years of study were more expensive than two. Its advertising circulars were ineffective: "All these students have come from direct personal influence," Emily noted. Even among enrolled students, there was a feeling "that the school is more respected than liked, that students feel more at home in the more easy indulgent and coddling tone of the Phil[adelphia] school," she continued. "It seems to me that, as usual, we have done more by stirring & forcing others on, than by our own success." Were the college's expectations too rigorous for undisciplined Americans?

Elizabeth, relieved to be free of the daily toil of hospital work—"I would sink the whole thing in the bottom of the Sound, rather than come back to it," she wrote—exhorted Emily to follow her to England. In Elizabeth's opinion, the new college would thrive best without either of its founding sisters. "It is, at present, the Blackwell College," she wrote, "and it won't succeed as long as it is, as a thoroughly American college." She advised Emily to stay only as long as it took to lay aside a bit more money, then leave the institution to grow up American, free of the austere "Blackwell element."

Emily agreed that the college needed to work on its public image. "I can see very well that what is really wanted is to bring in more of the popular American element, something which neither you nor I have ever been able to fully give," she told Elizabeth. "If I can get that I believe we shall neither of us be absolutely essential." She was eager to "build up a little group on whom I can devolve the burden of the Institution"— but she also intended to stay with the ship they had launched and to find the crew that would help her steer it. Emerging at last from Elizabeth's shadow, Emily would sustain the work of the New York Infirmary for Women and Children and its Woman's Medical College for the next thirty years—ironically ensuring the persistence of her sister's legacy in America.

Emily reached the end of April 1870 in a rush of lectures, examinations, inpatients, house calls for trustees' children with scarlet fever and pneumonia, and the college's first graduation ceremony—for which she wrote a last-minute speech when one speaker canceled the night before. "It seemed as though everything came to a climax, and burst upon me at once," she wrote. But just as she reached the end of her strength, she was surprised to find board members stepping forward to help, taking over the details of the ceremony, reception, and supper to follow. Perhaps she was not quite as alone as she had thought. "Everyone felt as though the whole affair was a success," she wrote with unaccustomed satisfaction. And more help was on the way. Mary Putnam had promised to join the college's faculty as soon as she finished her Paris degree. Surely she would bring some of the "popular American element" that was lacking—a combination of determined "push," scientific brilliance, and the adamantine faith in women's potential that Margaret Fuller had put into words a generation earlier.

Emily was moved when the class valedictorian made "a graceful & entirely spontaneous little tribute 'to our absent professor.'" For all that Emily had craved distance from Elizabeth, it was bittersweet to witness this milestone in their work without her. But Kitty, who attended the graduation "with great glee and interest," was struck more by Emily's presence than Elizabeth's absence. "Aunt Emily made her appearance on the occasion, in a black velvet dress with a train," she reported to young Alice. "I heard a good many people in the audience speak of her as 'a fine looking woman.'" She beamed with pride as she watched "the conferring of diplomas on the first five graduates of Aunt Emily's College."

~(

CHAPTER 17

DIVERGENCE

The story of Elizabeth and Emily Blackwell, pioneering and collaborating sister doctors, ends here. But each of their own stories, lived an ocean apart, continued for another forty years.

Elizabeth's trajectory flattened in England. Her confidence that the rising generation of British medical women—led by Elizabeth Garrett and Sophia Jex-Blake—would welcome her as their mentor and colleague was misplaced. "Miss Garrett, though outwardly pleasant, is bristling with distrust and anxiety," Elizabeth wrote to Emily from London. Over the next three years, Garrett would score a series of triumphs: the completion of her degree at the Sorbonne in 1870; the expansion of her Marylebone dispensary into the New Hospital for Women in 1872; the respect of physicians including Sir James Paget and the support of powerful philanthropists like Lord Shaftesbury; and the love of a Scottish shipping magnate, James Skelton Anderson, who not only approved of his bride's career but bought her a carriage as a wedding gift to facilitate it. She had also learned her predecessor's lesson—to hold other women at arm's length, lest they reflect poorly on herself—only too well.

Sophia Jex-Blake was achieving a different sort of recognition. Refusing to seek her medical degree on the continent, she pursued admission at the University of Edinburgh. When the faculty insisted it could not allow such disruption for the sake of one woman, she recruited four more. On November 2, 1869—a year to the day after the opening of the Blackwells' college—Jex-Blake's group, which later grew to seven, became the first women to join a class of men at a British university. "I do indeed congratulate you undergraduates with all my heart," Elizabeth wrote, beaming in their reflected light. "I feel as if I *must* come up to Edinburgh to see and bless the class!" But the Edinburgh Seven, as they became known, looked to Jex-Blake for leadership, and her take-no-prisoners style was the antithesis of Elizabeth's measured, understated approach. Opposition in Edinburgh reached an ugly climax a year later when the women were pelted with garbage and epithets as they entered Surgeons' Hall for an anatomy examination. The university eventually prevailed in preventing the women from completing their degrees, but the "Surgeons' Hall Riot" generated enormous publicity for the cause of women in medicine. Though her confrontational approach alienated many—including Garrett Anderson—Jex-Blake led the way to the founding of the London School of Medicine for Women in 1874.

Elizabeth would serve in ceremonial roles as a consultant to Garrett Anderson's hospital and on the faculty of Jex-Blake's college, but these public endorsements masked an unsettling degree of personal antipathy. "Neither Miss Putnam, Miss Garrett, nor Miss Jex-Blake will ever be doctors, that as a woman I feel in the slightest degree proud of," Elizabeth told Emily. "They are all hard, mannish, soulless; and though they are all doing excellent service as pioneers, and I am happy always to praise them . . . as women physicians such as we wish to see as a permanent and valuable feature of society, I think them not only useless but objectionable." Such women physicians as Elizabeth wished to see were formed in her own image, devoted to health education rather than clinical practice, and inspired by right living rather than scientific advancement. It did not help that the British often confused her with another notable American doctor, Mary Walker, who had served as both a surgeon and a spy during the Civil War, spent months in a Confederate prison, and received the Medal of Honor. Even more memorable than Walker's swashbuckling deeds was her personal style—she cut her hair short and wore trousers and frock coats. "I could not have imagined how very wide-spread and profound a mischief that little humbug could have done," Elizabeth complained bitterly. "I am constantly addressed by her name, in mistake."

Elizabeth found herself companionless, especially when the Bodichons decamped to Algiers and Barbara's lively intellectual circle disbanded. She missed Kitty, who had grown from daughter-servant into something more like the proverbial angel in the house. "You can help me so much by taking charge of all my things and telling where they are and reading and occasionally stitching for me and doing errands and keeping my rooms in first rate order and above all loving me very much," Elizabeth wrote to her in a plaintive rush. Kitty, deeply attached to Henry and Lucy's daughter Alice, was quietly devastated to leave America behind, but her first loyalty was to Elizabeth; a year after her departure, she joined her in London.

Elizabeth might have spent her life fighting to open a profession to women, but she made it clear that neither career nor marriage was an option for Kitty, who remained suspended outside class or category—a young woman prematurely old, with graying hair, weak eyesight, and compromised hearing. Perhaps to compensate for the life Kitty had been denied, Elizabeth arranged to foster a baby in the fall of 1870, just as Kitty joined her in London. The child—the illegitimate son of the sculptor Susan Durant, a well-connected acquaintance—would be Kitty's joy for the two years he remained with them.

Bolstered by Kitty's generous steadfastness—as Alice would later say, Kitty "fitted herself into all Dr. Elizabeth's angles like an eiderdown quilt"—Elizabeth continued her public quest. Medicine had always been just a pathway toward a morally perfect world, and the world remained far from perfect. She might be the only woman on the British Medical Register, but she had little success—or even interest—in attracting patients. She invested more active energy in the formation, in 1871, of the National Health Society, an organization devoted to the promotion of sanitary practice. Its motto—"Prevention is better than cure"—set hygiene firmly above the arts of diagnosis, pharmacology, and surgery. Over the next three decades, Elizabeth skipped from one cause to the next, always happiest when leading the way toward a better world. Her days were full of committee meetings and long stretches at her writing desk, churning out pamphlets and articles for publication. And though she was no longer spending much time healing the human body, she was no less preoccupied with it. As a physician and a moralist, she saw it as her responsibility to address the corrupting influence of sex.

Elizabeth had arrived in London days before the passage of the third and final Contagious Diseases Act, a measure—intended to curb the rampant spread of syphilis, especially in the military—that inflamed reform-minded women across Britain. The acts placed the burden of public health not on the soldier, whose need for sex was considered natural, but on the prostitute, who could now be arrested, forcibly examined, and confined to hospital if she was found to be infected. Elizabeth was outraged twice over: Not only did the law hold men and women to wildly different standards of sexual behavior, it also failed to condemn the evil of prostitution, punishing its victims instead of eliminating its causes. After her sojourns on the syphilis ward in Philadelphia and among the indigent women of Paris, London, and New York, Elizabeth understood how promiscuity and poverty converged in "that direful purchase of women which is really the greatest obstacle to the progress of the race." She would leave the issue of eradicating poverty to others, but she was determined to make war on promiscuity. The repeal of the Contagious Diseases Acts became a clearly defined battle.

In the world Elizabeth envisioned, children would learn to venerate chastity at their mother's knee, growing into men and women who honored the sanctity of procreation. Sanctity, indeed, had eclipsed science in the formulation of her opinions. Louis Pasteur's recent experiments confirming the concept of germ theory had not yet convinced the general public, including Elizabeth, who could not embrace the idea that amoral microbes might be responsible for disease. Germ theory detached health from virtue—but for Elizabeth the two were inseparable. As a student she had written that ship fever found its victims among the fearful; now she refused to relinquish the conviction that venereal disease was caused by licentious behavior. In order to break the cycle of depravity, it was critical that parents teach the paramount importance of sexual propriety. And therein lay a paradox: in order to promote purity, Elizabeth insisted that parents should talk to their children about sex.

The book she eventually wrote on the topic—*Counsel to Parents on the Moral Education of their Children in Relation to Sex*—had nothing to do with the reproductive anatomy, though its subject remained incendiary enough that the publisher marketed it as a medical text. Her point was simply that men and women needed to live according to the same sexual standards, prizing the "exquisite spiritual joys" of marital intercourse over the "slavery of lust," and teaching their children to understand and value the difference. Though *Counsel to Parents* did touch upon the dangers of autoerotic "self abuse," its content was otherwise remarkably innocuous. "It might almost be read aloud in mixed company," Emily wrote, shaking her head at the delicate sensibilities of British publishers. The book, released in 1879, would become the most widely read of Elizabeth's works.

For nearly ten years, Elizabeth moved restlessly, with Kitty dutifully packing and unpacking in each new lodging, nursing her guardian through repeated attacks of undefined gastric illness, and accompanying her on extended convalescent trips to Europe. It became clear that London was not a healthy home for either of them, and with Elizabeth employing her pen far more than her stethoscope, they had no reason to stay. They settled at last in the seaside town of Hastings, in a trim brick cottage known as Rock House, perched on the edge of the English Channel and close enough to London that Elizabeth could remain active in organizations including the Social Purity Alliance, the National Vigilance Association, and the Moral Reform Union, all of them devoted to the cause of upright sexual conduct. Eventually Anna and Marian would join Elizabeth in Hastings, in a double house with two entrances that allowed them both proximity and distance. The Blackwells, to the end, loved and annoyed each other in equal measure.

Though Elizabeth's primary message was one of chaste restraint, emphasizing the virtuous influence of wives and mothers in elevating the baser instincts of husbands and sons, she made detours into more eyebrow-raising areas, using her medical credentials to deflect criticism. In a pamphlet entitled *The Human Element in Sex*, she declared it "a well-established fact" that for happily married women, "increasing physical satisfaction attaches to the ultimate physical expression of love." Furthermore, she insisted, "a repose and general well-being results from this natural occasional intercourse, whilst the total deprivation of it produces irritability." It's tempting to see this as a bracingly direct statement about female libido, but Elizabeth's point reached straight back to the antique orthodoxy

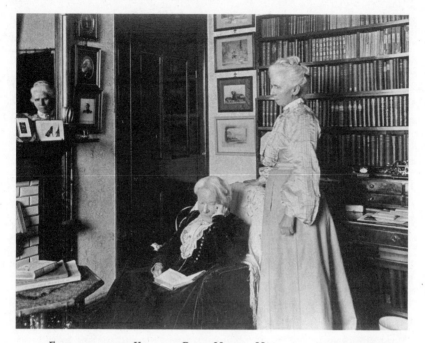

ELIZABETH AND KITTY AT ROCK HOUSE, HASTINGS, CIRCA 1905.
COURTESY SCHLESINGER LIBRARY, RADCLIFFE INSTITUTE, HARVARD UNIVERSITY

of Hippocrates and Galen. *Furor uterinus,* wandering womb, hysteria, nym-
phomania: since the dawn of medicine, men had been blaming female
ailments on the unsatisfied uterus. "Let her marry, and the sickness will
disappear," went the ancient adage. In this as elsewhere, Elizabeth did not
include herself among the women she counseled. She never ascribed her
own irritability to her unmarried state, and never acknowledged that her
authority on the health benefits of wifely sex might be questionable.

Though she endorsed the good-wife-wise-mother ideal, Elizabeth's
work among the poor had made it obvious that there was such a thing
as too many children, a point she made in a speech entitled "How to
Keep a Household in Health," delivered just after her return to England.
Procreation, she declared, "is largely under the control of established
physiological laws, which should be known to parents." Critics assumed
she was endorsing artificial contraception—in the form of condoms
(by this time made from rubber as well as animal intestine) or vinegar-

soaked sponges—but to Elizabeth, protected sex was just as degenerate as masturbation. The only moral way to limit family size, in her view, was to restrict intercourse to the infertile days of a woman's menstrual cycle. "From the outset of marriage the wife must determine the times of union," Elizabeth later wrote. "Through the guidance of sexual intercourse by the law of the female constitution, the increase of the race will be in accordance with reason." Her serene confidence that a righteous woman could regulate her husband's sexual needs remained, like much of Elizabeth's thinking, on a level too idealized for most flawed humans to find useful. Interestingly, in the same pamphlet, she defined a problem few acknowledged: marital rape. "A man who commits rape in marriage is even a meaner criminal than one who exposes himself to the just punishment which is attached to violence outside marriage," she wrote. She offered no suggestions for women on how to avoid it.

Elizabeth's moral crusading extended beyond the domestic sphere to the professional one. As her reform work led her further from the laboratory, she began to campaign *against* scientific advances she found morally questionable. Vaccination, for one. In New York. she had once lost an infant patient whose constitution was not strong enough to withstand the injection of the attenuated virus. "To a hygienic physician thoroughly believing in the beneficence of Nature's laws," she wrote in her memoir, "to have caused the death of a child by such means was a tremendous blow!" Wasn't the first duty of a physician to do no harm? She developed a similar horror for vivisection. In England, she and Kitty grew attached to a series of canine companions, which explained her condemnation of experimentation on animals, but her objections increasingly included what she perceived as unnecessary surgery on human patients as well. For a woman who had come to prize prevention over cure, the idea of resorting to a scalpel seemed like mutilation, a presumptuous trespass on the divine design of the human body.

The one area in which Elizabeth was actively interested in scientific experimentation was, ironically, the realm of spiritualism. As she approached old age, and as new truths clashed unnervingly with her own understanding of the world, she may have craved the kind of existential comfort Anna had always sought in the supernatural. Though she had never shared Anna's devoted faith in Mesmer's magnetism or Baron du Potet's séances—a faith her sister shared with many of the most prominent intellectuals of the era—she had never entirely dismissed it. Confidence in life after death, Elizabeth insisted as she entered her eighties, was "really of tremendous practical importance." So she devised a plan: she would write down specific memories and seal them away, and after her death her friends would convene to see if her spirit could convey the hidden information to them. She failed to muster much interest in her experiment but followed through with her end of it just in case: "My 'Test' is written and safely put away."

From the beginning, Elizabeth had seen medicine as a tool for showing people how to live: first in terms of opening the profession to women, and later as a way of teaching hygiene, both physical and moral. The girl who had refused to admit when she was sick grew into a woman who refused to accept human imperfection. The quest to transcend it fueled her, but her determination often hardened into a rigidity that drove potential allies away. "Doubt is disease," she had proclaimed, but to dismiss doubt was to reject all opinions other than one's own. Her refusal to compromise was the key both to her achievement and to her chronic isolation. She had dreamed of living in her own communal phalanx, but she never found people perfect enough to join her there.

~

For Emily, the period following Elizabeth's departure was not easy. In addition to overseeing the details of the infirmary and the college, she needed to reassure her board, staff, and faculty that Elizabeth's indefinitely extended absence did not signal their imminent failure. In the brief calm after the college's first commencement in the spring of 1870, she despaired at the prospect of another year alone. "I am utterly unwilling to be so overworked and harassed with detail," she wrote to Elizabeth, "to live in the midst of students & patients—the interests of my practice and the school interfering & clashing, and my personal life entirely suppressed." But she saw no alternative.

Soon afterward, in the heat of August, Hannah Blackwell died, her long decline accelerated at the end by gangrene in her foot. Emily, suspended uncomfortably between the roles of daughter and physician, bound Hannah's jaw with a handkerchief for her laying out. "I cannot describe the shock it gave me to perform that last office," she wrote to Elizabeth. "The visible family link seemed broken in her loss." Though they had never provided her with much emotional support, Hannah and Elizabeth had been fixed stars for her to steer by, one the center of the family circle, the other the driving force of her career. Now one was dead and the other distant. As she reached her mid-forties, Emily began for the first time to make her own choices.

Coming to her aid at last was Mary Putnam, her graduation from the Sorbonne having been delayed by the impact of the Franco-Prussian War. Emily had yearned for a competent colleague who shared her commitment to rigorous medical education; Putnam, having triumphed in the vibrant academic atmosphere of Paris, was if anything a more demanding instructor than Emily. Appalled by the caliber of the students she found at the Woman's Medical College, Putnam caused an uproar by immediately expanding the scope of the curriculum. "I do not know whether she can adapt herself to circumstances and learn to be a good teacher for an American class studying after American modes," Emily worried. Putnam seemed equally doubtful, dashing off an aggrieved letter to Elizabeth in which she announced the "thorough contempt" in which she held her new students. From England, Elizabeth attempted to mediate, advising Putnam to take things slowly. "It is utterly impossible to attempt to teach unless you are thoroughly in accord with your pupils," Elizabeth wrote. "Do, my dear Mary, be very prudent and patient!"

Mary Putnam Jacobi—as she was soon to be known after her marriage to the pioneering German-Jewish pediatrician Abraham Jacobi—would become both a passionate scientist and a highly respected physician: a practitioner like Emily rather than a proselytizer like Elizabeth. She stayed on as Emily's colleague at the college, always pushing for higher standards, and she eventually created a dedicated children's ward at the infirmary. She wrote scores of respected articles, including one—"The Question of Rest for Women During Menstruation"—that debunked the conventional wisdom and won Harvard's Boylston Prize. She became the first female fellow of the New York Academy of Medicine in 1880. Nearly two decades after Elizabeth's departure, having reached a professional height from which she could regard her former mentor as a peer, she addressed Elizabeth with characteristic candor. "It is your mind that conceived the idea of women physicians in modern life, and on a plane at which few have ever thought of it," she wrote, giving Elizabeth her due. But: "You never really descended from your vision, into the sphere of practical life within which that vision, if anywhere, must be realized. You left that for others to do."

With Putnam Jacobi and a growing cohort of promising students to help realize the vision, for the first time Emily had space to consider her own domestic happiness. She began to construct a new family for herself. In the fall of 1870, immediately following her mother's death, she adopted a baby girl and named her Hannah—"Nannie" within the family. "She is a bright sociable affectionate little thing and a wonderful pet," Emily wrote to Kitty. "She is not exactly a pretty child, but she has pretty eyes." As an infant, Nannie slept in a nest of cushions on Emily's examining table; as a curly-blond "chatterpye" toddler, she stood clutching the banister rails and watching the carriages roll by in the street when Emily returned at the end of the day. While Kitty never addressed her guardian as anything but Dr. Elizabeth, Nannie called Emily "Mama," and as an older child, she signed her affectionate letters with rows of kisses. She would go on to marriage and motherhood and would delight Emily with a quartet of towheaded grandsons.

The youngest Blackwell sister, Ellen, who had shelved her painterly aspirations and now served as Emily's rather haphazard housekeeper, also adopted a baby: Cornelia, or "Neenie." Nannie and Neenie would grow up together, often left in Ellen's charge when Emily was preoccupied at the infirmary and supported mostly by Emily when Ellen—who had a large-hearted but short-sighted habit of accumulating stray orphans—ran short of money.

A hospital was not a good place to raise children. Now that Emily had a child, she could justify a house of her own. In 1873 she moved to 53 East Twentieth Street, a few steps from Gramercy Park, with room for her office, a nursery for Nannie and Neenie, and accommodations for Ellen, Marian, and George. It was a profound relief to be able to leave the infirmary for a home at last. As the moving cart loaded with furnishings rumbled away toward Twentieth Street in the dusk, Emily paused for a moment on the hospital steps, remembering the day that she and Elizabeth had first mounted the brass plate with their two names beside the door. Now it would hang at the new address; even as Emily became head of her own household, Elizabeth's presence persisted. But the quiet delight with which Emily described the smallest details of her new home was palpable. "They have put down in the hall a sort of oilcloth called Linoleum," she wrote to Elizabeth. "Mine has a dark red brown ground with a small red & black figure, very neat and harmonious with the carpets." She planned to invite Henry and Sam and their families for Christmas, reuniting all the siblings who remained in America.

George would soon find a wife—Lucy Stone's niece, Emma—and start a family of his own; Ellen would escape the city to spend extended periods with Nannie and Neenie at Blackwell properties in the suburbs. But Emily was not alone for long. In 1870 a new student had arrived at the Woman's Medical College. Elizabeth Cushier, ten years younger than Emily, had come to medicine late, constrained by the care of her younger siblings after the death of their mother. Having spent a disappointing term at Clemence Lozier's New York Medical College for Women, she found the level of seriousness she sought at the "Blackwell college" under the tutelage of Emily and Mary Putnam Jacobi. Cushier received her degree in 1872, and with the exception of eighteen months of further study in Europe, she never again left Emily's side. She became an accomplished gynecological surgeon—eventually bringing J. Marion Sims's fistula repair technique to the infirmary—and taught both obstetrics and surgery at the college as the only female clinical professor. In Cushier, Emily recognized a kindred spirit: an independent woman who approached her responsibility both to her family and to her career with good-natured, unfussy pragmatism and skill. And even as she graduated from Emily's student to her colleague and then her closest friend, Cushier preserved the deep respect she had initially felt for her first medical mentor.

In the fall of 1882, Elizabeth Cushier moved in with Emily on East Twentieth Street. In her relationship with this new Elizabeth—as senior rather than junior partner—Emily found a steady source of something that had always been scarce: contentment. The two women were as compatible sharing a home as they were sharing an operating theater, and Cushier's sister Sophie became a more competent helpmeet than flighty Ellen had ever been. "You ought to have a partner like Dr Cushier," Emily wrote jovially to her niece Alice, "who has just superintended the making of my cloth suit, as she was not content with the unaided efforts of my dressmaker." Emily was even more admiring of Cushier's facility with a surgical needle. The two doctors, swathed in blue and white pinafores—"like a butcher's apron, but a little more dandy"—performed operations at the infirmary regularly, sometimes with a double row of students as an audience. "Dr Cushier is really a skillful surgeon," Emily wrote, "and very ambitious in that line." It was her highest praise.

Even the formidable Mary Putnam Jacobi approved. Cushier was "a remarkably lovely woman, spirited, unselfish, generous and intelligent," she wrote to Elizabeth in England. "I do not know what Dr. Emily would do without her. She absolutely basks in her presence; and seems as if she had been waiting for her for a lifetime." When Elizabeth—feeling displaced?—clucked over Emily's isolation from the rest of the Blackwell clan, especially when Emily suffered a bout of ill health, her sister set her straight. "No one could be more kind, devoted, and helpful than Dr Cushier was," Emily retorted. "There is not one of my own family who could or would have done so much for me." Cushier, she told Elizabeth, "is like a younger sister or elder daughter to me."

Emily's partnership with Elizabeth Cushier was warmed by love. "The last days have been busy ones dearest," Cushier wrote while Emily was visiting Henry and Lucy. In Emily's absence, Cushier was not only managing their patients but also having the house painted and polished. "Much as I want to see you dear, I am not sorry you will not be here until next week, for I do not wish you to come into an unsettled house," Cushier wrote. "By this time next week you will be quietly settled in just what will then be the nicest little house in the world & my own dear doctor what a happy winter we shall have! Shall we not?" They lived together for the last three decades of Emily's life.

The years passed rhythmically, with hospital practice and college instruction punctuated by summer escapes, first to Henry Blackwell's property on the south shore of Martha's Vineyard, and later to Emily and Cushier's own retreat at York Cliffs, on the coast of Maine. The infirmary and college prospered; in 1876 the hospital moved to new quarters on Livingston Place, on the edge of Stuyvesant Square Park, leaving more room for the college on Second Avenue, and in 1888 the college moved as well, around the corner from the hospital on East Fifteenth Street, to create a more compact campus for its students. The financial strains of the early days faded as generous patrons relieved Emily of the burden of fund-raising; there was even the beginning of an endowment. Two of Sam and Nettie's daughters, Edith and Ethel, received medical diplomas under Aunt Emily's supervision.

One April afternoon in 1897, Emily—in her seventies, but still serving as dean of the college—took the opportunity of a quiet Sunday to start a letter to Elizabeth. The city was on holiday; the distant sounds of a parade celebrating the completion of General Grant's tomb filtered toward them from uptown. "The doorbell has rung but once today, an unheard of calm," Emily wrote. It had been nearly half a century since her sister sat idle on University Place, wishing desperately for patients to arrive.

It was typical of Emily to bury catastrophe in the middle of home news and the weather. Days earlier a messenger had woken the household in the middle of the night: the college was on fire. Construction debris from the installation of a new boiler had ignited, and the flames had climbed an airshaft to the roof. The building was gutted, all its equipment lost. "On the top floor was a dissecting-room, in which there were several corpses, which were cremated," the *Tribune* noted ghoulishly. But the infirmary next door was unharmed, and discipline among the resident staff was so strong that many of the patients slept through the emergency.

"We have taken the next house, and made the best arrangements we can," Emily wrote. "We shall go to work at once to rebuild." She had stood by the institution from the beginning; she would not abandon it now. Neither would her trustees, who immediately printed a new appeal. "Women students need as much space to work in and as good material to work with as men do," the pamphlet insisted. It was in the interests of both skeptics and progressives that the college, "which represents the life work of Elizabeth and Emily Blackwell, is so equipped and endowed, and its standards kept so high, that its diploma represents the best that can be had in medical education." In the name of both Blackwells, then—the long-absent symbol and the present and active leader—the college was rebuilt and expanded, welcoming an unusually large class the following year. What had once been dubbed "the woman doctors' college"—"at first in derision, and, later, with respect," noted *The Sun*—had achieved a reputation sturdy enough to survive the blaze.

CODA

On a Tuesday evening in May 1899, a reporter from the *New-York Tribune* arrived at Emily's house on East Twentieth Street and asked for an interview. Was the rumor true, he wanted to know, that the Woman's Medical College was about to close its doors forever?

"I understand that is the intention," Emily said.

Warming to his scoop, the reporter asked, "Will the students of the institution enter the Cornell Medical College?"

"The students of the school have the right to go where they choose" came the tart reply. She would say no more.

The world was catching up to the Blackwells. In 1893, Johns Hopkins University in Baltimore had opened a medical school that included women in its first class; in 1898, in New York City, Cornell did likewise. "They have a million and a half dollars to start with, and will have more if they need it," Emily told Elizabeth. "So far they seem inclined to treat their women students fairly." Cornell was allowing women to teach as well and to serve as trustees. "This is very encouraging, for Coeducation means both sexes represented above as well as below," Emily added. Thirty years earlier the Blackwells had reluctantly decided to open a women's college because the best medical schools remained closed to women, but now that was changing. "The Infirmary is really a beautiful and admirably managed little Hospital, and I don't believe it will ever be closed," Emily wrote. She was right: the New York Infirmary for Women and Children would anchor the eastern edge of

Stuyvesant Square until 1981.* The college, on the other hand, had ful-
filled its purpose.

Two nights after the interview, thanks to the *Tribune*'s reporting, the
assembled graduates and guests at the thirtieth commencement exercises were not as shocked as they might have been at the announcement
that the Woman's Medical College of the New York Infirmary would
close. The truth was, Cornell had already been luring students away.
"The graduates think they inspire more confidence in the public, and can
more quickly procure a practice, if they can show that they have attended
the same lectures and passed the same examinations in all things as the
men," the *Tribune* explained. Which was precisely the logic Elizabeth and
Emily had used fifty years earlier.

The graduates sat on the platform, dignified in black academic caps
and gowns over white skirts and shirtwaists, as their venerable dean, Dr.
Emily Blackwell, took the stage to address them. The news of the college's closing was sudden, it was true, but the decision had been carefully considered, and she had faith that even those who doubted it would
come to understand its wisdom. The Woman's Medical College "had held
open the door for women until broader gates had swung wide for their
admission," she told the audience. And the ranks of women in medicine were growing: "In every city, and almost every town, and scattered
throughout the country, they are making their way." Of the eighteen
women receiving degrees that evening, five would continue to work at the
infirmary as interns and sanitary visitors, four more were headed to New
England hospitals, two were planning to work in China, and another in
Constantinople.

In the years since the Blackwells had received their own diplomas,
most women who pursued medicine had done so at women's colleges.
Now the lecture halls from which they had been barred were opening to

---

* In 1981 the infirmary merged with Beekman Downtown Hospital to create the
first community hospital in Manhattan's Financial District, on William Street.
Downtown Hospital is now part of New York–Presbyterian and is known as Lower
Manhattan Hospital.

them at last, a triumph but also a new challenge. "You will be brought in contact with the working ways of men," Emily told them. "Get from this new companionship all that is good, but do not lose in it a particle of what is truly and desirably your own." There was no one who could speak those words with more authority. Emily had wrested a medical degree from institutions that had tried to withhold it from her; she had studied with male mentors who learned to see her as a doctor first. She had felt doubt and learned to transcend it, and she had overseen the growth of an institution that would endure, even without its college. And where her sister had come to see women as a special category of physician, uniquely equipped to teach, Emily placed medical skill over sex. "It is for us to do our part," she concluded, "that hereafter the old and time-honored profession may be proud of her daughters as of her sons."

There was another reason to close the Woman's Medical College without delay. Emily was seventy-three years old. It was past time for her to lay down her professional responsibilities, but—with the exception of Elizabeth Cushier, who she hoped would retire with her—she had never found a woman she respected enough to name as her successor. "I am glad to feel that I stood at my post until the victory was gained," she told Elizabeth, "and did not have to leave the work to be carried on by uncertain hands."

~

On January 25, 1911, hundreds of well-dressed New Yorkers—most of them women or physicians, many of them both—filled every seat of stately Hosack Hall, the elegant auditorium of the New York Academy of Medicine on West Forty-third Street. Here at the heart of the city's medical establishment, they gathered to celebrate the lives of Elizabeth and Emily Blackwell, who had died within months of each other the previous year, Elizabeth at eighty-nine, at the end of a long decline in Hastings, and Emily a month short of eighty-four, after a sudden illness at her summer home in Maine.

A procession of notables eulogized Elizabeth with respect but also with distance, the inevitable result of her forty years absence. Of Emily they spoke with more personal warmth. "I remember how I trembled with awe before that very kind and harmless lady, Dr. Elizabeth," said Alice Stone Blackwell, now the editor of the *Woman's Journal*, the suf-

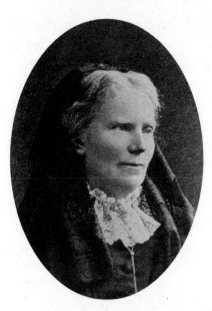

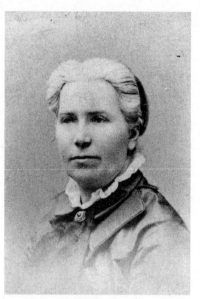

ELIZABETH.
*COURTESY SCHLESINGER LIBRARY, RADCLIFFE
INSTITUTE, HARVARD UNIVERSITY*

EMILY.
*COURTESY NEW YORK ACADEMY OF
MEDICINE*

fragist paper founded forty years earlier by her parents. Elizabeth, she remembered, had always seemed taller than her actual height. "I was not quite so much afraid of Dr. Emily—she used to give me chocolate drops."

Elizabeth, having fallen in love with Scotland on holiday travels, was buried there in the tiny lochside village of Kilmun, under a tall Celtic cross that announces her achievements as the first woman to earn a medical degree and to be placed on the British Medical Register. "It is only when we have learned to recognize that law for the human body is as sacred as—nay, is one with—God's law for the human soul, that we shall begin to understand the religion of health," reads one inscription, quoting Elizabeth's own writing. "Love seeketh not her own," reads another. "The pure in heart shall see God." It is a fitting monument to a woman who never doubted her understanding of God's intentions, or that it was her duty to explain them to the world. After her death, Kitty returned to America and her beloved Alice. She died in 1936, nearly ninety herself, and requested that her ashes be buried in Scotland, with Elizabeth.

Emily's grave is on Martha's Vineyard, close to the windswept, wave-battered coastline where the Blackwell family continued to summer for generations after her death. Her headstone is sturdy and square, inscribed with her name and dates, and otherwise unadorned.

~

In 1910, when the Blackwell sisters died, there were more than nine thousand women doctors in the United States, about six percent of all physicians. Today thirty-five percent of physicians—and slightly more than half of all medical students—are female.

ACKNOWLEDGMENTS

I t seems fitting that a book about pioneering women should have many godmothers. Cornelia Small let me tag along to the Sophia Smith Collection at Smith College, where I first encountered Emily Blackwell. Julie Quain appeared like the answer to a wish I hadn't yet made, opening doors and joining me on treasure hunts. Jane Carey Blackwell Bloomfield welcomed me into the story of her family. Mary Wright gave me two unforgettable days in Bristol, as well as her friendship, which will last much longer. Jill Platner invited me inside her home at the corner of Bleecker and Crosby to spend time with the ghosts. Darcy Fryer brought her brilliance as a reader and a historian to every page and made me think harder, as the best teachers do.

Profound thanks to the archivists and guardians who let me in and helped me out: Jane Kamensky, Sarah M. Hutcheon, and Diana Carey, Schlesinger Library, Radcliffe Institute for Advanced Study; Arlene Shaner, New York Academy of Medicine; Alan Hawk, National Museum of Health and Medicine; Patrick Kerwin, Library of Congress; Nina Couzin and Jeremy Tavaré, Elizabeth Blackwell Institute, University of Bristol; Jacqueline Cahiff, Royal College of Surgeons, Edinburgh; Kate Jarman and Amanda Engineer, St. Bartholomew's Hospital Archive, London; Gillian Murphy, Women's Library, London School of Economics; Father Franck Derville and Patricia Tailhades, La Maternité, Paris; Glenn Horowitz and Hayley Setear, Dobkin Family Collection of Feminism; Harry Bubbins and Ariel Kates, Greenwich Village Society for Historic Preservation; Lisa Mix and Elizabeth Shepard, Weill-Cornell Medical

Center Archives; Kim Turchin and Connie Wu, New York–Presbyterian Lower Manhattan Hospital; Tommy Rodecki, Green-Wood Cemetery; Frances Rosenfeld and Emily Chapin, Museum of the City of New York; Tricia McEldowney and Brandon Moblo, Hobart and William Smith College Archive; Martin Dornbaum, Health Professions Education Center, Hunter-Bellevue School of Nursing; and Carolyn Waters, Catherine McGowan, Barbara Bieck, and the entire staff of the New York Society Library, my second home.

For close reading, and close friendship: Elisabeth Gitter, Jessica Francis Kane, Gail Marcus, Caroline Rodoni, and Zanthe Taylor.

For good medicine, in so many forms: Fredi Pomerance, Leslie and Eric Slocum, Stacy Schiff, Megan Marshall, Ellen Feldman, Dr. Abigail Ford Winkel, Toby Cox, Yuko Uchikawa, Karina Yan Glaser, Daniel Clarke, Elise Cappella, Elisha Cooper, Peggy Sturdivant, Dr. Flavia Golden, Dr. Ana Alzaga Fernandez, Matthew Warnes, Maryann Parker, Linda Schapiro, J.C. Hallman, Samuel B. Jones, Jr., Betty Bayer, Steve O'Malley, Ted Aub, and the sisterhood of Women Writing Women's Lives.

In 2017 I was honored to receive a Public Scholar grant from the National Endowment for the Humanities. Any views, findings, conclusions, or recommendations expressed in this book do not necessarily reflect those of the NEH.

I am privileged to work with the best book people imaginable. Few editors are as incisive and farseeing as Alane Salierno Mason: thank you for pushing me further. I could not do this work at all without Rob McQuilkin's warmth and faith. Michael Taeckens and Whitney Peeling are gifted at telling the story of a book; I am lucky this book is one of their stories. At W. W. Norton, I'm grateful for Mo Crist, Janet Biehl, Yang Kim, Chris Welch, Michelle Waters, and Erin Lovett.

Last and first, to Yoji, Clare, and David Nimura, who make everything possible.

NOTES

PROLOGUE

2 **"This institution"**: "New York Infirmary for Women and Children," *New York Daily Herald*, May 13, 1857, 3.

2 **"The full thorough education"**: Ibid.

3 **"There are none less able"**: Ibid.; "Opening of the New-York Infirmary for Women and Children," *New-York Tribune*, May 13, 1857, 4; "Infirmary for Women and Children," *New-York Times*, May 13, 1857, 8.

3 **"There is certainly nothing"**: Emily to Elizabeth, 1852 or 1853, Folder 163, Collection MC411, SL.

CHAPTER I: BRISTOL—NEW YORK—CINCINNATI

5 **"There lived as my story says"**: Elizabeth, undated notebook, Reel 45, LC.

6 **"Little Shy"**: Anna, "Early Life of the Blackwells," 169, Reel 72, LC.

6 **"I was fitted"**: Hannah, dictated to Henry, Reel 75, LC.

7 **"sky parlour . . . parapet"**: Anna, "Early Life of the Blackwells," 129, Reel 72, LC.

8 **"Anna, Bessy, & Polly!"**: Ibid., 130.

8 **"There was a dreadful scene"**: Ibid., 113.

8 **"The pretty baby"**: Ibid., 12.

8 **"shabbily dressed"**: Ibid., 151.

9 **"poor starveling aunts"**: Ibid., 57.

9 **"natural lady"**: Ibid., 55–56.

9 **"very small . . . Greek"**: Ibid., 57.

9 **"very well-meaning"**: Ibid., 50.

9 **"disagreeable . . . broomstick"**: Ibid., 50.

9 **"putting forth . . . Grandpapa"**: Ibid., 23.

10 **"We children"**: Ibid., 134.

10 **"great feathers"**: Ibid., 135.

11 **eventually committed**: Ibid., 52.

10 **Bristol shipping firm:** Joelle Million, "Samuel Blackwell: Sugar Refiner and Abolitionist," *New York History Review,* June 14, 2017.

12 **"active dollar-getting":** Samuel Sr., "Two Years in New York," 1835, Folder 3, Collection A145, SL.

12 **"If people will":** Elizabeth's journal, June 30, 1837, Reel 39, LC.

13 **"How gay":** Ibid., March 17, 1837.

13 **"I fear":** Ibid., March 6, 1837.

13 **"The Greek oration":** Ibid., October 3, 1837.

13 **"How I do long":** Ibid., March 14, 1838.

13 **abstinence pledge:** Ibid., February 27, 1838.

13 **"I wish":** Ibid., January 31, 1838.

13 **"poor, foolish":** Anna, "Early Life of the Blackwells," 48, Reel 72, LC.

13 **"Just as I was getting":** Elizabeth's journal, April 4, 1837, Reel 39, LC.

14 **"into partnership":** Ibid., May 2, 1837.

14 **"I wonder":** Ibid., September 16, 1837.

14 **"Mamma, Anna, Marian":** Sam's journal, January 1, 1836, Folder 88v, Collection A77, SL.

15 **"the bumpy science":** Elizabeth's journal, January 28, 1837, Reel 39, LC.

15 **"Not disposed to trifle":** Elizabeth, notes on phrenology, January 28, 1837, Folder 61, Collection MC411, SL.

16 **"to plead the cause":** *Proceedings of the Anti-Slavery Convention,* 9.

16 **"very ill advised":** Elizabeth's journal, May 11, 1837, Reel 39, LC.

16 **"The spirit of Slavery":** Samuel Sr. to Kenyon, September 27, 1836, Folder 5, Collection MC411, SL.

16 **"A colored man":** Elizabeth's journal, December 29, 1837, Reel 39, LC.

17 **"What a dearth":** Ibid., July 18, 1837.

17 **"How ardently":** Ibid., July 24, 1837.

17 **"I hope Papa":** Ibid., February 6, 1837.

17 **"make some experiments":** Sam's journal, March 25, 1837, Folder 88v, Collection A77, SL.

18 **"Tell dear Washy":** Samuel Sr. to Hannah, March 5, 1838, Folder 5, Collection MC411, SL.

18 **"I suppose":** Elizabeth's journal, May 12, 1838, Reel 39, LC.

18 **Fanny Trollope:** Trollope, *Domestic Manners,* 51.

18 **"I saw some very":** Elizabeth's journal, May 13, 1838, Reel 39, LC.

19 **"If we cannot":** Marian to Elizabeth, June 16, 1838, Folder 32, Collection MC411, SL.

19 **"He is just the color":** Elizabeth's journal, August 6, 1838, Reel 39, LC.

20 **"I put my hand"**: Ibid., August 7, 1838.

20 **"Reading, Writing"**: School prospectus, Folder 82, Collection MC411, SL.

20 **"Aunt Mary"**: Elizabeth's journal, September 30, 1838, Reel 39, LC.

21 **"They don't know"**: Ibid., October 1, 1838.

21 **"After school"**: Ibid., March 20, 1839.

21 **"I have cut"**: Emily to Henry, June 14, 1841, Reel 74, LC.

22 **"I well remember"**: Blackwell, *Pioneer Work*, 13.

22 **"I'm sorry to say"**: Sam to Henry, January 14, 1841, Reel 76, LC.

CHAPTER 2: BETWEENITY

23 **"Madam . . . fire screen"**: Elizabeth to Blackwell family, March 5, 1844, Reel 42, LC.

23 **"I give as far"**: Elizabeth to Marian, March 19, 1844, Reel 76, LC.

24 **"Carlyle's name"**: Elizabeth to Marian, April 4, 1844, Folder 61, Collection MC411, SL.

24 **"I had many offers"**: Elizabeth to Hannah, 1844, Reel 42, LC.

24 **"To live . . . whisper"**: Elizabeth to Marian, April 4, 1844, Folder 61, Collection MC411, SL.

24 **"I feel independent"**: Elizabeth to Marian, 1844, Reel 76, LC.

24 **St. Ann's Hall**: "St. Ann's Hall, Flushing, Long Island, New-York," *Southern Literary Messenger*, February 1843, 127–28.

25 **"very fond . . . my hand"**: Emily to Elizabeth, 1844, Reel 74, LC.

25 **"*Go by all means*"**: Elizabeth to Emily, June 1844, Folder 45, Collection MC411, SL.

25 **"'crack' Greek pupil"**: Anna to Elizabeth, May 11, 1845, Reel 71, LC.

25 **"Alas!"**: Sam's journal, November 10, 1844, Folder 89v, Collection A77, SL.

25 **"pretty busily"**: Emily to Henry, May 11, 1845, Reel 71, LC.

25 **"Her progress"**: Anna to Sam, March 9, 1845, DF.

26 **"the manifold uncomfortablenesses"**: Anna to Elizabeth, May 11, 1845, Reel 71, LC.

26 **inaugural Annual**: Christmas Annual 1844, Reel 50, LC.

26 **"a lady friend"**: Blackwell, *Pioneer Work*, 27.

26 **"gross perversion"**: Ibid., 30.

27 **"My favourite studies"**: Ibid., 28.

27 **"I think women need"**: Fuller, *Woman in the Nineteenth Century*, 159.

28 **"I believe that"**: Ibid., 158.

28 **"If I had some noble"**: Sam's journal, November 3, 1844, Folder 89v, Collection A77, SL.

28   "Eliz. is thinking": Ibid., May 3, 1845.

28   "common malady . . . heart": Blackwell, *Pioneer Work*, 28.

29   "highly useful": Ibid., 31.

30   "The idea of winning": Ibid, 76.

30   "drunken drivers": Elizabeth to Emily, July 2, 1845, Folder 45, Collection
      MC411, SL.

30   "Miss Student . . . puns": Ibid.

31   "goblin groans": Sam's journal, June 16, 1845, Folder 89v, Collection A77, SL.

31   "Shall I say": Elizabeth to Emily, July 2, 1845, Folder 45, Collection MC411, SL.

31   "country boobies . . . hospitality": Elizabeth to Marian, June 29, 1845, Reel
      76, LC.

31   "I had many causes": Elizabeth to Henry, April 12, 46, Folder 61, Collection
      MC411, SL.

32   "I *knew* that": Blackwell, *Pioneer Work*, 35.

32   "my first professional cure": Elizabeth to Hannah, July 27, 1845, Reel 42, LC.

32   "a great treat . . . known": Elizabeth to Marian, December 4, 1845, Reel 76, LC.

32   "determined . . . principles": Elizabeth to Hannah, July 27, 1845, Reel 42, LC.

33   "strong electric . . . alone": Elizabeth to Henry, August 17, 1845, Reel 50, LC.

33   "I feel very wakeful": Elizabeth to Hannah, July 27, 1845, Reel 42, LC.

33   "It is so painful": Anna to Sam, July 27, 1845, DF.

33   "I assure you": Emily to Sam, July 27, 1845, DF.

33   "A most unscrupulous": Henry's journal, August 12, 1845, Reel 50, LC.

34   "He thrust his hand": Paul Trapier, *A Narrative of Facts Which Led to the Pre-
      sentment of the Rt. Rev. Benj. T. Onderdonk, Bishop of New-York* (New York:
      Stanford & Swords, 1845), 51.

34   "reading," Elizabeth reported: Elizabeth to Sam, April 5, 1846, DF.

34   "Your letters always": Elizabeth to Emily, February 14, 1846, Folder 45, Collec-
      tion MC411, SL.

34   "So our young giantess": Elizabeth to Marian, May 15, 1846, Folder 61, Collec-
      tion MC411, SL.

35   "The more . . . important one": Elizabeth to Sam, March 8, 1846, DF.

35   "I trace out": Elizabeth to Sam, April 5, 1846, DF.

35   "whether I . . . at night": Elizabeth to Marian, November 1, 1846, Reel 76, LC.

35   "Do listen": Elizabeth to Hannah, February 28, 1847, Reel 42, LC.

36   "the famous Trojan": Elizabeth to Sam, March 8, 1846, DF.

36   "I did not know . . . lives": Elizabeth to Sam, April 5, 1846, DF.

36   "I beg thee": Elizabeth to Hannah, February 28, 1847, Reel 42, LC.

37   "thin as an aspen leaf": Anna to Blackwell family, August 3, 1845, Reel 71, LC.

38 **"a thinking talking couple"**: Elizabeth to Marian, June 22, 1847, Reel 76, LC.

38 **"Poor A"**: Sam's journal, May 19, 1847, Folder 90v, Collection A77, SL.

38 **Elizabeth sought interviews**: Blackwell, *Pioneer Work*, 60.

38 **"You cannot expect"**: Ibid., 61.

39 **"It was to my mind"**: Ibid., 62.

39 **"I cannot tell you"**: Elizabeth to Emily, 1847, Reel 76, LC.

39 **"The beauty of the tendons"**: Blackwell, *Pioneer Work*, 59.

40 **"to purchase a black baby"**: Elizabeth to Sam, August 5, 1847, DF.

40 **"I determined not"**: Ibid.

40 **"I must accomplish"**: Elizabeth to Emma Willard, May 24, 1847, Reel 44, LC.

CHAPTER 3: ADMISSION

41 **"most extraordinary request"**: Stephen Smith, "The Medical Co-Education of the Sexes," in Blackwell, *Pioneer Work*, 256.

42 **Of the 113 students**: *Register of Geneva College, for the Academical Year 1847–48* (Geneva: Merrell & Dey, 1848).

42 **"At the instant"**: Stephen Smith, "A Woman Student in a Medical College," in *In Memory of Dr. Elizabeth Blackwell*, 5–7.

43 **"For the first time"**: Smith, "Medical Co-Education," in Blackwell, *Pioneer Work*, 257.

43 **letter from Geneva**: Charles Lee to Elizabeth, October 20, 1847, Reel 46, LC.

44 **"Dear Milly"**: Elizabeth to Emily, October 27, 1847, Folder 45, Collection MC411, SL.

44 **"though not surprise"**: Blackwell, *Pioneer Work*, 64.

45 **"The weather"**: Elizabeth to Marian, November 9, 1847, Reel 76, LC.

45 **"Think of the cases"**: Ibid.

46 **"the utmost friendliness"**: Blackwell, *Pioneer Work*, 68.

46 **"Oh, this is the way"**: Ibid., 70.

46 **"Today when I"**: Elizabeth to Marian, November 9, 1847, Reel 76, LC.

46 **"The little fat Professor"**: Blackwell, *Pioneer Work*, 70.

46 **"a pretty little specimen"**: "Females Attending Medical Lectures," *Boston Medical and Surgical Journal* 37 (December 15, 1847): 405.

46 **"Nothing has transpired"**: "Female Physicians," *Boston Medical and Surgical Journal* 37 (January 12, 1848): 506.

46 **"inexpedient"**: Hunt, *Glances and Glimpses*, 217–18.

47 **"special branches . . . present"**: "Female Physicians," *Buffalo Medical Journal* 3, no. 8 (January 1848).

47   "We admire MISS BLACKWELL": "A Medical Maiden," *Punch* 14 (1848): 117.

47   "flat, heavy feeling": Blackwell, *Pioneer Work*, 69.

47   "In the amphitheatre": Ibid., 73.

48   "See the one in pink!": Ibid.

48   "I believe the professors": Ibid., 69.

48   "as at a curious animal": Ibid., 70.

48   "I told him . . . desire": Ibid., 72.

49   "He could hardly": Ibid., 71.

49   "Dr. Webster, who": Ibid., 72.

49   "saying . . . gods": Smith, "Woman Student," in *In Memory of Dr. Elizabeth Blackwell*, 11.

49   "The lectures on anatomy": Blackwell, *Pioneer Work*, 259.

51   "some respectable practitioner": *Catalogue of the Medical Institution of Geneva College, Session of 1846–47* (Rochester, N.Y.: Jerome & Brother, 1846), 15.

52   "Medicine is always": Elizabeth's lecture notes, Reel 46, LC.

52   "blood is the fuel": Ibid.

53   "The human body": Ibid.

53   "'Twas a horrible": Blackwell, *Pioneer Work*, 72.

54   "[Elizabeth] says": Sam's journal, January 16, 1848, Folder 90v, Collection A77, SL.

54   "they treated me": Blackwell, *Pioneer Work*, 74.

54   intricate diagrams: Elizabeth's lecture notes, Reel 46, LC.

54   "tracing out": Blackwell, *Pioneer Work*, 74.

56   "It cheered me": Ibid., 75.

56   "I suppose they were": Ibid.

56   "They talked over": Ibid., 76.

57   "Maiden of earnest thought": William H. C. Hosmer, "To Miss B., A Candidate for Medical Honors," *Western Literary Messenger* 10, no. 3 (February 19, 1848): 33.

57   clarify his stance: William Hosmer, *Appeal to Husbands and Wives in Favor of Female Physicians* (New York: George Gregory, 1853).

CHAPTER 4: BLOCKLEY ALMSHOUSE

58   thirteen and eighteen degrees: Lawrence, *Almshouses and Hospitals*, 165–66.

58   This ice: Croskey, *History of Blockley*, 131.

58   Cholera and puerperal: Ibid., 59–60.

58   Wealthy visitors: Ibid., 47–48.

59 **"Blockley is the microcosm"**: Ibid., 133.

59 **"all were prepared"**: Blackwell, *Pioneer Work*, 77.

59 **"Resolved that permission"**: Blockley admission, Reel 46, LC.

59 **"I feel disposed"**: Elizabeth to Marian, March 1848, Reel 76, LC.

60 **"Most of the women"**: Blackwell, *Pioneer Work*, 79.

60 **"It was thought"**: Ibid., 77.

60 **"the hideousness"**: Ibid., 79.

60 **"Within one week"**: Elizabeth to George, June 1848, Folder 51, Collection MC411, SL.

61 **"I see a great deal . . . wrong"**: Elizabeth to Emily, April 16, 1848, Folder 45, Collection MC411, SL.

61 **"Today, for the first time"**: Elizabeth to Marian, March 1848, Reel 76, LC.

61 **"stepping out"**: Elizabeth to Emily, April 16, 1848, Folder 45, Collection MC411, SL.

61 **"When I walked"**: Blackwell, *Pioneer Work*, 80.

61 **"the very loveliest"**: Ibid., 78.

61 **"I glean a little"**: Elizabeth to Emily, April 16, 1848, Folder 45, Collection MC411, SL.

62 **"I find that some . . . physician"**: Elizabeth to Marian, March 1848, Reel 76, LC.

62 **"Ensconced in her armchair"**: Blackwell, *Pioneer Work*, 78.

62 **"I drank tea"**: Elizabeth to Henry, August 20, 1848, Folder 61, Collection MC411, SL.

63 **"mere *hands*"**: Elizabeth to Marian, March 1848, Reel 76, LC.

63 **"voice as gentle"**: Blackwell, *Pioneer Work*, 78.

63 **"one, 'Letters from Ireland"**: Elizabeth to Henry, September 8, 1848, Folder 61, Collection MC411, SL.

63 **"fear predisposes"**: Elizabeth's lecture notes, Reel 46, LC.

63 **"Without employment"**: Elizabeth's thesis ms on Ship Fever, Folder 61, Collection A145, SL.

64 **"In truth we know"**: Ibid.

64 **"The eyes were bloodshot"**: Ibid.

65 **"well worthy"**: Ibid.

65 **"the practise of washing"**: Elizabeth Blackwell, "Ship Fever: An Inaugural Thesis, submitted for the degree of M.D. at Geneva Medical College, Jan. 1849," *Buffalo Medical Journal and Monthly Review* 4, no. 9 (February 1849): 530, DF.

65 **"I am not afraid"**: Elizabeth to Marian, March 1848, Reel 76, LC.

66 "There are a few strong ones": Elizabeth to Emily, April 16, 1848, Folder 45, Collection MC411, SL.

66 "As I learnt to realize": Elizabeth to Anna, May 20, 1848, Folder 61, Collection MC411, SL.

67 "so there seems . . . earnestness": Elizabeth to Emily, 1848, Reel 74, LC.

67 "[W]omen will . . . effort": Ibid.

68 "a history of repeated injuries": Stanton, *History of Woman Suffrage*, 70.

68 "persevering and independent": Ibid., 809.

68 "I don't sympathize": Elizabeth to Henry, August 20, 1848, Folder 61, Collection MC411, SL.

68 "full of enthusiastic": Ibid.

69 "The study and practice": Elizabeth to Emily Collins, August 12, 1848, in Stanton, *History of Woman Suffrage*, 90.

69 "I have curious glimpses": Elizabeth to Henry, August 20, 1848, Folder 61, Collection MC411, SL.

70 "dreamy & indifferent": Elizabeth to Henry, September 8, 1848, ibid.

70 "They form . . . object": Ibid.

70 "As I watched": Blackwell, *Pioneer Work*, 81.

CHAPTER 5: DIPLOMA

71 "while all around . . . prevailed": Elizabeth to Emily, October 15, 1848, Folder 45, Collection MC411, SL.

72 "People still gossip": Elizabeth to Sam, December 27, 1848, DF.

72 "I've never met": Ibid.

72 "He is to me utterly": Elizabeth to Marian, December 1848, Reel 76, LC.

72 "Your life . . . our college": Elizabeth to Emily, October 15, 1848, Folder 45, Collection MC411, SL.

73 "I did more laughing": Blackwell, *Pioneer Work*, 82.

73 "the accomplishment . . . utterance": Ibid., 83.

73 "How little they know": Ibid., 84.

74 "Believe me, brother mine": Elizabeth to Henry, December 17, 1848, Folder 61, Collection MC411, SL.

74 "told everybody": Elizabeth to Sam, December 27, 1848, DF.

74 "pretty blind girl": Blackwell, *Pioneer Work*, 84.

74 "a constant concert . . . exposed": Elizabeth to Marian, January 19, 1849, Reel 76, LC.

74 "the very thought": Elizabeth to Emily, October 15, 1848, Folder 45, Collection MC411, SL.

75 **"I have the strengthening"**: Elizabeth to Marian, December 1848, Reel 76, LC.

75 **"the examinations . . . circumstances"**: Elizabeth to Marian, January 19, 1849, Reel 76, LC.

75 **"Nothing but a vast"**: Margaret Munro Delancey to Josephine Delancey, January 29, 1849, Museum of the City of New York.

76 **"I can neither disgrace"**: Elizabeth to Blackwell family, in Anna Blackwell, "Elizabeth Blackwell," *English Woman's Journal* 1, no. 2 (April 1858): 91.

76 **"for the purpose of striking . . . suppose it wouldn't"**: Henry to Blackwell family, January 23, 1849, Reel 50, LC.

77 **"A silence deep as death"**: "Geneva Medical College Commencement," *Geneva Gazette*, January 26, 1849.

77 **"Sir, I thank you"**: Blackwell, *Pioneer Work*, 87; Henry to Blackwell family, January 23, 1849, Reel 50, LC; *Geneva Gazette*, January 26, 1849; Margaret Munro Delancey, January 29, 1849.

77 **"feeling more thoroughly"**: Blackwell, *Pioneer Work*, 87.

78 **"You have learned how"**: Lee, *Valedictory Address*, 5–6.

78 **"It has been said"**: Ibid., 13.

78 **"who would be better employed"**: Ibid., 23.

78 **"witches and impostors"**: Ibid., 26.

78 **"ministering angel . . . admiration"**: Ibid., 27–28.

78 **"would have more practice"**: Margaret Munro Delancey to Josephine Delancey, January 29, 1849, Museum of the City of New York.

79 **"to the great astonishment"**: Henry to Blackwells, January 23, 1849, Reel 50, LC.

79 **"I was glad"**: Blackwell, *Pioneer Work*, 87.

79 **"Beloved Relations"**: Henry to Blackwell family, January 23, 1849, Reel 50, LC.

79 **"God be with our dear"**: Sam's journal, January 24, 1849, Folder 90v, Collection A77, SL.

79 **"has thousands"**: Marian to Charles and Eliza Lane, February 14, 1849, Folder 21, Collection A145, SL.

80 **"I trust her life"**: Hannah to Charles and Eliza Lane, February 12, 1849, ibid.

80 **"But oh what a life"**: Hannah to Henry, February 12, 1849, Reel 75, LC.

80 **"affection & sympathy"**: Elizabeth to Hannah, February 25, 1849, Reel 42, LC.

80 **"partly to give"**: Elizabeth to Sam, December 27, 1848, DF.

80 **"When the laws of health"**: Elizabeth Blackwell, "Ship Fever: An Inaugural Thesis, submitted for the degree of M.D., at Geneva Medical College, Jan. 1849," in *Buffalo Medical Journal and Monthly Review* 4, no. 9 (February 1849): 523–31, DF.

80 "glowing . . . research": "Doctress in Medicine," *Boston Medical and Surgical Journal* 40, no. 1 (February 7, 1849): 26.

81 A writer signing himself D.K.: "The Late Medical Degree to a Female," *Boston Medical and Surgical Journal* 40, no. 3 (February 21, 1849): 58–59.

81 A letter in response to D.K.: "The Late Medical Degree at Geneva," *Boston Medical and Surgical Journal* 40, no. 4 (February 28, 1849): 87.

81 startling footnote: Lee, *Valedictory Address*, 28.

83 "Dr Lee . . . invited": Elizabeth to Henry, February 20, 1849, Folder 61, Collection MC411, SL.

83 "My mornings": Ibid.

83 "rubbing up my French": Elizabeth to Hannah, February 25, 1849, Reel 42, LC.

84 "Is Emily teaching": Ibid.

84 "Obstacles overcome": Sam's journal, April 19, 1849, Folder 90v, Collection A77, SL.

84 "I could not keep down": Blackwell, *Pioneer Work*, 95.

CHAPTER 6: PARIS

86 "I gave myself . . . to the heart": Elizabeth to Blackwell family, May 2, 1849, Reel 42, LC.

88 "all manner of drugs . . . doors & windows": Elizabeth to Blackwell family, May 10, 1849, Reel 42, LC.

89 "I parted from Portway": Elizabeth to Blackwell family, May 17, 1849, Reel 42, LC.

89 "the lung of a frog . . . power of working": Ibid.

90 "He must be no longer": Elizabeth to William Elder, May 1849, Reel 43, LC.

90 "He would neither": Elizabeth to Anna, May 22, 1849, Reel 71, LC.

91 "I have not time": William Elder to Blackwell family, May 28, 1849, Folder 204, Collection MC411, SL.

91 "I cannot give": Elizabeth to Anna, May 22, 1849, Reel 71, LC.

91 "où allez-vous": Blackwell, *Pioneer Work*, 112.

91 "miserable little town": Elizabeth to Anna, May 22, 1849, Reel 71, LC.

91 "launched boldly": Blackwell, *Pioneer Work*, 113.

91 "I am utterly . . . very much": Elizabeth to Anna, May 22, 1849, Reel 71, LC.

92 "I have great trouble . . . headdress": Elizabeth to Blackwell family, May 1849, Reel 43, LC.

93 students at the École de Médecine: McCullough, *Greater Journey*, 106–7.

93 "Well," she sighed: Elizabeth to Emily, June 1849, Reel 42, LC.

93   "Some of them are certain": "An American Doctress," *Daily Union* (Washington), July 27, 1849, 1.

93   "hung round with": Elizabeth to Blackwell family, October 22, 1849, Reel 42, LC.

94   "I am obliged": Ibid.

94   "He will pursue": Elizabeth to Marian, June 5, 1849, Reel 42, LC.

94   "ignorant and degraded . . . in the world": Ibid.

95   "fearful descent . . . in the world": Elizabeth to Kenyon, June 22, 1849, Reel 42, LC.

95   "We passed through": Blackwell, *Pioneer Work*, 121.

96   "Young ladies all": "An M.D. in a Gown," *Punch* 16 (1849): 226.

96   "funniest little cabinet": Elizabeth to Hannah, July 1, 1849 Reel 42, LC.

97   "tremendous projecting teeth": Elizabeth to Howard, July 1849, Reel 42, LC.

97   "with the injunction": Elizabeth to Hannah, July 1, 1849, Reel 42, LC.

97   "a large wooden stand . . . very droll": Ibid.

98   "I almost fainted": Blackwell, *Pioneer Work*, 143.

98   Her *dortoir*: Elizabeth to Hannah, July 1, 1849, Reel 42, LC.

98   "Of course I lie": Elizabeth to Blackwell family, August 1849, Reel 42, LC.

99   "I am learning to take wine": Elizabeth to Hannah, July 1, 1849, Reel 42, LC.

99   "we have every variety": Elizabeth to Blackwell family, August 1849, Reel 42, LC.

100   "deliciously reposing": Ibid.

100   "I have been handling": Elizabeth to Hannah, July 1, 1849, Reel 42, LC.

100   "a very intelligent . . . affection": Elizabeth to Blackwell family, August 1849, Reel 42, LC.

100   "Shall I describe": Elizabeth to Henry, 1849, Reel 50, LC.

101   "he colours": Ibid.

101   "His sentiments": Blackwell, *Pioneer Work*, 146.

101   "I think he must have been": Ibid., 144.

102   "and it sounded": Elizabeth to Hannah, July 1, 1849, Reel 42, LC.

102   "Everything delights them": Blackwell, *Pioneer Work*, 140.

102   "promenading the bedsteads": Elizabeth to Henry, 1849, Reel 50, LC.

102   "He wished I would": Blackwell, *Pioneer Work*, 144.

103   "I am actually": Elizabeth to Marian, 1849, Reel 76, LC.

103   "the pleasure of looking": Elizabeth to Blackwell family, October 22, 1849, Reel 42, LC.

103   "a woman of great experience": Elizabeth to Blackwell family, August 1849, Reel 42, LC.

103   "I imagined a whole romance": Blackwell, *Pioneer Work*, 147–48.

CHAPTER 7: SETBACK

104 "a little grain of sand": Blackwell, *Pioneer Work*, 154.

105 a pharmacopeia: James Rennie, *A New Supplement to the Pharmacopoeias of London, Edinburgh, Dublin, and Paris* (London: Baldwin, Cradock & Joy, 1826), 76ff.

106 "For the first few days . . . poor E's eye": Anna to Blackwell family, November 22, 1849, Reel 72, LC.

106 "if the portion mortified": Ibid.

106 "The pupil presents": Anna to Blackwell family, December 13, 1849, Reel 72, LC.

107 "She is even sometimes . . . symptoms creates": Anna to Blackwell family, November 22, 1849, Reel 72, LC.

107 "I do admire": Blackwell, *Pioneer Work*, 156.

108 *en congé illimité*: Registre d'entrée des Élèves Sages-Femmes, Cours de 1849 à 1850, La Maternité.

108 "I felt very weak": Blackwell, *Pioneer Work*, 157.

108 "as through thick mist": Sam's journal, February 3, 1850, Folder 90v, Collection A77, SL.

108 "I suffered according to": Elizabeth to Blackwell family, January 15, 1850, Reel 42, LC.

109 *"son excellente conduit"*: Paul Antoine Dubois, April 29, 1850, Reel 46, LC.

109 "as soon as I can": Elizabeth to Blackwell family, c. January 21, 1850, Reel 72, LC.

109 "a real sororal gem": Sam to Emily, February 20, 1850, Folder 96, Collection MC411, SL.

109 *"son noble caractère"*: Hippolyte Blot to Blackwell family, February 15, 1850, Reel 43, LC.

109 "I regard her course": Marian to Charles and Eliza Lane, January 15, 1850, Folder 21, Collection A145, SL.

109 Currer Bell's *Shirley*: Sam's journal, December 27, 1849, Folder 90v, Collection A77, SL.

110 "Everyone will be prepared": Elizabeth to Blackwell family, March 7, 1850, Reel 42, LC.

110 Henderson's discomforts: Emily to Sam, March 31, 1850, Folder 180, Collection MC411, SL.

110 "I think I never": Emily to Sam, April 7, 1850, Reel 74, LC.

110 "Farewell embryo Esculapius!": Henry to Emily, April 27, 1850, Folder 96, Collection MC411, SL.

110 "infernal regions . . . free state": Emily to Sam, April 7, 1850, Reel 74, LC.

111 "I can imagine you": Elizabeth to Emily, June 5, 1850, Reel 74, LC.

111 "I have been placed": Ibid.

111 "My intention": Ibid.

112 "My kind young physician . . . roses": Ibid.

112 "I beg Uncle": Elizabeth to Charles and Eliza Lane, 1850, Folder 22, Collection MC411, SL.

113 "The most beautiful picture": Elizabeth's journal, July 3, 1850, Reel 47, LC.

114 "I wrote to him": Ibid., June 25, 1850.

114 "only the embrace": Ibid., July 3, 1850.

114 "feeling decidedly blue": Elizabeth to Blackwell family, June 1850, Reel 42, LC.

114 "the High Priest of water": Elizabeth to John Dickson, December 15, 1850, Reel 42, LC.

114 "honest & good . . . things with you": Elizabeth to Blackwell family, June 1850, Reel 42, LC.

114 "something like one of our cotton manufactories . . . swallow it": Ibid.

115 "Everybody seems . . . demands of the place": Ibid.

115 "The *abreibung*": Elizabeth's journal, June 26, 1850, Reel 47, LC.

115 "too stimulating": Blackwell, *Pioneer Work*, 163.

116 "It is a sad business": Anna to Eliza Lane, August 31, 1850, Folder 22, Collection MC411, SL.

116 "That poor only eye": Sam to Emily, October 21, 1850, Folder 96, Collection MC411, SL.

CHAPTER 8: LONDON

117 "I must go to bed": Emily's journal, June 5, 1851, Folder 80, Collection A77, SL.

117 "served up with its legs": Emily to George, October 29, 1850, Folder 179, Collection MC411, SL.

117 "I wish I could acquire": Emily's journal, August 20, 1850, Folder 80, Collection A77, SL.

117 "I certainly have": Ibid., August 24, 1850.

118 "If I get anything . . . of my disposition": Ibid., June 15, 1851.

119 "You will be greatly pleased": Henry to Elizabeth, May 5, 1851, Folder 134, Collection MC411, SL.

120 "terrible discharging tumour": Emily's journal, March 24, 1851, Folder 80, Collection A77, SL.

120   "I have been teaching": Ibid., June 18, 1851.

120   "the dingy look": Elizabeth to Blackwell family, October 20, 1850, Reel 42, LC.

120   "I will not speak of him": Ibid.

121   "a charming young Parisienne": Anna to Eliza Lane, August 31, 1850, Folder 22, Collection MC411, SL.

121   "A little dark figure": Blackwell, *Pioneer Work*, 169.

121   sounds, sights, and smells: "Twenty-four Hours in a London Hospital," *Household Words* 2, no. 46 (February 8, 1851): 457–64.

122   terms of Elizabeth's admission: St. Bartholomew's Hospital Medical Council minutes, May 23, 1850, 37, St. Bartholomew's Hospital Archive.

122   "Auscultation shows": Elizabeth's notes at St. Bartholomew's, November 22, 1850, Reel 46, LC.

123   "Well we have our 'Lady Doctor' ": Paget, *Memoirs of Paget*, 168–69.

123   "gentlemanly fellows": Elizabeth to Blackwell family, October 20, 1850, Reel 42, LC.

123   "Women so dressed out": Ibid.

123   "I am prepared": Blackwell, *Pioneer Work*, 170.

123   "Here there is no excitement": Elizabeth to Samuel Dickson, December 15, 1850, Reel 42, LC.

123   "I must confess": Elizabeth to Blackwell family, October 20, 1850, Reel 42, LC.

124   "neither hydropathy . . . rational course?": Elizabeth to Emily, November 20, 1850, Reel 74, LC.

124   "that bedside knowledge": Elizabeth to Samuel Dickson, December 15, 1850, Reel 42, LC.

124   "All the gentlemen . . . the boys": Elizabeth to Emily, November 20, 1850, Reel 74, LC.

124   "people whose position": Ibid.

125   "She is really": Ibid.

125   "Such a tale!": Bessie Parkes to Barbara Leigh Smith, November 13, 1850, CU.

126   "I cannot sympathise": Elizabeth to Marian, December 24, 1850, Reel 76, LC.

126   "grand moral army . . . fetter them": Elizabeth to Samuel Dickson, December 15, 1850, Reel 42, LC.

126   "I have forgotten": Elizabeth to Marian, December 24, 1850, Reel 76, LC.

127   "with the most hearty": Elizabeth to Emily, April 4, 1851, Reel 74, LC.

127   "Dear Lady Byron": Elizabeth to Lady Byron, March 4, 1851, Reel 42, LC.

128   "My earliest ideal": Lady Byron to Elizabeth, March 31, 1851, Reel 42, LC.

128   "But I do not desire": Lady Byron to Elizabeth, March 27, 1851, Reel 42, LC.

128   "The oneness of dependency": Lady Byron to Elizabeth, March 31, 1851, Reel 42, LC.

128 **"Life opens to me"**: Elizabeth to Emily, April 4, 1851, Reel 74, LC.

129 **"To be nailed"**: Gill, *Nightingales*, 228.

129 **Embley Park**: Ibid., 78.

129 **"Walked much"**: Blackwell, *Pioneer Work*, 185.

130 **"Woman stands askew"**: *The Institution of Kaiserswerth on the Rhine, for the Practical Training of Deaconesses, Under the Direction of the Rev. Pastor Fliedner . . .* (London: London Ragged Colonial Training School, 1851), 6.

130 **"Do you know . . . true communion"**: Blackwell, *Pioneer Work*, 185.

130 **"My own mind"**: Elizabeth to Emily, April 4, 1851, Reel 74, LC.

131 **"zeal and assiduity"**: George Burrows, testimonial, July 16, 1851, Reel 46, LC.

131 **"They have learned"**: Blackwell, *Pioneer Work*, 187.

131 **"I very nearly astounded"**: Bessie Parkes to Elizabeth, July 22, 1851, Reel 43, LC.

CHAPTER 9: PRACTICE

132 **"Miss Elizabeth Blackwell"**: *New-York Daily Tribune*, September 12, 1851, 4.

134 **"I think I have mentioned"**: Elizabeth to Marian, March 8, 1846, Reel 46, LC.

134 **"I do not think"**: Anna to Eliza Lane, October 3, 1851, Folder 22, Collection MC411, SL.

134 **"TO MARRIED WOMEN"**: *Sun* (New York), March 18, 1839.

135 **"FEMALE PILLS"**: *Sun* (New York), May 9, 1839.

136 **"a monster"**: Gunning S. Bedford, "Vaginal Hysterotomy," *New York Journal of Medicine and the Collateral Sciences* 2, no. 5 (1844).

136 **"Nature is appalled"**: *Wonderful Trial of Caroline Lohman*, 5.

136 **"She has made enough money"**: *New-York Tribune*, March 26, 1844, 2.

137 **"this noted 'Doctress'"**: "Madame Restell, and Some of Her Dupes," *New-York Medical and Surgical Reporter* 1, no. 10 (February 21, 1846): 158.

138 **"The gross perversion"**: Blackwell, *Pioneer Work*, 30.

138 **"horrible cupidity"**: *New-York Tribune*, April 30, 1841, 2.

138 **"This announcement"**: *New-York Daily Tribune*, September 12, 1851, 4.

138 **"Blackwell Elizabeth, physician"**: *The Directory of the City of New-York, for 1852–1853* (New York: John F. Trow, 1852), 510.

139 **"insolent letters"**: Blackwell, *Pioneer Work*, 190.

139 **"I imagine you"**: Emily to Elizabeth, September 28, 1851, Folder 163, Collection MC411, SL.

139 **"I fear this stupid"**: Emily's journal, August 29, 1851, Folder 80, Collection A77, SL.

139   **"I am convinced"**: Elizabeth to Lady Byron, March 2, 1852, Reel 42, LC.

140   **"Now though it might"**: Elizabeth to Emily, September 27, 1851, Folder 45, Collection MC411, SL.

140   **"I must tell you"**: Emily to Elizabeth, September 28, 1851, Folder 163, Collection MC411, SL.

140   **"I came home tired"**: Emily's journal, October 4, 1851, Folder 80, Collection A77, SL.

141   **"though the large majority"**: Ibid., December 9, 1851.

141   **"the Faculty deems it"**: Frederick C. Waite, "Dr. Nancy E. (Talbot) Clark: The Second Woman Graduate in Medicine to Practice in Boston," *New England Journal of Medicine* 205, no. 25 (December 17, 1931): 1195–98.

141   **"I ask myself often"**: Ibid., November 23, 1851.

141   **"with higher objects"**: Ibid., January 6, 1852.

141   **"I think often my intense"**: Ibid., January 8, 1852.

141   **"It gives a wonderful zest"**: Ibid., June 22, 1852.

142   **"Send me a scrap"**: Elizabeth to Emily, February 8, 1852, Folder 45, Collection MC411, SL.

143   **"The mother, forgetful"**: Blackwell, *Laws of Life*, 78.

143   **"physical conditions"**: Ibid., 145.

143   **"I believe that the chief source"**: Elizabeth to Hannah Darlington, May 27, 1852, Reel 42, LC.

144   **"These lectures"**: Blackwell, *Laws of Life*, 5.

144   **"She certainly has"**: Emily's journal, March 23, 1852, Folder 80, Collection A77, SL.

144   **"Oh dear"**: Elizabeth to Emily, 1852, Folder 45, Collection MC411, SL.

144   **"By the bye"**: Elizabeth to Emily, May 9, 1852, ibid.

145   **"A most extraordinary case!"**: Blackwell, *Pioneer Work*, 195.

146   **"That experience has been"**: Marian to Emily, March 23, 1852, Folder 45, Collection MC411, SL.

146   **"his clear perception"**: Elizabeth to Emily, May 9, 1852, ibid.

147   **"I have marked out"**: Emily's journal, July 9, 1852, Folder 80, Collection A77, SL.

147   **"So Milly is actually"**: Elizabeth to Sam, July 18, 1852, Folder 62, Collection MC411, SL.

CHAPTER 10: ADMISSION, AGAIN

148 **glass prosthetic glinted:** Sam's journal, June 4, 1852, Folder 1.3, Collection M715, SL.

148 **"From Wednesday noon":** Emily's journal, July 24, 1852, Folder 80, Collection A77, SL.

148 **"Her visit gave me":** Elizabeth to Lady Byron, August 5, 1852, Reel 42, LC.

149 **"The men did not wear":** Emily's journal, August 3, 1852, Folder 80, Collection A77, SL.

149 **"a different country":** Ibid., July 24, 1852.

150 **"Why Milly":** Ibid., August 11, 1852.

150 **"I like the room":** Elizabeth to Emily, May 9, 1852, Folder 45, Collection MC411, SL.

150 **"warehouse for the destitute":** Oshinsky, *Bellevue*, 51.

150 **"Now my dear":** Emily's journal, September 1, 1852, Folder 80, Collection A77, SL.

151 **"Yesterday I had . . . operation, & me":** Emily to George, September 2, 1852, Folder 120, Collection A145, SL.

151 **"I shall certainly find":** Emily's journal, September 2, 1852, Folder 80, Collection A77, SL.

151 **"Rather different kind":** Emily to George, September 2, 1852, Folder 120, Collection A145, SL.

151 **"The young Drs":** Emily's journal, October 1852, Folder 80, Collection A77, SL.

152 **"They are all willing":** Emily to Elizabeth, October 30, 1852, Folder 165, Collection MC411, SL.

152 **"I have introduced":** Emily's journal, October 1852, Folder 80, Collection A77, SL.

152 **"I have today completed":** Emily to George, November 27, 1852, Folder 168, Collection MC411, SL.

153 **"dirty little Chicago":** Emily to Elizabeth, undated, Folder 163, Collection MC411, SL.

153 **"external generative organs":** Emily's journal, November 7, 1852, Folder 80, Collection A77, SL.

153 **"I like Dr Brainard":** Emily to George, November 27, 1852, Folder 168, Collection MC411, SL.

153 **"Doctor, you don't":** Emily's journal, December 1, 1852, Folder 80, Collection A77, SL.

154 **"The Dr has no other":** Emily to Henry, December 5, 1852, Folder 180, Collection MC411, SL.

154 **"And so two weeks":** Emily's journal, December 15, 1852, Folder 80, Collection A77, SL.

154 **"I examined them":** Emily to Elizabeth, December 20, 1852, Folder 163, Collection MC411, SL.

155 **"would I believe admit":** Emily to Elizabeth, December 25, 1852, ibid.

155 **"has liked me thoroughly":** Ibid.

155 **"I would choose":** Emily's journal, December 19, 1852, Folder 80, Collection A77, SL.

155 **"I have come . . . carry them out":** Ibid., January 9, 1853.

156 **"nothing more ghostly":** Sam's journal, December 26, 1852, Folder 1.3, Collection M715, SL.

156 **"Her letters often":** Emily's journal, January 14, 1853, Folder 80, Collection A77, SL.

156 **"I do hope":** Emily to Elizabeth, 1853, Folder 163, Collection MC411, SL.

157 **"He said any young":** Emily to Elizabeth, December 25, 1852, ibid.

157 **a dispensary: a free clinic:** "Report on the Condition of the Dispensaries of the State of New York," in *Annual Report of the State Board of Charities for the Year 1897* (New York: Wynkoop Hallenbeck Crawford Co., 1898), 1:616–54.

157 **"say, the New York Institution . . . it's true":** Emily to Elizabeth, December 25, 1852, Folder 163, Collection MC411, SL.

158 **"I have often thought":** Emily's journal, June 16, 1853, Folder 80, Collection A77, SL.

158 **"He told me the trustees":** Ibid., May 7, 1853.

158 **oyster supper:** Henry to Sam, May 8, 1853, Folder 134, Collection MC411, SL.

158 **"We had quite a merry":** Emily's journal, May 8, 1853, Folder 180, Collection A77, SL.

158 **"I do not feel perfectly":** Ibid., June 9, 1853.

158 **"nervous oppressive discomfort":** Ibid., January 14, 1853.

159 **"The future lies black":** Ibid., October 8, 1853.

159 **"I find I shall have":** Ibid., November 27, 1853.

159 **"It is too absurd":** "Throw Physic to the Dogs, I'll None of It," *Chicago Tribune*, November 30, 1853, 2.

159 **"In behalf of":** "Letter to the Editor," *Chicago Tribune*, December 3, 1853, 2.

160 **"I am beginning to feel":** Emily's journal, December 11, 1853, Folder 80, Collection A77, SL.

160 **"That is the only student":** Sam's journal, February 26, 1854, Folder 1.3, Collection M715, SL.

160 **"it was not often that roses"**: Emily's journal, February 17, 1854, Folder 80, Collection A77, SL.

160 **"Emily is now Dr. Emily"**: Anna Blackwell, "Elizabeth Blackwell," *English Woman's Journal* 1, no. 2 (April 1858): 98.

160 **"The Principles Involved"**: Ibid.

160 **"not only successfully"**: Sam's journal, February 26, 1854, Folder 1.3, Collection M715, SL.

CHAPTER II: EDINBURGH

161 **"Judging from the fine"**: Emily to Blackwell family, March 30, 1854, Folder 180, Collection MC411, SL.

161 **Steamship *Arabia***: "The Royal Mail Steam-Ship 'Arabia,'" *Illustrated London News*, January 8, 1853, 29.

161 **"a little solitary"**: Emily to Blackwell family, April 1, 1854, Folder 180, Collection MC411, SL.

162 **"The design of this institution"**: *First Annual Report of the New York Dispensary for Indigent Women and Children*, 1855, Folder 50, Collection A145, SL.

162 **"medical practitioners of either sex"**: "The New York Infirmary for Indigent Women & Children, Minutes of the Board of Managers, Dec 1853 . . . ," Weill Cornell Archive.

162 **tacked a card**: Elizabeth to Emily, April 20, 1854, Folder 45, Collection MC411, SL.

163 **"pecuniary . . . for a time"**: *First Annual Report of the New York Dispensary for Indigent Women and Children* (1855), Folder 50, Collection A145, SL.

163 **"the people struck me . . . hedgerow"**: Emily to Blackwell family, April 1, 1854, Folder 180, Collection MC411, SL.

164 **"another Dr. Blackwell . . . *sérieux*"**: Emily to Blackwell family, April 15, 1854, ibid.

164 **"The hills grew . . . touched with grey"**: Emily to Blackwell family, May 10, 1854, ibid.

166 **head of Zeus**: McCrae, *Simpson*, 63.

167 **"There was one . . . carriage"**: Emily to Blackwell family, May 10, 1854, Folder 180, Collection MC411, SL.

168 **"surrounded by"**: Ibid.

168 **"I believe I shall"**: Ibid.

168 **"fast set"**: Emily to Elizabeth, June 20, 1854, Folder 163, Collection MC411, SL.

169 **"most decent"**: Emily to Blackwell family, June 24, 1854, ibid.

170 **"I looked grave"**: Emily to Elizabeth, June 2, 1854, ibid.

170   "He makes a physical": Ibid.

170   "He has made in this way": Emily to Elizabeth, June 20, 1854, Folder 163, Collection MC411, SL.

171   "I have not seen": Emily to Elizabeth, July 1854, ibid.

171   "Through August": Emily to Blackwell family, July 7, 1854, Folder 180, Collection MC411, SL.

171   "Period generally": Anna to Emily, September 12, 1854, Folder 27, Collection MC411, SL.

171   gynecological remedies: Lady Northesk, 1850, Royal College of Surgeons Edinburgh archive.

171   "galvanic pessary": Emily to Elizabeth, May 15, 1854, Folder 163, Collection MC411, SL.

172   "I have yet to be": Emily to Elizabeth, June 2, 1854, ibid.

172   he performed frequently: Emily to Elizabeth, July 24, 1854, ibid.

172   He inserted it: Sims, "On the Surgical Treatment," 55.

173   "forthwith quitted": "A Female M.D.," *Caledonian Mercury*, September 25, 1854, 2.

173   "I wish while they": Emily to Blackwell family, October 1, 1854, Folder 180, Collection MC411, SL.

173   "ineffaceable hostility": Elizabeth to Emily, August 11, 1854, Reel 74, LC.

173   "a joke which appeared": Emily to Blackwell family, August 22, 1854, Folder 180, Collection MC411, SL.

173   "He rather likes the novelty": Emily to Elizabeth, September 4, 1854, Folder 163, Collection MC411, SL.

174   "The whole case": Elizabeth to Emily, January 23, 1855, Folder 65, Collection A145, SL.

174   "I believe it has made": Emily to Blackwell family, January 1, 1855, Folder 180, Collection MC411, SL.

174   "made a Dr of me": Emily to Elizabeth, January 29, 1855, Folder 163, Collection MC411, SL.

174   "as I shall not": Emily to Elizabeth, November 5, 1854, ibid.

174   "She will probably thus": Elizabeth to Emily, November 13, 1854, Reel 74, LC.

174   "It seems strange": "From a Correspondent in England," *Una* 3, no. 1 (January 1855): 10.

175   "in which article": Emily to Blackwell family, November 27, 1854, Folder 180, Collection MC411, SL.

175   "I do think you have assumed": Lovejoy, *Women Doctors*, 52.

CHAPTER 12: NEW FACES

177   "This medical solitude": Elizabeth to Emily, May 12, 1854, Reel 74, LC.

177   "With few talents": Vietor, *Woman's Quest*, 3.

177   "I thanked him": Dall, *Practical Illustration*, 105.

178   "She knows far more": Elizabeth to Emily, May 22, 1854, DF.

179   "My sister has just": Vietor, *Woman's Quest*, 113.

179   "Yesterday little Mrs. Clark": Elizabeth to Emily, April 20, 1854, Folder 45, Collection MC411, SL.

179   "Would her companionship": Ibid.

179   "I don't want her": Emily to Elizabeth, c. July 6, 1854, Folder 163, Collection MC411, SL.

179   "A more ignorant": Emily to Elizabeth, June 2, 1854, ibid.

179   "I fancy she's": Elizabeth to Emily, August 11, 1854, Reel 74, LC.

180   "much grander": Elizabeth to Emily, May 22, 1854, DF.

180   "You must settle": Ibid.

181   "My Dispensary business": Elizabeth to Emily, July 24, 1854, Folder 65, Collection A145, SL.

181   "I look on the little": Emily to Elizabeth, July 24, 1854, Folder 163, Collection MC411, SL.

181   filling the margins: Emily to Elizabeth, July 14, 1854, ibid.

181   "She cried oh": Elizabeth to Emily, August 11, 1854, Reel 74, LC.

182   "I found my mind": Boyd, *Excellent Doctor Blackwell*, 174.

182   "Infant Congress": W. H. Davenport, "The Nurseries on Randall's Island," *Harper's New Monthly Magazine* 36, no. 11 (December 1867): 8–24.

182   "great depot": Elizabeth to Barbara Bodichon and Bessie Parkes, June 3, 1856, Folder 2, MS#0124, CU.

183   "I must tell you": Elizabeth to Emily, October 1, 1854, Reel 74, LC.

183   "She is a sturdy": Ibid.

183   "Oh nice God": Sam's journal, November 19, 1854, Folder 1.3, Collection M715, SL.

183   "Doctor," she exclaimed: Blackwell, *Pioneer Work*, 198.

183   "I have had, and I shall": Elizabeth to Barbara Bodichon and Bessie Parkes, June 3, 1856, Folder 2, MS#0124, CU.

183   "Oh Doctor": Ibid.

184   "very pleasant-voiced": Kitty, "Reminiscences," Folder 650, Collection MC411, SL.

185   "I decidedly prefer": Henry to Sam, June 2, 1853, Reel 50, LC.

186   "I think you will like": Henry to Lucy Stone, June 13, 1853, in Wheeler, *Loving Warriors*, 36.

186   "If both parties": Henry to Lucy Stone, July 2, 1853, ibid., 45.

186   "I am very glad": Lucy Stone to Henry, September 10, 1854, ibid., 98–99.

187   "You shall choose": Henry to Lucy Stone, December 22, 1854, ibid., 109.

187   "Lucy, I wish": Henry to Lucy Stone, January 3, 1855, ibid., 116.

187   "We view life": Elizabeth to Henry, December 27, 1854, Reel 50, LC.

187   "morbid craving": Elizabeth to Emily, September 15, 1854, Reel 74, LC.

187   "We must absolutely": Elizabeth to Emily, January 23, 1855, Folder 65, Collection A145, SL.

187   "I hope that intercourse": Emily to Elizabeth, January 29, 1855, Folder 163, Collection MC411, SL.

187   "Sam says": Marian, quoted in Elizabeth to Emily, January 23, 1855, Folder 65, Collection A145, SL.

188   "She has very good taste": Henry to Lucy Stone, February 13, 1855, in Wheeler, *Loving Warriors*, 122.

188   "I protest against": Elizabeth to Henry, February 22, 1855, Reel 50, LC.

188   "this act on our part": "Protest Published by Lucy Stone and Henry B. Blackwell, on their Marriage, May 1st 1855," DF.

189   "putting Lucy Stone": Lucy Stone to Antoinette Brown, March 29, 1855, in Wheeler, *Loving Warriors*, 128.

189   "a young woman of strange": Quoted in Wheeler, *Loving Warriors*, 16.

190   Henry had tried: Henry to Antoinette Brown, April 16, 1855, Reel 50, LC.

190   "I forgot my drenched": Sam's journal, November 8, 1854, Folder 1.3, Collection M715, SL.

190   "The love of her": Ibid., December 16, 1855.

190   "They are for you": Antoinette Brown to Sam, December 22, 1855, in Hays, *Extraordinary Blackwells*, 122.

190   "spirited miscellaneous kissing": Sam's journal, March 2, 1856, Folder 1.3, Collection M715, SL.

190   "alone of all men": Lucy Stone to Antoinette Brown, January 20, 1856, in Hays, *Extraordinary Blackwells*, 122.

191   "You are a little wretch": Lucy Stone to Susan B. Anthony, in Wheeler, *Loving Warriors*, 142–43.

191   "Would you like to see": Kitty, "Reminiscences," Folder 650, Collection MC411, SL.

192   "Thanks to our judicious": Sam's journal, November 9, 1856, Folder 1.3, Collection M715, SL.

192   **"I have experienced"**: Emily to Elizabeth, March 23, 1855, Folder 163, Collection MC411, SL.

192   **"ardent love"**: Anna Blackwell, "Elizabeth Blackwell," *English Woman's Journal* 1, no. 2 (April 1858): 99.

193   **"The surname of the lady"**: "Physicians in Muslin," *Punch*, April 5, 1856, 133.

193   **"The European hospitals"**: Emily to Elizabeth, September 16, 1855, Folder 163, Collection MC411, SL.

193   **"old fogies"**: Emily to Elizabeth, June 1855, Folder 165, Collection MC411, SL.

194   **"As things have turned out"**: Anna to Blackwells, April 14, 1856, Folder 22, Collection MC411, SL.

CHAPTER 13: INFIRMARY

195   **"I have no turn"**: Elizabeth to Henry, December 23, 1855, Folder 62, Collection MC411, SL.

195   **"Dr. Sims has never called"**: Elizabeth to Emily, 1855, Reel 74, LC.

196   **"Women have always presided"**: Blackwell, *Medical Education of Women*, 3.

196   **"The midwife must"**: Ibid., 5.

196   **"The grandest name"**: Ibid., 5–6.

197   **"their ignorance"**: Ibid., 8.

197   **"unnatural and monstrous"**: Ibid., 8.

197   **"bitter mortification"**: Ibid., 9.

197   **"utter want of delicacy"**: Ibid., 8.

197   **"There is but one way"**: Ibid., 14.

197   **"sound judgment"**: Ibid., 15.

198   **"There was scarcely any life"**: Vietor, *Woman's Quest*, 183.

198   **"If you must talk"**: Ibid., 197.

198   **"designed to meet"**: Circular, June 2, 1856, Folder 83, Collection MC411, SL.

198   **"I shall have an Art"**: Elizabeth to Emily, June 20, 1856, Folder 68, Collection MC411, SL.

199   **"This enterprise must not"**: *New-York Tribune*, December 15, 1856, 7.

200   **"manifested the capacity"**: "Female Physicians," *New-York Tribune*, December 5, 1856, 7.

200   **"Debauchery"**: Charles Dickens, *American Notes for General Circulation* (London: Chapman & Hall, 1842), 1:212.

200   **"She must have both"**: Florence Nightingale to Emily, May 12, 1856, Folder 70, Collection MC411, SL.

201   **"Beecher's theater"**: Applegate, *Most Famous Man*, 299.

202   **five thousand dollars:** Ibid., 291, 294.

202   **William Elder:** "New York Infirmary for Women and Children," *New York Daily Herald*, May 13, 1857, 3; "Opening of the New-York Infirmary for Women and Children," *New-York Tribune*, May 13, 1857, 4.

202   **"Elizabeth Blackwell seemed":** Boyd, *Excellent Doctor Blackwell*, 190.

203   **"fully respectable":** Vietor, *Woman's Quest*, 209.

204   **"It is a principle":** *Fourth Annual Report of the New York Infirmary for Indigent Women and Children for the Year 1857* (New York: Baker & Taylor, 1858), NYAM. *Fourth* counts from the founding of the dispensary in 1853; this was the first annual published after the founding of the infirmary.

205   **"What the Lady Doctors Are Doing":** "What the Lady Doctors Are Doing," *New-York Times*, July 24, 1857, 8.

205   **"I found that she also":** Vietor, *Woman's Quest*, 185.

206   **"Night after night":** *Sixth Annual Report of the New York Infirmary for Indigent Women and Children for the Year 1859* (New York: Baptist & Taylor, 1860), 7.

206   **"unpleasant annoyances":** Blackwell, *Pioneer Work*, 197.

206   **"killing women in childbirth":** Vietor, *Woman's Quest*, 219.

206   **"It was a sight":** Ibid., 227.

207   **"I informed him":** Elizabeth to Emily, July 11, 1857, Reel 74, LC.

207   **"I have been delighted":** Elizabeth to George, June 22, 1857, Folder 51, Collection MC411, SL.

207   **"the kindly, home-like way":** *Fourth Annual Report of the New York Infirmary*, 7.

208   **"Its funds have been":** "The Woman's Own Hospital," *New-York Times*, July 12, 1858, 4.

208   **"She sprang up":** Blackwell, *Pioneer Work*, 210.

208   **"When a woman has won":** "The Position of Women," *Philadelphia Press*, August 25, 1857.

208   **"Your kind thought":** Elizabeth to Lady Byron, December 27, 1857, Reel 42, LC.

CHAPTER 14: RECOGNITION

210   **"I am going to tell you":** Elizabeth to George, June 9, 1858, Folder 51, Collection MC411, SL.

210   **"I should not object":** Emily to George, August 25, 1857, Folder 168, Collection MC411, SL.

210   **"Life in New York":** Elizabeth to George, June 9, 1858, Folder 51, Collection MC411, SL.

211   **"Whatever happened":** Emily to Elizabeth, April 9, 1859, Folder 163, Collection MC411, SL.

211 **"very general misapprehension"**: Anna Blackwell, "Elizabeth Blackwell," *English Woman's Journal* 1, no. 2 (April 1858): 80.

211 **"incapable of resorting"**: Ibid., 94.

212 **"I think it very desirable"**: Elizabeth to George, June 9, 1858, Folder 51, Collection MC411, SL.

212 **"An agony of doubt"**: Emily's journal, June 20, 1858, Folder 80, Collection A77, SL.

213 **"She needs change"**: Emily to George, July 13, 1858, Folder 168, Collection MC411, SL.

213 **"throw Kitty overboard"**: Elizabeth to Emily, August 21, 1858, Reel 74, LC.

213 **"Dear Kittykin"**: Elizabeth to Kitty, October 1, 1858, Reel 42, LC.

214 **"Having read, small as I was"**: Kitty, "Reminiscences," Folder 650, Collection MC411, SL.

215 **"heartfelt welcome"**: Lady Byron et al. to Elizabeth, 1859, Reel 46, LC.

215 **"represents an exaggeratedly"**: Elizabeth to Emily, November 1858, Reel 74, LC.

215 **"You can hardly have . . . leech"**: Elizabeth, lecture draft, 1859, Reel 44, LC.

216 **"I cannot help thinking"**: Elizabeth to Emily, January 11, 1859, Folder 46, Collection MC411, SL.

217 **"She feels"**: Ibid.

217 **"She thinks moreover"**: Ibid.

217 **"She wishes, I see"**: Elizabeth to Barbara Bodichon, March 16, 1859, Folder 3, MS#0124, CU.

217 **"I remember my impression"**: Florence Nightingale to Elizabeth, February 10, 1859, in Boyd, *Excellent Doctor Blackwell*, 217.

218 **"FN's idea"**: Emily to Elizabeth, February 8, 1859, Folder 163, Collection MC411, SL.

218 **"Keep quietly clear"**: Emily to Elizabeth, April 9, 1859, ibid.

218 **"The most characteristic"**: Elizabeth to Emily, January 28, 1859, Folder 50, Collection MC411, SL.

218 **"I can hardly tell you"**: Ibid.

219 **"shriek of horror"**: Elizabeth to George, February 26, 1859, Folder 51, Collection MC411, SL.

219 **"about 150 people"**: Elizabeth to Emily, March 4, 1859, Folder 50, Collection MC411, SL.

219 **"Now, let us for a moment"**: "Lectures by a Lady-Doctor," *Chambers's Journal of Popular Literature Science and Arts*, no. 276 (April 16, 1859): 255–56.

219 **"something definite"**: Elizabeth Garrett to Emily Davies, March 23, 1861, *Autograph Letters of Dr. Elizabeth Garrett Anderson, 1860–1939*, ref. GB 106 9/10, Women's Library.

219   "Last night I saw": Elizabeth to Emily, June 17, 1859, Reel 74, LC.

219   "I remember feeling": Elizabeth Garrett to Emily Davies, March 23, 1861, *Autograph Letters of Dr. Elizabeth Garrett Anderson, 1860–1939*, ref. GB 106 9/10, Women's Library.

219   "There is an immense charm": Elizabeth to Emily, April 15, 1859, Reel 74, LC.

220   "I do not think you know": Florence Nightingale to Elizabeth, March 7, 1859, Reel 43, LC.

220   "They have got so completely": Emily to Elizabeth, November 21, 1858, Folder 163, Collection MC411, SL.

220   "a younger, less well known": Emily to Elizabeth, March 16, 1859, ibid.

220   "My liking is for Europe": Emily to Elizabeth, January 7, 1859, ibid.

221   "as her sister, Dr. Emily": "Passing Events," *English Woman's Journal* 3, no. 13 (March 1859): 72.

221   "In looking over the book": Emily to Elizabeth, October 1, 1858, Folder 163, Collection MC411, SL.

221   "She is evidently desirous": Emily to Elizabeth, October 15, 1858, ibid.

221   "Z doesn't even make": Emily to Elizabeth, January 7, 1859, ibid.

221   "The whole affair": Emily to Elizabeth, December 27, 1858, ibid.

222   "I felt that a larger": Vietor, *Woman's Quest*, 237.

222   "We can not make the hospital": Emily to Elizabeth, November 21, 1858, Folder 163, Collection MC411, SL.

222   "If ever I come": Emily to Elizabeth, April 9, 1859, ibid.

222   "one of those old": Ibid.

222   "I have had our names": Emily to Elizabeth, April 16, 1859, ibid.

222   "Blackwell Emily": *Trow's New York City Directory for the Year Ending May 1, 1859*, 78, Digital Collections, New York Public Library.

222   "Blackwell Elizabeth & Emily": *Trow's New York City Directory for the Year Ending May 1, 1860*, 81, Digital Collections, New York Public Library.

223   "get people to regard us": Emily to Elizabeth, April 16, 1859, Folder 163, Collection MC411, SL.

223   "half crazy": Elizabeth to Barbara Bodichon, May 7, 1859, MS#0124, CU.

223   "I confess I've had": Elizabeth to Emily, April 11, 1859, Folder 163, Collection MC411, SL.

223   "I have only one": Elizabeth to Emily, June 17, 1859, Reel 74, LC.

223   "Your registration": Emily to Elizabeth, July 5, 1859, Folder 163, Collection MC411, SL.

CHAPTER 15: WAR

224 "I wrote the above": Elizabeth to Barbara Bodichon, April 23, 1861, MS#0124, CU.

224 "the overbearing insolence": Elizabeth to Emily, June 20, 1856, Folder 68, Collection MC411, SL.

224 "I think it is much more": Elizabeth to Barbara Bodichon, April 13, 1861, MS#0124, CU.

225 "their true position": Elizabeth to Barbara Bodichon, June 23, 1860, MS#0124, CU.

225 "I do not look on a good": Elizabeth to Barbara Bodichon, April 13, 1861, MS#0124, CU.

225 "Doubt is disease": Elizabeth to Barbara Bodichon, undated, MS#0124, CU.

225 "She has taken an extreme": Elizabeth to Barbara Bodichon, December 2, 1860, MS#0124, CU.

225 "We are compelled": Elizabeth to Barbara Bodichon, April 23, 1861, MS#0124, CU.

226 "To the Women of New York": "An Appeal," *New-York Times*, April 28, 1861.

226 "God bless the women!": "Ladies' Military Relief Meeting at the Cooper Institute," *New-York Tribune*, April 20, 1861.

227 "Every woman is a nurse": Nightingale, *Notes on Nursing*, 3.

227 "There has been a perfect mania": Elizabeth to Barbara Bodichon, June 5, 1861, MS#0124, CU.

227 Emily even traveled: "A Fragment of Cousin Kitty's Reminiscences," dictated by Kitty to George H. Blackwell, August 1933, Collection of Martin Dornbaum and Patricia Simino Boyce, Health Professions Education Center, Hunter-Bellevue School of Nursing. A second, slightly different version was sent to me by Jane Carey Blackwell Bloomfield, daughter of George H. Blackwell and great-granddaughter of Elizabeth and Emily's youngest brother, George W. Blackwell.

227 "On the Selection": "Report Concerning the Woman's Central Association of Relief at New York to the U.S. Sanitary Commission at Washington, Oct. 12, 1861," *Sanitary Commission No. 32* (New York: Wm. C. Bryant & Co., 1861), 24–26.

228 "Girls of eighteen": "A Fragment of Cousin Kitty's Reminiscences," August 1933.

229 Bellows's proposal: "Report Concerning the Woman's Central Association of Relief at New York to the U.S. Sanitary Commission at Washington, Oct. 12, 1861," 20.

229 "to have anything to do": Elizabeth to Barbara Bodichon, June 5, 1861, MS#0124, CU.

229 "lest our name": Emily to Barbara Bodichon, June 1, 1861, MS#0124, CU.

229 "Of course as it is essential": Elizabeth to Barbara Bodichon, June 5, 1861, MS#0124, CU.

229 "Miss Dix, though in many": Emily to Barbara Bodichon, June 1, 1861, MS#0124, CU.

230 "The government has given": Elizabeth to Barbara Bodichon, June 5, 1861, MS#0124, CU.

230 "We completed the 100": Elizabeth to George, June 7, 1862, Folder 51, Collection MC411, SL.

230 "They were inclined": Emily to George, June 16, 1862, Folder 169, ibid.

230 "commutation": Hays, *Extraordinary Blackwells*, 151.

230 "I have given up": Emily to George, August 21, 1862, Folder 169, Collection MC411, SL.

231 "Our carpenter": Emily to George, September 1, 1862, ibid.

231 As Kitty remembered it: "A Fragment of Cousin Kitty's Reminiscences," dictated by Kitty to George, August 1933.

232 "The green flickering": Elizabeth to Barbara Bodichon, June 9, 1863, MS#0124, CU.

232 "villages of tents": Elizabeth to Emily and Kitty, June 6, 1864, Reel 55, LC.

232 "We have had charming": Elizabeth to Kitty, June 8, 1864, Reel 55, LC.

232 "making acquaintance": Ibid.

233 "Why don't you go up . . . quite in luck": Ibid.

234 "handsome dark eyed . . . young Doctor": Ibid.

CHAPTER 16: COLLEGE

235 "They have each quite": Elizabeth to Barbara Bodichon, January 14, 1861, MS#0124, CU.

235 "I am sick of the farce": Emily to Elizabeth, November 10, 1858, Folder 163, Collection MC411, SL.

235 "It is the old difference": Elizabeth to Barbara Bodichon, January 14, 1861, MS#0124, CU.

236 "sentimental air . . . doing": Emily to Elizabeth, May 10, 1859, Folder 163, Collection MC411, SL.

236 "If we could have joined": Elizabeth to Barbara Bodichon, June 9, 1863, MS#0124, CU.

236 "Being the first": *Second Annual Announcement and Constitution of the New York Medical College for Women and Hospital for Women and Children* (New York, 1864), 7.

236 **"The true plan"**: Elizabeth to Barbara Bodichon, June 9, 1863, MS#0124, CU.

237 **"a vulgar little class"**: Elizabeth to Barbara Bodichon, January 18, 1865, in Boyd, *Excellent Doctor Blackwell*, 236.

237 **"We believe that the time . . . kind of disease"**: Blackwell, *Medical Education of Women*.

238 **"It is knowledge"**: Ibid.

238 **"to enable the corporation"**: *Constitution and By-Laws of the New York Infirmary for Women and Children, and Woman's Medical College* (New York: Wynkoop & Hallenbeck, 1864).

238 **"the San Greal"**: Elizabeth to Barbara Bodichon, September 7, 1864, in Boyd, *Excellent Doctor Blackwell*, 237.

238 **"The great secret"**: Elizabeth to Barbara Bodichon, May 23, 1865, ibid., 240.

239 **"The circle is broken"**: Emily's journal, March 5, 1866, Folder 80, Collection A77, SL.

239 **"I had built"**: Anna to Blackwell family, March 20, 1866, Folder 22, Collection MC411, SL.

239 **"Whether I shall really"**: Anna to Elizabeth, April 2, 1866, Reel 71, LC.

239 **"a kind of 'social evil' "**: Elizabeth Garrett to Louisa Garrett Smith, November 22, 1862, Women's Library.

239 **"Science, at best"**: "Shall Women Be Doctors?" *Lancet* 2 (August 3, 1861): 117.

239 **"In Miss Garrett"**: "Medical News," *British Medical Journal* 2 (July 14, 1866): 62.

240 **"I have had an unexpected"**: Elizabeth to Marian, October 5, 1866, Reel 76, LC.

240 **"a very talented girl"**: Elizabeth to Barbara Bodichon, April 25, 1860, MS#0124, CU.

241 **"Little Miss Putnam"**: Elizabeth to Marian, October 5, 1866, Reel 76, LC.

241 **"a great Spiritualist"**: Mary Putnam to Victorine Putnam, October 21, 1866, in Putnam, *Life and Letters of Mary*, 99.

241 **"They will, as always"**: Emily to Elizabeth, July 21, 1866, Folder 163, Collection MC411, SL.

242 **"The Eye and its Appendages"**: Rebecca J. Cole, "The Eye and its Appendages, Submitted as a Thesis to the Faculty of Female Medical College of Pennsylvania," February 1867, Drexel University Archives and Special Collections.

242 **"carried on this work"**: Blackwell, *Pioneer Work*, 228.

242 **"the respectability of a household"**: Rebecca J. Cole, "First Meeting of the Women's Missionary Society of Philadelphia," *Woman's Era* 3, no. 4 (October 1896).

242 **"Emily . . . does grandly"**: Elizabeth to Barbara Bodichon, January 13, 1867, in Boyd, *Excellent Doctor Blackwell*, 245.

243   **"When you write"**: Emily to George, April 18, 1867, Folder 169, Collection MC411, SL.

. 243   **"True growth"**: Blackwell, *Address Delivered at the Opening*, 3–4, Reel 48, LC.

243   **board of examiners**: "The Women's Medical College of the New York Infirmary," 1st catalog/announcement, 1868, Reel 48, LC.

243   **"This school is the only one"**: Blackwell, *Address Delivered at the Opening*, 13.

244   **"keen intuition"**: "The Woman's Medical College," *New-York Times*, November 3, 1868, 8.

245   **"I'm afraid she won't"**: Elizabeth to Barbara Bodichon, October 28, 1868, CU, in Sahli, "Blackwell.: A Biography," 165.

245   **"If I am to be a doctor"**: Sophia Jex-Blake's journal, April 12, 1868, in Todd, *Life of Jex-Blake*, 200.

245   **"to which she instantly"**: Sophia Jex-Blake to Mary Jex-Blake, November 8, 1868, ibid., 206.

245   **"In 1869 the early"**: Blackwell, *Pioneer Work*, 241.

246   **"Partnership (of 10 years"**: Emily? Notes on partnership, 1869, Folder 191, Collection MC411, SL.

246   **"If you would take a peep"**: Kitty to Alice, July 10, 1869, Reel 55, LC.

247   **wrote a will**: Elizabeth's will, July 14, 1869, Folder 81, Collection MC411, SL.

247   **"They claim me"**: Elizabeth to Samuel Willetts, October 18, 1869, Folder 62, ibid.

247   **"I am settled"**: Elizabeth to Kitty, February 23, 1870, Reel 55, LC.

248   **"I did not indulge"**: Emily to Elizabeth, October 11, 1869, Folder 164, Collection MC411, SL.

248   **"I would sink"**: Elizabeth to Emily, January 4, 1870, Folder 46, ibid.

248   **"I can see very well"**: Emily to Elizabeth, 1869, Folder 183, ibid.

248   **"build up a little group"**: Emily to Elizabeth, April 13, 1870, Folder 164, ibid.

249   **"It seemed as though everything"**: Ibid.

249   **"a graceful & entirely"**: Ibid.

249   **"Aunt Emily made"**: Kitty to Alice, April 5, 1870, Reel 55, LC.

CHAPTER 17: DIVERGENCE

250   **"Miss Garrett"**: Elizabeth to Emily, August 20, 1869, Folder 46, Collection MC411, SL.

250   **"I do indeed congratulate"**: Elizabeth to Sophia Jex-Blake, in Todd, *Life of Jex-Blake*, 264.

251   **"Neither Miss Putnam"**: Elizabeth to Emily, August 1870, Folder 50, Collection MC411, SL.

251   **"I could not have imagined"**: Elizabeth to Emily, May 14, 1870, Folder 46, Collection MC411, SL.

252   **"You can help me so much"**: Elizabeth to Kitty, October 12, 1869, in Boyd, *Excellent Doctor Blackwell,* 280.

252   **"fitted herself into all"**: "In Memory of Dr. Elizabeth Blackwell and Dr. Emily Blackwell, January 25, 1911," NYAM, 12–13.

252   **"Prevention is better"**: Blackwell, *Pioneer Work,* 247.

253   **"that direful purchase"**: Ibid., 243.

254   **"exquisite spiritual joys"**: Blackwell, *Counsel to Parents,* 56.

254   **"It might almost be read aloud"**: Emily to Lucy Stone, January 29, 1879, LC, in Sahli, "Blackwell: A Biography," 235.

254   **"a well-established fact"**: Blackwell, *Human Element in Sex,* 51.

255   **"is largely under the control"**: Blackwell, *How to Keep a Household in Health,* 9.

256   **"From the outset of marriage"**: Blackwell, *Medical Address on Malthus,* 34.

256   **"A man who commits rape"**: Ibid., 28.

256   **"To a hygienic"**: Elizabeth, *Pioneer Work,* 239.

257   **"really of tremendous practical"**: Elizabeth to Annie Leigh Browne, April 1902, in Boyd, *Excellent Doctor Blackwell,* 293.

257   **"My 'Test'"**: Elizabeth to Emma Stone Blackwell, July 6, 1894, in Sahli, "Blackwell: A Biography," 341.

257   **"I am utterly unwilling"**: Emily to Elizabeth, June 15, 1870, Folder 164, Collection MC411, SL.

258   **"I cannot describe the shock"**: Emily to Elizabeth, August 25, 1870, ibid.

258   **"I do not know whether"**: Emily to Elizabeth, October 6, 1871, ibid.

258   **"It is utterly impossible"**: Elizabeth to Mary Putnam, December 31, 1871, in Putnam, *Life and Letters of Mary,* 307.

259   **"It is your mind"**: Mary Putnam Jacobi to Elizabeth, December 25, 1888, Reel 43, LC.

259   **"She is a bright"**: Emily to Kitty, November 14, 1871, Folder 180, Collection MC411, SL.

259   **clutching the banister**: Emily to Kitty, July 31, 1871, Reel 55, LC.

259   **rows of kisses**: Nannie to Emily, January 24, 1884, Folder 713, Collection MC411, SL.

260   **"They have put down"**: Emily to Elizabeth, November 25, 1873, Folder 164, ibid.

261   **"You ought to have a partner"**: Emily to Alice, January 14, 1884, Reel 73, LC.

261   **"like a butcher's"**: Emily to Alice, March 9, 1884, Reel 73, LC.

261   **"a remarkably lovely woman"**: Mary Putnam Jacobi to Elizabeth, December 25, 1888, Reel 43, LC.

261   **"No one could be more kind"**: Emily to Elizabeth, February 26, 1896, Reel
       74, LC.

261   **"The last days"**: Elizabeth Cushier to Emily, September 14, n.d., Folder 187,
       Collection MC411, SL.

262   **"On the top floor"**: "Woman's Medical College Burned," *New-York Tribune*,
       April 23, 1897, 4.

262   **"We have taken the next"**: Emily to Elizabeth, April 27, 1897, Reel 74, LC.

262   **"Women students need"**: "In Connection with the Burning of the College
       Building . . . ," pamphlet, NYAM.

263   **"at first in derision"**: "Woman Doctors' College Burned," *Sun* (New York),
       April 23, 1897, 8.

                                   CODA

264   **"I understand that is"**: "Institution May Close," *New-York Tribune*, May 24,
       1899, 5.

264   **"They have a million"**: Emily to Elizabeth, December 27, 1898, Reel 74, LC.

265   **"The graduates think"**: "Confirmed by Dr. Loomis," *New-York Tribune*, May
       25, 1899, 9.

265   **"had held open the door"**: Women's Medical College of the New York Infir-
       mary for Women and Children, 321 East 15th Street, Final Catalogue and
       Announcement, June 1899, 14.

265   **"In every city"**: Ibid., 15.

265   **Of the eighteen women**: "Its Last Commencement," *Sun* (New York), May 26,
       1899, 4.

266   **"You will be brought . . . her sons"**: Women's Medical College of the New York
       Infirmary for Women and Children, 321 East 15th Street, Final Catalogue and
       Announcement, June 1899, 18–19.

266   **"I am glad to feel"**: Emily to Elizabeth, December 13, 1899, Reel 74, LC.

266   **"I remember how I trembled"**: "In Memory of Dr. Elizabeth Blackwell and Dr.
       Emily Blackwell, January 25, 1911," NYAM, 23–24.

267   **"It is only when we have learned"**: Blackwell, *Religion of Health*, 22.

268   **In 1910**: Walsh, *"Doctors Wanted,"* 186.

268   **Today thirty-five percent**: Federation of State Medical Boards, "FSMB Cen-
       sus of Licensed Physicians in the United States, 2018," *Journal of Medical
       Regulation* 105, no. 2 (2018): 7–23, https://www.fsmb.org/siteassets/advocacy/
       publications/2018census.pdf

BIBLIOGRAPHY

Blackwell Family Papers, Schlesinger Library, Radcliffe Institute for Advanced Study, Harvard University (SL)
Blackwell Family Papers, Library of Congress (LC)
Elizabeth Blackwell Letters, Rare Book & Manuscript Library, Columbia University (CU)
Dobkin Family Collection of Feminism (DF)
New York Academy of Medicine (NYAM)
Samuel J. Wood Library, Weill Cornell Medicine
Women's Library, London School of Economics

PRIMARY SOURCES

Blackwell, Elizabeth. *Address Delivered at the Opening of the Woman's Medical College of the New York Infirmary, 126 Second Avenue, November 2, 1868*. New York: Edward O. Jenkins, 1869.

———. *Address on the Medical Education of Women, December 27th, 1855*. New York: Baker & Duyckinck, 1856.

———. *Counsel to Parents on the Moral Education of Their Children*. New York: Brentano's Literary Emporium, 1880.

———. *How to Keep a Household in Health: An Address Delivered Before the Working Women's College*. London: W.W. Head, 1870.

———. *The Human Element in Sex, Being a Medical Inquiry into the Relation of Sexual Physiology to Christian Morality*. London: J. & A. Churchill, 1894.

———. *The Laws of Life, With Special Reference to the Physical Education of Girls*. New York: George P. Putnam, 1852.

———. *A Medical Address on the Benevolence of Malthus, Contrasted with the Corruptions of Neo-Malthusianism*. London: T.W. Danks & Co., 1888.

———. *Pioneer Work in Opening the Medical Profession to Women*. New York: Longmans, Green, 1895.

———. *The Religion of Health*. Edinburgh: John Menzies & Co., 1878.

Boardman, Andrew. "An Essay on the Means of Improving Medical Education and Elevating Medical Character." Philadelphia: Haswell, Barrington, & Haswell, 1840.

Code of Ethics of the American Medical Association, Adopted May 1847. Philadelphia: T.K. & P.G. Collins, 1848.

Cushier, Elizabeth. "Autobiography of Elizabeth Cushier." In Kate Campbell Hurd-Mead, Medical Women of America: A Short History of the Pioneer Medical Women of America and of a few of their colleagues in England. New York: Froben Press, 1933.

Dall, Caroline, ed. A Practical Illustration of "Woman's Right To Labor"; or, A Letter from Marie E. Zakrzewska, M.D. Boston: Walker, Wise & Co., 1860.

Denis, Jules, Baron du Potet de Sennevoy. An Introduction to the Study of Animal Magnetism. London: Saunders & Otley, 1838.

Emmet, Thomas Addis. Incidents of My Life: Professional—Literary—Social, With Services in the Cause of Ireland. New York: G.P. Putnam's Sons, 1911.

———. Reminiscences of the Founders of the Woman's Hospital Association. New York: Stuyvesant Press, 1893.

Fuller, S. Margaret. Woman in the Nineteenth Century. New York: Greeley & McElrath, 1845.

Hunt, Harriot K., M.D. Glances and Glimpses; or Fifty Years Social, Including Twenty Years Professional Life. Boston: John P. Jewett & Co., 1856.

In Memory of Dr. Elizabeth Blackwell and Dr. Emily Blackwell. New York Academy of Medicine, 1911.

Lee, Charles A., M.D. Valedictory Address to the Graduating Class of Geneva Medical College at the Public Commencement, January 23, 1849. Buffalo, N.Y.: Jewett, Thomas & Co., 1849.

Nightingale, Florence. Notes on Nursing: What It Is, and What It Is Not. London: Harrisons, 1859.

Proceedings of the Anti-Slavery Convention of American Women, Held in the City of New-York, May 9th, 10th, 11th, and 12th, 1837. New York: William S. Dorr, 1837.

Sims, J. Marion. "On the Surgical Treatment of Stenosis of the Cervix Uteri." In Transactions of the American Gynecological Society. Vol. 3, For the Year 1878. Boston: Houghton, Osgood & Co., 1879.

Stanton, Elizabeth Cady et al., eds. History of Woman Suffrage. Vol. 1, 1848–1861. Rochester, N.Y.: Charles Mann, 1881.

Trollope, Frances Milton. Domestic Manners of the Americans. London: Whittaker, Treacher & Co., 1832.

Trial of Madame Restell, Alias Ann Lohman, for Abortion and Causing the Death of Mrs. Purdy . . . New York, 1841.

Wonderful Trial of Caroline Lohman, Alias Restell. New York: Burgess, Stringer & Co., 1847.

SECONDARY SOURCES

Abram, Ruth J., ed. *"Send Us a Lady Physician": Women Doctors in America, 1835–1920.* New York: W. W. Norton, 1985.

Antler, Joyce. "Medical Women and Social Reform—A History of the New York Infirmary for Women and Children," *Women and Health* 1, no. 4 (July–August 1976): 11–18.

Applegate, Debby. *The Most Famous Man in America: The Biography of Henry Ward Beecher.* New York: Doubleday, 2006.

Berry, Daina Ramey. *The Price for Their Pound of Flesh: The Value of the Enslaved, from Womb to Grave, in the Building of a Nation.* Boston: Beacon Press, 2017.

Boyd, Julia. *The Excellent Doctor Blackwell: The Life of the First Woman Physician.* Stroud: Sutton, 2005.

Browder, Clifford. *The Wickedest Woman in New York: Madame Restell, the Abortionist.* Hamden, Conn.: Archon Books, 1988.

Crawford, Elizabeth. *Enterprising Women: The Garretts and Their Circle.* London: Francis Boutle, 2002.

Croskey, John Welsh, ed. *History of Blockley: A History of the Philadelphia General Hospital from its Inception, 1731–1928.* Philadelphia: F. A. Davis, 1929.

Daniel, Annie Sturgis. "A Cautious Experiment: The History of the New York Infirmary for Women and Children and the Women's Medical College of the New York Infirmary; Also Its Pioneer Founders, 1853–1899," *Medical Woman's Journal* 46, no. 5 (May 1938) through July 1941.

Fancourt, Mary St. J. *They Dared to Be Doctors: Elizabeth Blackwell, Elizabeth Garrett Anderson.* London: Longmans, Green, 1965.

Fuchs, Rachel G. *Poor and Pregnant in Paris: Strategies for Survival in the Nineteenth Century.* New Brunswick, N.J.: Rutgers University Press, 1992.

Giesburg, Judith Ann. *Civil War Sisterhood: The U.S. Sanitary Commission and Women's Politics in Transition.* Boston: Northeastern University Press, 2000.

Gill, Gillian. *Nightingales: The Extraordinary Upbringing and Curious Life of Miss Florence Nightingale.* New York: Ballantine, 2004.

Hays, Elinor Rice. *Those Extraordinary Blackwells.* New York: Harcourt Brace, 1967.

Horn, Margo. "Family Ties: The Blackwells, a Study in the Dynamics of Family Life in Nineteenth Century America." Ph.D. diss., Tufts University, 1980.

Kinney, Janet. *Saga of a Surgeon: The Life of Daniel Brainard, M.D.* Springfield, Ill.: Southern Illinois University School of Medicine, 1987.

Lasser, Carol, and Marlene Deahl Merrill, eds. *Friends and Sisters: Letters between Lucy Stone and Antoinette Brown Blackwell, 1846–1893.* Chicago: University of Illinois Press, 1987.

Lawrence, Charles. *History of the Philadelphia Almshouses and Hospitals.* Philadelphia: Charles Lawrence, 1905.

Lovejoy, Esther Pohl. *Women Doctors of the World.* New York: Macmillan, 1957.

Manton, Jo. *Elizabeth Garrett Anderson.* New York: E. P. Dutton, 1965.

Marshall, Megan. *Margaret Fuller: A New American Life.* New York: Houghton Mifflin Harcourt, 2013.

McCrae, Morrice. *Simpson: The Turbulent Life of a Medical Pioneer.* Edinburgh: John Donald, 2010.

McCullough, David. *The Greater Journey: Americans in Paris.* New York: Simon & Schuster, 2011.

McGregor, Deborah Kuhn. *From Midwives to Medicine: The Birth of American Gynecology.* New Brunswick, N.J.: Rutgers University Press, 1998.

Morantz-Sanchez, Regina Markell. *Sympathy and Science: Women Physicians in American Medicine.* New York: Oxford University Press, 1985.

Oshinsky, David. *Bellevue: Three Centuries of Medicine and Mayhem in America's Most Storied Hospital.* New York: Doubleday, 2016.

Paget, Stephen, ed. *Memoirs and Letters of Sir James Paget.* London: Longmans, Green, 1901.

Putnam, Ruth, ed. *Life and Letters of Mary Putnam Jacobi,* New York: G.P. Putnam's Sons, 1925.

Rossi, Alice S. "The Blackwell Clan." In Alice S. Rossi, ed., *The Feminist Papers: From Adams to de Beauvoir.* New York: Columbia University Press, 1973.

Rothstein, William G. *American Physicians in the Nineteenth Century: From Sects to Science.* Baltimore: Johns Hopkins University Press, 1972.

Sahli, Nancy. "Elizabeth Blackwell M.D.: A Biography 1821–1910." Ph.D. diss., University of Pennsylvania, 1974.

———. "A Stick to Break Our Heads With: Elizabeth Blackwell and Philadelphia Medicine." *Pennsylvania History* 44, no. 4 (October 1977): 335–47.

Starr, Paul. *The Social Transformation of American Medicine: The Rise of a Sovereign Profession and the Making of a Vast Industry.* New York: Basic Books, 1982.

Todd, Margaret, M.D. *The Life of Sophia Jex-Blake.* London: Macmillan, 1918.

Vietor, Agnes Caecilia. *A Woman's Quest: The Life of Marie E. Zakrzewska, M.D.* New York: D. Appleton, 1924.

Walsh, Mary Roth. *"Doctors Wanted: No Women Need Apply": Sexual Barriers in the Medical Profession, 1835–1975.* New Haven, Conn.: Yale University Press, 1977.

Wheeler, Leslie, ed. *Loving Warriors: Selected Letters of Lucy Stone and Henry B. Blackwell, 1853–1893.* New York: Dial Press, 1981.

INDEX

Page numbers in *italics* refer to illustrations. The letter *n* after a page number refers to a footnote.